T0314573

ART THERAPY
& THE NEUROSCIENCE OF
RELATIONSHIPS,
CREATIVITY & RESILIENCY

The Norton Series on Interpersonal Neurobiology
Louis Cozolino, PhD, Series Editor
Allan N. Schore, PhD, Series Editor, 2007–2014

Daniel J. Siegel, MD, Founding Editor

The field of mental health is in a tremendously exciting period of growth and conceptual reorganization. Independent findings from a variety of scientific endeavors are converging in an interdisciplinary view of the mind and mental well-being. An interpersonal neurobiology of human development enables us to understand that the structure and function of the mind and brain are shaped by experiences, especially those involving emotional relationships.

The Norton Series on Interpersonal Neurobiology provides cutting-edge, multidisciplinary views that further our understanding of the complex neurobiology of the human mind. By drawing on a wide range of traditionally independent fields of research—such as neurobiology, genetics, memory, attachment, complex systems, anthropology, and evolutionary psychology—these texts offer mental health professionals a review and synthesis of scientific findings often inaccessible to clinicians. The books advance our understanding of human experience by finding the unity of knowledge, or consilience, that emerges with the translation of findings from numerous domains of study into a common language and conceptual framework. The series integrates the best of modern science with the healing art of psychotherapy.

A NORTON PROFESSIONAL BOOK

ART THERAPY & THE NEUROSCIENCE OF RELATIONSHIPS, CREATIVITY & RESILIENCY

SKILLS AND PRACTICES

NOAH HASS-COHEN
JOANNA CLYDE FINDLAY

Forewords by Louis J. Cozolino and Frances Kaplan

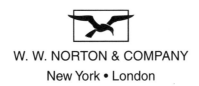

W. W. NORTON & COMPANY
New York • London

For information about permission to reproduce selections from this book,
write to Permissions, W. W. Norton & Company, Inc.,
500 Fifth Avenue, New York, NY 10110

For information about special discounts for bulk purchases, please contact
W. W. Norton Special Sales at specialsales@wwnorton.com or 800-233-4830

Manufacturing by Edwards Brothers Malloy
Production manager: Christine Critelli

ISBN 978-0-393-781074-8

W. W. Norton & Company, Inc.
500 Fifth Avenue, New York, N.Y. 10110
www.wwnorton.com

W. W. Norton & Company Ltd.
Castle House, 75/76 Wells Street, London W1T 3QT

1 2 3 4 5 6 7 8 9 0

Dedicated to our families

Amit, Nimrod, Lina, & Hamutahl
Cohen

and

Andrew, Leo & Laura
Findlay

Contents

Chapter 11
Transformative Integrating: Creating, Mentalizing,

Chapter 12

Chapter 13

Chapter 14
Reflections on the Love of Art Therapy: An Epilogue on Art,

Expanded Contents

Chapter 4

Chapter 5

Chapter 6

Chapter 7
Expressive Communicating: Accessing Emotions and the
Creative Unconscious   171

Chapter 8
Expressive Communicating: Interpersonal Touch and Space   205

Foreword

by Louis J. Cozolino

THE SYNERGY OF DIVERSE DISCIPLINES, a defining principle of interpersonal neurobiology, necessitates that we stand back and take a broader and more thoughtful view of the complexity of human experience. It challenges us to see human brains as social organs that can only be understood in the contexts of evolution, biology, epigenetics, and relationships. The broad and integrative perspective offered here by Noah Hass-Cohen and Joanna Clyde Findlay takes up the challenge of interpersonal neurobiology, revealing the magic of art therapy in high definition.

Art forms and art making mirror our experience while at the same time stimulating new ways of seeing, feeling, and thinking. For those of us stuck in ill-fitting and painful ways of being, new images are capable of generating maps to liberation. To heal, we need both these mirrors to help us to see more clearly and to serve as transformative portals to new possibilities. The transformative power of art is beyond question.

In the chapters ahead, the authors weave their extensive experience as art therapists with neurobiology, attachment theory, memory, and mindfulness into a fascinating and informative tapestry of wisdom. In the process, they provide ample evidence for the power of "art-in-relationship" as a living matrix for the connection of minds, brains, and hearts across the social synapse. Their work makes it clear that there is magic in art, magic in human connection, and an even greater magic when the two combine to heal suffering. Once the connection is made, the client-therapist brain can "fire together" in the service of regulating affect, creating new avenues of expression, and enhancing neural connectivity. Pretty good magic.

As a child I found the world to be a giant canvas; brilliant white clouds passing through the dark branches of bare trees, the tone of the afternoon light in southern New England, and the shimmering of the thousands of small ocean waves at sunset. Somewhere along the way, I forgot to look up; my vision became more limited, less embodied, more abstract—little of this for the better. Later, art woke me up. A self-portrait by van Gogh glowing green in the corner of a room at the Fogg museum at Harvard stopped me in my tracks and held me captive for an hour. Years later, innocently stopping in the Museo Reina Sofia of Madrid to see Picasso's Guernica, only to spend the day transfixed by the images and overwhelmed by the emotions it evoked.

For some of those who come to therapy, day-to-day experience can be a straightjacket, which they desperately need to escape from and change. Here is where art's transformative powers, directed by a skillful guide and companion, can save souls and lives. Within the six principles of their "CREATE" art therapy relational neuroscience model, the authors weave together a living framework of therapist-client collaboration in the service of self-discovery and social emotional learning. They leverage the power of art through a methodology of connection that supports and encourages insight and growth.

During primate evolution, our primitive executive center—the amygdala—has shifted its attention from olfactory to visual information in a dramatic way. We know that visual information now possesses a fast track to the amygdala ten times faster than conscious awareness. The information superhighway of visual information to the amygdala may be one of the reasons for art's raw emotional power and its ability to "shake us" into seeing things in new ways. A good deal of early learning is also directed by shared gaze, making one wonder how much of the impact of art therapy is multiplied by the activation of this primitive bonding reflex during the co-creation of art.

Happily, we are moving beyond the modern-day phrenology of locating specific functions in particular regions of the brain. Understanding how the brain evolved and exploring the networks of connectivity throughout the brain is providing important insights into how our brains are shaped, organized, and function. Our brains were shaped like coral reefs with newer structures being built upon and interwoven with older structures. This is why our sense of emotional balance and our ability to achieve affect-regulation relies upon our vestibular balance, coordination, and our sense of self in space. We are learning that our executive systems are not limited to our frontal lobes, but reside in broader systems that combine systems in both hemispheres and at all levels of the neuraxis in how our brains construct space-time and the sensorial world.

In the process of creation, art provides us with an avenue into the implicit-unconscious, which, combined with our creative imaginations, can reveal inner meanings, personal truths, and pathways to connection and healing. While much of this process must necessarily be intuitive on the part of both client and therapist, the authors provide deep insights into the mechanisms of action at the level of brain and mind that provide the practitioner with a way of understanding and explaining their practice. For beginning students, these explanations can broaden their perspectives and help conceptually grasp the process along the way to embodying its essential wisdom. The multidisciplinary perspective here also calls to art therapists, in fact all therapists, to go beyond simplistic or manualized versions of our craft.

Fields of therapy related to processes such as art, sensory-motor processing, drama, and other activities have been traditionally kept out of the mainstream by the medicalization of healing. Their positions have not been aided by their lack of attention to their underlying mechanisms of action. Our new and expanded notions of brain functioning from interpersonal neurobiology and its allied scientific fields are providing evidence that these "fringe" treatments are actually biological interventions. We now know that relationships themselves are biological interventions. It is indeed ironic that a field that requires double-blind pharmacological studies that pay homage to the power of the mind to impact our reaction to drugs completely ignores the healing impact of doctors' attitudes. By definition, art therapists acknowledge the value of the clients' perspectives by using the clients' work as the central tool of their work.

Every form of therapy generates some form of narrative. All therapists provide a perspective of illness and health and ways of being and thinking that gets translated into language and becomes part of our personal life story. We have learned from research in attachment that our ability to generate a coherent narrative that is clearly comprehensible to others is a complex achievement that correlates with the quality of our early relationships. Clearly, the art grounds and provides a coherent foundation for this explicit narration. The discovery of the world in collaboration with articulate, attuned, and compassionate parents and then therapists and trusted others allow our brains to develop and integrate in ways that enhance emotional regulation, intimacy with others, and self-esteem.

This work uses art as a matrix for the co-construction of integrated implicit and explicit self and, by association, the ability to deeply and fully connect with others. In essence, Noah Hass-Cohen and Joanna Clyde Findlay have created a framework that parallels our best guess at what are the optimal contexts for interpersonal plasticity throughout the life span. This is a rich and synthetic work that will both challenge and reward the reader. Over and over, the arts and therapeutic art making have the power to awaken us from our slumber to new possibilities of ourselves and the world. My recommendation is that if you take a deep breath and dive deeply, you will be well rewarded. Good magic indeed.

Los Angeles, California, October 2014

Foreword

by Frances F. Kaplan, MPS, DA, ART-BC

Science . . . in partnership with art, has much to offer art therapy. It offers a means to establish proof of worth. More important, it offers the prospect of revealing the secrets of art and art making and, as a consequence, of developing a true theory of art therapy. (Kaplan, 2000, p. 17)

IF YOU HAVE EVER WONDERED exactly how art therapy, creativity, and interpersonal neurobiology work together, wonder no more. Noah Hass-Cohen and Joanna Clyde Findlay's book describes art therapy processes and art making in a relational setting, discusses attachment theory, and relates both topics to what is currently known about the workings of the brain and clinical neuroscience. In undertaking this project, the authors have provided a text containing a wealth of information. Furthermore, the text is instructional on a number of levels.

In essence, *Art Therapy & the Neuroscience of Relationships, Creativity, & Resiliency* is a substantial revision and elaboration of the first author's Art Therapy Relational Neuroscience (ATR-N) model for art therapy (Hass-Cohen, 2008; Hass-Cohen, Clyde Findlay, Carr, & Vanderlan, 2014). The model comprises six CREATE principles: Creative Embodiment, Relational Resonating, Expressive Communicating, Adaptive Responding, Transformative Integrating, and Empathizing and Compassion. As Hass-Cohen stated, "CREATE emerged from the search for an understanding of how the functional entrainment and synchronization of bodily systems—the nervous, immune, endocrine, sensory, visual and motor systems—express in art therapy processes" (2008, p. 283).

The various instructional levels, then, involve stimulation of creativity, therapeutic technique regarding interpersonal relationships, theoretical aspects of attachment, and the neurobiology underlying all of these areas. Thus, the book can be approached from the point of view of different angles facilitating readers' access to the complexity of the material. For example, the ATR-N directives can be utilized to good effect without fully considering the details of the related neuroscience. Likewise, the neuroscience can be explored without in-depth presentations of art directives. Finally, the introduction section of each chapter and the last application section can be read together, establishing a foundational knowledge of the integration of CREATE with psychological theory. This has the interesting consequence of allowing readers to create their own reading sequence as well as making this book several texts in one.

There is no doubt that an integration of art and science is involved here. Indeed, this is how it should be to achieve a more complete understanding of art therapy. As science philosopher Paul Churchland has stated, "From a neurocognitive point of view, the differences [between art and science] are superficial" (1995, p. 297). Naturally, this work takes a particular approach to the integration of art and science. It emphasizes brain science, that exciting new and rapidly developing area of science that has only been in the forefront of scientific research since the latter part of the 20th century. This is no surprise because in both the art and art therapy communities there has long been acceptance of the notion that visual imagery is in and of itself a cognitive process (Arnheim, 1969). What is surprising has to do with the fact that many art therapists cannot make the (small) leap from there to embracing science. It is as though they perceive science as somehow doing violence to the art part of the art-science equation. Hass-Cohen and Clyde Findlay's work has considerable potential to move things along toward greater acceptance of science.

Around the 1980s and 1990s when interest in the brain was taking hold, I remember telling students that we knew the brain and the mind were connected but we didn't yet know how to think about this connection. Previously, we tended to think about the mind—when we thought about the connection with the brain at all—as something parallel to but outside the brain. That is, a kind of synchrony between mind and brain, between thoughts, behavior, and external occurrences, was involved (Calvin, 1996; Jung, 1965). Psychologists and therapists talked about the "mind-brain problem." As time passed, however, my thinking along these lines became clearer. I decided that there is no mind-brain problem, and that the mind is what the brain does, a point of view supported by Nobel Prize laureate Eric Kandel (2006). Although some neuroscientists see the mind as bigger than the brain (Siegel, 2012), it seems that most embrace Kandel's general idea that the brain is responsible for the existence of the mind, either in whole or in part. Hass-Cohen and Clyde Findlay's work takes this attitude for granted and builds from there.

It would be a bit much for the authors to cover all of brain science. The primary focus of the neuroscience-art amalgam here is the interface of creativity, attachment theory, and resilience. In basing their work on relevant attachment theory and clinical neuroscience research, the authors devised original art therapy techniques that are informed by the efforts of established investigators such as Daniel Siegel (2012), Louis Cozolino (2010), Vittorio Gallese (2003), Marco Iacoboni, (2009), Peter Fonagy (1998) and a growing group of art therapists whom the authors credit in the introduction and throughout the chapters. However, Hass-Cohen and Clyde Findlay's ATR-N approach differs from those of their art therapy peers as they provide an encompassing neuroscience framework for art therapy. Relationally focused, the authors have also expanded the interpersonal neurobiology approach (Siegel, 2006) to include interpersonal space, movement, and touch.

The ART-N model is designed to teach about the workings of the brain, as well as how to use this learning with clients. The art directives have the goal of being both instructive and therapeutic in terms of promoting repair and resiliency when attachment disruptions are present. The names of the ATR-N directives alert the reader to how these psychological benefits might be accessed and processed. Examples include attachment albums, autobiographical timelines, making a collage of personal resources, drawing a stressful moment, drawing moving toward others, and so on. These ATR-N directives engage sensory, relational, affective, and verbal and nonverbal cognitive transitional processes. Furthermore, the ATR-N directives and art making reinforce positive rather than negative processes, contributing to optimism and resiliency (Hass-Cohen et al., 2014).

The art therapy directives are presented to art therapists through practice-based experientials, which allow them not only to practice relating but also to explore their own typical ways of relating, with all the positives and negatives that implies. The major triumph of this book, then, is that it presents a highly innovative program of relational neuroscience directives that can teach, treat, and promote critical thinking in an area where clinicians of all stripes should be well versed.

To conclude, the state of neuroscience makes much of this book theoretical even though it provides a hearty helping of clinical applications and facts. That is a significant contribution because a solid, up-to-the-minute theory of art therapy is sorely needed. That aside, to suggest that art therapy—or any other therapy for that matter—is the best way to achieve certain results, or to achieve them at all, has yet to be tested through well-designed research. Hass-Cohen and Clyde Findlay have taken an important step in supporting the likelihood that empirical studies will demonstrate what at this point is hypothetical. I can only hope that as findings from neurobiological science continue to emerge, these excellent writers will provide us with the next step.

Therefore, having found the present text more than worthwhile, I anticipate that an updated edition will follow. Of course, art therapists and art therapy educators need to steep themselves in this initial book in order to become conversant with what is to follow.

Oregon City, Oregon, May 2014

REFERENCES

Arnheim, R. (1969). *Visual thinking*. Berkeley, CA: University of California Press.

Calvin, W. H. (1996). *How brains think: Evolving intelligence, then and now*. New York, NY: Basic Books.

Churchland, P. M. (1995). *The engine of reason, the seat of the soul: A philosophical journey into the brain*. Cambridge, MA: MIT Press.

Cozolino, L. (2010). *The neuroscience of psychotherapy: Healing the social brain* (2nd ed.). New York, NY: Norton.

Fonagy, P., & Target, M. (1997). Attachment and reflective function: Their role in self organization. *Development and Psychopathology, 9*, 679–700.

Gallese, V. (2003). The roots of empathy: The shared manifold hypothesis and the neural basis of intersubjectivity. *Psychopathology, 36,* 171–180.

Hass-Cohen, N. (2008). CREATE: Art Therapy and Relational Neuroscience principles (ATR-N). In N. Hass-Cohen & R. Carr (Eds.), *Art therapy and clinical neuroscience*. Philadelphia, PA: Jessica Kingsley.

Hass-Cohen, N., Clyde Findlay, J., Carr, R., & Vanderlan, J. (2014). "CHECK, change and/or keep what you need": An Art Therapy Relational Neurobiological (ATR-N) trauma intervention. *Art Therapy, 31*(2), 69–78.

Iacoboni, M. (2009). Imitation, empathy, and mirror neurons. *Annual Review of Psychology, 60*(3), 653–670.

Jung, C. G. (1965). *Memories, dreams, reflections* (R. Winston & C. Winston, Trans.). New York, NY: Vintage.

Kaplan, F. F. (2000). *Art, science and art therapy: Repainting the picture*. Philadelphia, PA: Jessica Kingsley.

Kandel, E. R. (2006). *In search of memory: The emergence of a new science of mind*. New York, NY: Norton.

Siegel, D. J. (2006). An interpersonal neurobiology approach to psychotherapy: Awareness, mirror neurons, and neural plasticity in the development of well-being. *Psychiatric Annals, 36*(4), 248–256.

Siegel, D. J. (2012). *Pocket guide to interpersonal neurobiology: An integrative handbook of the mind*. New York, NY: Norton.

Acknowledgments

WE WANT TO EXPRESS OUR heartfelt appreciation for the wonderful participants in our creative milieu: clients, faculty, alumni, and students who have taught us so much over the years. Many thanks to those who directly contributed to this publication: Kristen Anastasia, Veronica Avalos, Rebecca Bokoch, Celine Elise Briggs, Autumn Cade, Tamara Cates, Lisa Cerrina, Jonathan Chris, Jean Clyde, Maggie Fong, Sylvia Garcia, Irit Ivey, Marta Gordon Martinez, Norma Y. Guerrero-Lewis, Lauryn Hunter, Elise Jones, Lisa Kandaros, Anna Louisa Kingston, Jennifer Klein, Marguerite Lathan, Andrea Lewis, Patty Lewis, Ilene Lopez, Margaret McSwain, Jessica Tress Masterson, Kazuko Numata, Jennifer Ostin, Jessica Plotin, Zainab Pirbhai, Linda Ross, Patti Russell, Maribel Sandoval, Robin Shanon, Lisa Smith, Louise Smith, Emily Skelton, Olivia Stern, Janine Stuppel, Channie Thal, Rachel Tate, and Kara Wahlin for their contributions, illustrations, and art. Thank you to Natasha Lewis Harrington for research support; Pauline Lazari, Rebecca Lee, and Selina Mangassarian for editorial assistance; and to Jessa Forsythe-Crane for her never-ending support.

We gratefully thank Richard Carr for reviewing this book, Frances Kaplan for her splendid foreword, and Sylvia Cary for her excellent editing. Much appreciation to Lou Cozolino, who recommended us to W. W. Norton and Co. and warmly invited us to be part of the interpersonal neurobiology family of publications. This project would have not been possible without the support of the Norton team, especially that of Nathan Cohan. We are very appreciative of Sheryl Rowe from Bytheway Publishing Services who has gone out of her way to make this book possible. We are grateful for her positive support, attention to detail, and expertise.

Finally, our deepest thanks go to our families for seeing us through the many long hours of writing and editing throughout the years of teaching and writing. Looking forward, we are indebted to the researchers whose ever-unfolding data and expositions invite us and others to gain insight into the integration of expressive arts practices and relational neuroscience.

Noah Hass-Cohen   Joanna Clyde Findlay

2014

ART THERAPY
& THE NEUROSCIENCE OF
RELATIONSHIPS,
CREATIVITY & RESILIENCY

CHAPTER 1

The Framework:
The Art Therapy Relational
Neuroscience Model

In short, the revolution in neuroplasticity has shown that the brain can change as a result of two distinct outputs. It can change as a result of the experiences that we have in the world—how we move and behave and what sensory signals arrive in our cortex. The brain can also change in response to purely mental activity, ranging from meditation to cognitive-behavior therapy, with the result that when the activity is specific circuits can increase or decrease. (Davidson & Begley, 2012, p. 175)

THIS BOOK INTEGRATES ART THERAPY practice and creativity with interpersonal neurobiology topics and relational neuroscience-based research. The purpose is to highlight and demonstrate how an Art Therapy Relational Neuroscience (ATR-N) approach can support resiliency. The ATR-N approach is comprised of six principles, captured by the acronym CREATE: Creative Embodiment, Relational Resonating, Expressive Communicating, Adaptive Responding, Transformative Integrating, and Empathizing and Compassion (Hass-Cohen, 2008a). Use of verbs for the principles' names, such as Relational Resonating, rather than Relational Resonance, is a symbolic reference to the dynamic and plastic nature of the human nervous system and humans' potential for change. The chapters are organized according to the six CREATE principles, and each one begins with an overview of the associated principle and established interpersonal neurobiology (IPNB) topics as well as those of motion and touch, which we have added. A description and discussion of ATR-N directives is then illustrated by the art therapy group members' artwork and intrapersonal reflections and insights. In each chapter, we focus on how these ATR-N directives and art-based dialogues create a contagious social energy and a supportive, sensorial group experience. We hope that readers, whether art therapists, mental health providers, or artists, can envision themselves partaking in the art therapy experientials and engaging with the written reflections and clinical topics. This kind of guided learning highlights clients' participatory meaning-making experiences. The experientials build upon the clinical experience of the authors and their teaching. Experiential art making also assists in learning the relevant neurobiological information. Salient relational neuroscience research is then discussed, followed by a clinical skills application section, which further integrates the chapter's material with all the CREATE principles. Throughout, selected readings in clinical and interpersonal neuroscience, art therapy, and psychology are referenced to illustrate how the ATR-N principles are grounded in widely accepted research and theory. The information provided can be used for the purposes of professional development, enhancing clinical treatment skills, teaching, or developing research protocols.

Throughout this book, expressive visual approaches provide gateways to learning the complexities of neuroanatomy, IPNB topics, and relational neuroscience research tenets. Learning about our bodies and ourselves through the arts is a time-honored tradition that can be traced back to Michelangelo and Leonardo da Vinci. In fact, most people gather and process information visually. Visual acuity influences how we learn about our world and how we react to others (Kalat, 2012). This is most likely because visual dominance provides humans with an evolutionary advantage when faced with novel situations, such as learning and change. Furthermore, the unique properties of the visual system provide us with an integrated image of the world (Zeki & Bartels, 1998). In our method, art-based expressions, such as drawing, painting, and sculpting, serve as meaningful social-emotional roadways for learning the brain's structures, localized functions, and their implications for ATR-N practices. Creating two-dimensional charts and images often successfully conveys what can essentially be a confusing three-dimensional world. However, this example should not be construed as either straightforward or simple. For the art therapist, drawing and sculpting the brain brings up basic internal conflicts associated with self-judgment, criticism, and a quest for knowledge. Thus engaging with art processes helps people decipher the functional mystery of our relational nervous system, enhances cognitive abilities, and increases the motivation to learn novel concepts and participate socially (Petitto, 2008; Posner, Rothbart, Sheese, & Kieras, 2008). Understanding our environment is made possible by an inclusion of many ways of knowing that range from the abstract and theoretical to the imaginative, aesthetic, sensory, and kinetic. From a clinical perspective, it is not sufficient to rely on visual processing. Other multi-modal sensory processes, namely touch, sound and movement are critical for successful treatment (Perry, 2006).

Our participants' reflective narratives promote learning and integration within this intersubjective and creative matrix (Gerber et al., 2012). For the most part each reflection is accompanied by illustrated artwork examples. Storied written reflections engage higher brain regions that are responsible for social and cognitive function, and the regulation of midbrain emotions (Cozolino, 2013). Such reflections and art-based inquiry support creativity, which has been associated with divergent thinking and ingenuity (Jung, Mead, Carrasco, & Flores, 2013).

Research shows that effective change and learning must include hands-on experiential practices that address both emotional and intellectual aspects (Kolb & Kolb, 2005). Experiential learning theory defines learning as experiences that are transformed into knowledge (Kolb, 1984). There are two dialectical forms of learning (Kolb & Kolb, 2005). One form involves concrete, active experiences, such as our ATR-N experientials and the ensuing artwork. The second form of learning involves abstract processing, mental conceptualization of information, and a reflection on what the learning is. Opportunities to engage in the second kind of learning are found in chapter sections that review the IPNB topics, relational neuroscience, and the CREATE, ATR-N principles. This book integrates both types of learning. Consequently, we recommend that readers adapt our offerings to best fit their own learning styles: some may prefer to start by reading the theory and neuroscience research, while others may prefer to first approach the experiential ATR-N practices or focus on the clinical CREATE applications. Our approach cultivates what Gerber has called the artistic interpersonal matrix: "The interaction of self-knowledge and knowledge of the other expressed through the dynamic art process as it emerges within the interpersonal matrix is not only necessary for clinical art therapy but also is an essential component of an epistemology for art therapy" (2014, p. 106).

RELATIONAL NEUROSCIENCE

Relational neuroscience focuses on self-internal working models of relationships, the interactions between people, and more broadly on social-self interfaces with one's environment. Triggered by an outpouring of attachment theory research, this clinically helpful information has come to focus on the development of the relational self throughout the life span, emphasizing a variety of contexts: positive, such as creativity, or difficult, such trauma.

The central idea is that the mind emerges from the interactions between intrapersonal and interpersonal mind-body exchanges (Siegel, 2006, 2012). Importantly, significant relationships can shape the flow and synchronicity of energy and information between people, and within each person (Badenoch,

2008; Wallin, 2007). Such ongoing experiences shape the genetically pro-grammed maturation of the nervous system and develop the individual mind (Underwood & Rosen, 2011). Based on animal and human brain-based studies, the associated human research on fear, emotion, cognition, memory, and empathy is defining the impact of socialization and relationships on the mind-brain (Meaney, 2001; Panksepp & Biven, 2012). Throughout the life span new experiences, relationships, ideas, behaviors, and information change the landscape of people's lives and brains, increasing or decreasing their abil-ity to cope and relate to their communituies (Davidson & Begley, 2012).

Some of brain understanding started developing in the nineteenth cen-tury as phrenologists believed attitudes and temperaments responsible for certain behaviors and moods could be located via bumps on a skull's surface. Later, scientists more accurately mapped localized functional brain regions (Carter, 2010), including the frontal speech motor production area, discov-ered by Pierre Broca in 1861, and the temporal language comprehension area, discovered by Carl Wernicke a decade later (Carlson, 2013). Evolution-ary theory, which also took shape in the mid-19th century, signaled the beginning of the contemporary understanding of neuroplasticity. Darwin contended that environment shapes development. For example, biological changes in the beaks of finches that lived on different Galapagos islands could be traced to their food sources; longer beaks developed so birds could access food lodged between rocks. While Darwin's study of finches demonstrated the workings of natural selection, the notion of individual neuroplasticity, adaptations in neural pathways and synapses emerging as a result of behav-ioral and environmental changes, did not gain wide acceptance until after the 1960s (Klein & Thorne, 2006).

Whereas earlier the human brain was believed to be immutable after crit-ical developmental periods in childhood, research now supports that neuro-plasticity exists throughout life (Fox, Levitt, & Nelson, 2010). An inquiry into the renewable brain has gained significant momentum since the discov-ery that new neural cells are born through neurogenesis. New neurons are born in the adult hippocampus and lateral ventricles, which are areas respon-sible for memory (Altman, 1969; Eriksson et al., 1998; Gross, 2000; Kays, Hurley, & Taber, 2012). It is also now known that the human adult brain shows the ability to grow neurons in the olfactory blub, an area for the detec-tion of odor, which is associated with survival functions. However, there are many outstanding questions, the most important ones being: Is the central nervous system able to regenerate neurons elsewhere? What are the qualities of these neurons? How do they connect to existing neural pathways, and what are their effects on the brain? Do they replace neurons that die and are they physiological expressions of resiliency? (Ming & Song, 2011). Some very interesting emerging research suggests that neurogenesis which emerges from the acquisition of new information assists in coping with stress (Schoenfeld, & Gould, 2012). Thus new neurons increase the person's ability to regulate anxiety and stress.

From birth onward, changes on the level of neuronal connections result in increased capacities for memory learning. Psychologically, the regeneration of neurons in memory is of special interest as the formation of memories is the foundation of self and change. Yet neuroplasticity, as we discuss in our beginning chapters, extends beyond the confines of development and the formation of memories to both brain growth and brain reorganization throughout the life span. When these changes arise from positive experiences, such as voluntarily engaging in enriching and novel experiences, they most likely contribute to resiliency (Bekinschtein, Oomen, Saksida, & Bussey, 2011).

The mind can change in two ways. One is dubbed bottom-up change, meaning neurobiological changes that occur in response to sensory inputs to the mind; these changes reorganize brain functionality. As described in Chapter 2, upper regions of the brain, such as the feeling strip, also called the somatosensory strip, can change their function according to repeated inputs such as need, and practice. Across-lobe-modalities changes also occur, as when the visual cortex of people with blindness assumes responsibility for processing auditory and tactile information, whereas the auditory cortex in people with deafness seems to respond to peripheral visual cues (Collignon et al., 2013; Pascual-Leone & Hamilton, 2001; Stevens & Neville, 2009). As demonstrated by stroke rehabilitation research, these changes are not limited to congenital birth deficits but also occur later in life (Taub et al., 2006). Readers may at this point ask themselves how this information pertains to this book and the field of art therapy. First, in art therapy, sensory inputs mediate dynamic mind-body interactions. The manipulation of art media and the weekly generation of new creations in a supportive interpersonal context target sensory-emotive-cognitive processing areas of the brain that are needed for psychological transformation. Furthermore, the conditions that are needed for these kinds of changes, are dependent on movement, social interactions, novelty, attention, and voluntary intention (Bekinschtein et al., 2011; van Praag et al., 2002), and prevail in the creative clinic and therapeutic milieu. While our mind-brains are ever changing, it is these conditions that engender resiliency and coping, which are thought to be critical for the generation and survival of new neurons. Although neurons are continuously and rather rapidly generated in some areas, a novel enriched environment is necessary for new neurons to survive and migrate to the hippocampus; this context allows them to effectively link to existing networks and to become functional (Kempermann, Kuhn, & Gage, 1997, 1998).

Speaking of attention and intention, the second way that the brain changes is from the top down. For example, the representation in a person's mind of playing a five-finger piano exercise, a mental image, stimulates some similar brain regions and may have effects similar to the direct action itself (Pascual-Leone et al., 1995; Hamamé, 2012). Human thoughts, emotions, intentions, and targeted efforts are required in order to maximize positive impacts of bottom-up influences. Although nonmaterial and nontangible, they change the mind. Startlingly, the abundance of mindfulness research suggests that mindfulness, intentional attention, and reflection support brain changes, not only engendering affect regulation, relational security, and compassion but also changing the mind-brain in a variety of ways. Attentional and cognitive changes as well as stress reduction, which are associated with mindfulness practices, are expressed as thickened cortical mass. Neuroplasticity in regions of the brain that control emotions, the stress response, cognitions, and empathic responses contributes to psychological well-being (Farb, Segal, & Anderson, 2013; Singleton et al., 2014). What seems to be critical in mediating the top-down effects of mindfulness is a process of de-identification, not only with emotions but also with thoughts (Ives-Deliperi, Solms, & Meintjes, 2011). Process art therapy procedures, typical for our field, that emphasize creativity by detachment from the final product may be linked to such benefits.

The therapeutic creative milieu inspires intentionality, a sense of community, and a combination of reflective and action-based practices. With demonstrated growth in empirical research, our clinical practices and studios seem to offer such environments and conditions. The art therapy creative office or studio offers social opportunities for intentional encounters with novel expressions and considerable symbolic and actual movement.

During the last few decades, research regarding the interplay between life events, social experiences, mentalized intentions, and neurobiology has also greatly expanded our understanding of what kind of psychological approaches are needed (Cozolino, 2010). Over the lifetime of an individual, the effects of neglect, stress, and declining social, emotional, and physical health also contribute to a chronic imbalance of central nervous system and immune system functions (Perry, Pollard, Blakley, Baker, & Vigilante, 1995; Sapolsky, 2004). Although many of the ill effects of early childhood severe deprivation are spontaneously reversible, it seems that such early impacts may permanently change social, brain-based functions; for example, even three years after adoption, levels of oxytocin, the bonding hormone do not rise in adopted children when cuddled by loving adoptive mothers (Wismer Fries, Ziegler, Kurian, Jacoris, & Pollak, 2005). As reviewed by Kravits (2008a), studies of relationally deprived Romanian orphans have revealed further detrimental interactions between the orphans' genetic makeup and the environment. In fact, throughout the life span, childhood and adult chronic stress are clearly implicated as risk factors for negative neuroplasticity (Kays et al., 2012), necessitating different and novel kinds of early childhood interventions

The cross-fertilization of neuroscience research and psychotherapy (Cozolino, 2010; Schore, 1994; Siegel, 2006) has led to three key efforts: attachment- and IPNB-based treatment, trauma-informed work, and mindfulness compassionate practices. These efforts have all included a focus on relational neurological communication as the basis for facilitating therapeutic change. The work of John Bowlby (1999) which sparked the investigation of the effect of attachment relationships on social and emotional development has instigated the first focus. Emphasizing attachment, IPNB, learns from studies on the neurobiology of secure attachment and advances a clear understanding of the mechanisms of affect regulation, delineating the crucial mechanisms of reciprocal early adult-infant interactions throughout the lifetime. Mentalizing treatment provides a systemic platform for working with dyads and families (Asen, & Fonagy, 2012; Harel, Kaplan, Avimeir-Patt, & Ben-Aaron, 2006). Intersubjective work postulates that positive therapeutic change occurs during attuned and attuning relationships (Bowlby, 1988; Fonagy, & Target, 1998; Hesse, 1999; Main & Solomon, 1990; Schore, 1994; Siegel, 2012; Stern, 1985; Wallin, 2007). IPNB also provides an understanding of how the therapist's and the client's nervous systems can fire together, coregulate, and support security, interpersonal change, and development. The second approach, trauma treatment, involves an investigation of fear, stress, memory, and adaptation. These areas of investigation have deepened insights into developmental theory as well as complex post-traumatic stress disorders (Allen, 2001; Bremner, 2002; Foa, Keane, Friedman, & Cohen, 2009; Fonagy, Gergely, Jurist, & Target, 2002; Herman, 1997; van der Kolk, 2001). The neuroscience research on fear and negative emotion shows that impacted neural pathways influence the construction of the social self (Damasio, 2005). Active efforts are also being made to harness the advantages that mindfulness and compassionate practices can contribute to the amelioration of the pain that trauma clients suffer (Brier & Scott, 2012). Conversely, brain plasticity can extend to learning happiness and compassion, resulting in resiliency (Davidson, 2004). In other words, both positive and negative experiences affect transformations in the brain over a person's lifetime.

Mindfulness-based practices, which have demonstrated the possibility for resilient brain function and well-being provide innovative treatment for pain, stress, trauma, and aging-related disorders (Baer, 2006; Germer, Siegel, & Fulton, 2005; Segal, Williams, & Teasdale, 2002; Siegel, 2006). Notable mindfulness based approaches incorporating awareness, and acceptance include acceptance and commitment therapy, developed in the early 1990s by Steven Hayes, Kirk Strosahl, and Kelly Wilson (2003); dialectical behavioral therapy, developed by Marsha Linehan (1993a, 1993b); mindfulness based stress reduction, started in the 1980s by Jon Kabat-Zinn (2005); mindfulness based cognitive therapy, developed by Zindel Segal, Mark Williams, and John Teasdale in 2002 and others which we describe later. For the most part these third-wave therapies, which were inspired by Buddhist traditions do not espouse mindfulness for mindfulness sake. Instead mindfulness practices are the foundation of compassion toward self and others (Neff, 2011). To all of these progenitors, and to others referenced in our chapters, we are deeply indebted.

Situated at the crossroads of these three foci, the ATR-N approach, enables art therapists to better understand the potential effectiveness of art therapy interventions. In recent years, art therapy book editors and authors have joined us in navigating these oceanic waters of art therapy and clinical neuroscience (Belkofer, Van Hecke, & Konopka, 2014; Bat-Or, 2010; Chapman, 2014, Gantt & Tinnin, 2007, 2009; Gavron, 2013; 2014a; Franklin, 2010; Kaiser & Deaver, 2009; Klorer, 2005, 2014; Kruk, 2004; Hinz, Lusebrink (2004); Malchiodi, 2011; Peterson, 2014; Rappaport, 2014; Sarid & Huss, 2011; Talwar, 2007; Tripp 2007). These and other colleagues, to whom we have referred throughout this book, have all identified important art therapy–based relational neuroscience points of contact and have contributed to our epistemologies. Some, like Frances Kaplan (2000), have pioneered the way for innovative thinking about our field, and others are continuing to map the way (King, 2015). We hope that the understanding of relational neurological communications articulated in the six CREATE ATR-N principles will provide our field with a broad theoretical foundation and support an effective facilitation of psychotherapy change. Unique to CREATE is the emphasis on social and relational implications of clinical neuroscience. This work also differs from others in that it provides an overall encompassing interpersonal neurobiology framework for art therapy

THE ATR-N MODEL

The CREATE principles map the ATR-N model, thus constructing an interpersonal neurobiology art therapy theory and expressive practices approach (Hass-Cohen, 2008a). As stated earlier, CREATE is an abbreviation for Creative Embodiment, Relational Resonating, Expressive Communicating, Adaptive Responding, Transformative Integrating, and Empathizing and Compassion. The CREATE principles assist in conceptualizing how the interpersonal neurobiology of emotion, cognition, and action are expressed

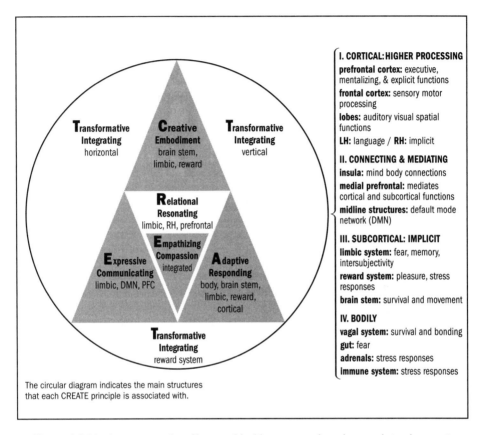

The circular diagram indicates the main structures that each CREATE principle is associated with.

Figure 1.1 The dynamic interplay of brain and bodily systems and art therapy relational neuroscience principles. The diagram demonstrates the centrality of Relational Resonating. Transformative Integrating to all six principles and the vertical and horizontal integration of all neurobiological systems. The circulation of the reward system's neurochemistry provides additional integration routes. Within the diagram, each principle is associated with the primary cortical, subcortical, and bodily regions. On the right, their structures and related functions are listed in a hierarchal order.

in the dynamic interplay of brain and bodily systems during art therapy (Figure1.1)

Supported by the act of art making, ATR-N practices incorporate sensory and perceptual foci into therapeutic interventions. However, as demonstrated in the figure above an integrated involvement of cortical, subcortical, bodily and connective structures and functions occurs at all levels of art making. For example, as demonstrated by EEG measurements, there are significant differences between cortical activities when artists versus non-artists create art. There were also significant differences between pre- and post EEG recordings (Belkofer, Van Hecke & Konopka, 2014).

The CREATE framework suggests that an attuned, mindful, compassionate, and integrated state of mind can emerge during the novel sensory experiences of creating art in the therapist's presence in the art therapy creative space. ATR-N underscores the neurological underpinnings of art therapy interventions and change, assisting art therapists in fine-tuning their clinical, teaching, and research practices.

Creative Embodiment represents the creative manifestation of human senses, experiences, and expression. These include feeling, thinking, talking, seeing, touching, and so on. In this publication Creative Embodiment highlights the potential therapeutic effects of kinesthetic art making, movement, play and touch. The therapeutic significance of purposeful and rhythmic movement is a complex and broad topic that ranges from the basic literal physical movements needed for art expression, pain relief, and bodily function to the perceived, anticipated and symbolized motions involved in adaptive responses and empathic resonance. Movement has become a locus of investigation in the past century for its central role in social, cognitive, and emotional function. Although fine motor and perceived movements have traditionally been expressive components of art therapy, we suggest both cognitive and emotional advantages to incorporating motion into the interpersonal space and to exploring images of actual and implied action. Movement and motor system pathways, including mirror neuron functions strengthen beneficial links between emotion, and cognition. As an example, the motor system coordinates with the planning system and emotive-social system. This enables the integration of actions, emotions, and thoughts, promoting increased motivation, reduced inactivity, and social interaction. The creative process enhances new-found freedom from constricting affect and contributes to the co-construction of safe interpersonal experiences.

Relational Resonating represents the importance of attuned therapeutic relationships and communication that promote stable internal and flexible psychobiological states and interpersonal interactions. Social exchanges and their ensuing mental representations have the potential to stabilize affect regulation, update autobiographical memories, and contribute to earned attachment. Collaborative and coherent art therapy relationships can increase experiences of positive affect and help disengage from negative feelings. Relational Resonating infuses the ATR-N creative environment, be it an office or studio setup, media choices, art engagement, and relational interactions. Examples of such experiences include offering and sharing media, touching others' art, working together, and representing an image of a loved one or beloved objects. These interpersonal exchanges and representations have the potential to activate and mend attachment wounds, alter attachment states, stabilize affect regulation, and update autobiographical memories. Perhaps more than any of the other CREATE principles, Relational Resonating has the potential to transform our field. Over the lifetime, aversive experiences such as early childhood developmental trauma, may negatively impact the maturation of critical linkages in the brain related to the development of secure internal working memories of attachment. Positive experiences, such as those within attuned relationships, can transform relational insecurity to security. ATR-N practices easily engage emotive-implicit and cognitive-explicit functions and nonverbal right-to-right hemispheric communication they are particularly suitable to achieve these ends. We contend that it is both the sharing of art with others, and the making of art in the presence of others that most contribute to therapeutic change. We stress that the significance of relationships for the ever-changing and growing mind and self are carried throughout all our art therapy practices.

Expressivity has always been an art therapy staple, and Expressive Communicating reflects how motivation and emotion are stimulated and used in an art therapy environment. It is likely that this activation also charges our neurological reward circuitry and helps maintain a dynamic balance between excitation, pleasure, and tranquility. Excitation can also facilitate affect regulation and increase the cognitive capacity to tolerate emotional frustration and experience joy, satisfaction, and relational security. The ability to express and regulate emotions develops from birth and is critical to the development and connectivity of sensory, emotional, and cognitive regions. In a relational context, expressivity is central to the ability to communicate what is often difficult or too embarrassing to discuss. The vivid and sensory qualities of art media alongside the inherent ambiguity of the art making processes may evoke strong emotions and present an opportunity to express, communicate, and regulate. Although not always pleasurable, usually some satisfaction is involved in the completion of art and a relief in exchanging emotional states.

Adaptive Responding to stress is necessary for a continued sense of safety, control, acceptance, and resiliency. To develop Adaptive Responding, art therapists use color, diverse materials, and demonstrative therapeutic interventions that balance and support optimal arousal, and expressivity. The simultaneous experience of these states contains the tangible representations of trauma, desensitizes emotions and memories, and generates solutions. Dynamic balancing of arousal and avoidance supports well-being, while stimulating emotional networks and activating cognitive responses. Thus, ATR-N practices foster optimal neural firing, repeated synchronized activation of neural networks with repetitive coping and success. This approach involves simultaneous art making, meaning making, and contextual memory processing. Furthermore, through the completion of art pieces, a sense of satisfaction and control is promoted; through interpersonal exchange and consolidation of emotional states, art making fosters relief.

The CREATE principles of Creative Embodiment, Relational Resonating, Expressive Communicating and Adaptive Responding serve as doorways to Transformative Integrating. These capacities are essential to an integrated self. The internal space which integration opens can give rise to pro-social empathizing, the last CREATE principle. For example, Transformative Integrating can occur over time with the repeated association of secure affective experiences and sensory expression. The exploration of kinesthetic expression and visual conveyance of meaning, experienced with non-verbal affirmation and verbal discussion, allow for functional integration. Attribution of new meanings and gaining new responses, a functional integration of the interpersonal self, are supported by cycles of ATR-N experientials, group discussions, therapeutic connections, and individual reflective writing. Under therapeutic conditions, symbol-making and verbalization of art making can re-organize and re-structure implicit emotional memories. Translating implicit bodily memories into explicit conscious narratives supports the vertical integration of the emotional and cognitive centers of the brain. Thus, a negative memory may be reinterpreted as a positive experience through comprehension, action, and acceptance (i.e., integrated brain function). This can contribute to a transformed sense of self and renewed autobiographical memories. Besides, as therapeutic goals are consistently met, ATR-N CREATE oriented therapy may activate integrated changes across brain areas, contributing to a sense of hope, well-being, flexibility, stability, and overall wellness. Adaptive Responding requires demonstrative therapeutic interventions that balance and support optimal arousal, safety, and expressivity. Dynamic balancing of arousal and avoidance, supports well-being while stimulating emotional networks and activating cognitive responses. The simultaneous experience of these states helps to contain the tangible representation of stress and trauma, desensitize difficult emotions and intrusive memories, and generate new solutions

The sixth CREATE principle, Empathizing and Compassion, involves the development of insight and compassion toward oneself and others as well as toward the art product. Empathizing, or empathic attention, provides a gateway to compassion, as well as kindness and nurturing in the desire to relieve another's suffering.

Interpersonally, empathic and compassionate responses are linked to the capacity for affect regulation, as they assume the allowance for and the acceptance of one's own self and the selfhood of others. Deliberately monitoring and shifting thoughts, feelings, and perceptions as well as adopting kindness-based values is thus linked to the transformation of the self-other dialectic; self-awareness deepens and joining with others, emerges as a new and differentiated "we." We also suggest that empathic compassion forms the basis for a universal understanding of the arts and unites art therapists in the love of their work.

FOUNDATIONS

We emphatically agree that participation in art making forms the most critical foundation for the self-development of a skillful art therapist (Moon, 2009; Waller, 2014). Within a creative arts environment, the budding and the seasoned therapist learn how clients react to art therapy materials, art making, and direction from the therapist. Most importantly, this is where the client and art therapist work toward change. Personal art making also provides an opportunity for the therapist to identify personal issues that may interfere with client work, as well as an opportunity to experience artistic and other dimensions of personal growth (Jensen, 2001). Multifaceted experiences and discussions keep the imagery alive, continuing to infuse them with meaningful content (McNiff, 1992).

Creative processes and intrapersonal work are a special focus of art therapy (Allen, 1995; Malchiodi, 1998a). Still, the art therapy clinic is also a social laboratory where the process of art making provides participants with the opportunity to experience, understand, and develop a felt sense of others and of interpersonal security (Kapitan, 2010). Openness, awareness, and acceptance of others' artwork create a climate of felt vulnerability to expressed emotions, thoughts, and beliefs. As such, the art-based environment offers a therapeutic opportunity for art to be safely witnessed by others (Allen, 1995). Functioning as affirmations, verbal and nonverbal responses from an audience can reduce the inner artistic critic and create space for empathic interpersonal communication (Allen, 1995; McNiff, 1992). Moreover, the interpersonal process of sharing a secure creative space can nurture increased awareness and mindfulness.

When we make art, we deeply engage with the reality of our images. The raw, elemental qualities of media, such as sticky glue or damp clay, and the kinesthetic actions of art making, such as sweeping a brush loaded with paint across a surface, can give rise to a host of emotions (Malchiodi, 1998a). Some art making may be pleasant or neutral, while other labors may trigger anxiety or fear of the unknown (Allen, 1995). This art making contributes to personal integration and growth as it is likely that sensory-emotional investment combined with relationship bonding command the attention of the emotional brain center and help shape cognitive responses. These subcortical structures, which connect to the thinking brain, are attuned to novel experiences that may trigger threatening memories (LeDoux, 2003b). Because older mammalian brain structures responsible for the brain's alarm and emotional responses are also very receptive to visual and tactile stimuli the art making becomes significant (Hass-Cohen & Carr, 2008). Thus as the art makers receive and exchange attuned and empathic responses, the experiential practices offer opportunities for affect expression and regulation, social sharing, the repairing of relational vulnerabilities, and the development of flexible mentalizing, trust and hope. The well-rounded benefits of the arts can be used to assist the development of emotionally balanced and cognitively flexible people, because "the arts have strong positive cognitive, emotional, social, collaborative, and neurological effects" (Jensen, 2001, p. 68). Thus, the key clinical aspect is that art making provides safe and secure opportunities for ATR-N processing.

We propose that the creative clinic also provides an advantageous framework for therapists wishing to master the ATR-N approach and the CREATE principles. It is an ideal setting for didactic learning of clinical neuroscience information, experiential engagement with specific art directives, and mindful reflection. Thus we expand the traditional uses of creative spaces, which invite the creator to spontaneously engage with art media, to include specific ATR-N directives. This learning approach also aids in exploring various methods and media that allow artistic competence to develop, while at the same time helping therapists meet the varied needs of clients (McNiff, 1986). Accordingly, the ATR-N environment supports an integrated balance between personal artistic expression, professional development, and clinical work (Allen, 1995).

CREATE PRINCIPLES AND CLINICAL APPLICATIONS

Application or clinical skills refer to therapist ATR-N competencies that are integral to therapeutic change. They include implicit and explicit sets of process-based skills needed for meeting clients, gathering clinical data, goal setting, implementing therapeutic interventions, and terminating with clients (Ivey & Ivey, 2007). The two foundations of clinical abilities are nonverbal and verbal skills. Nonverbal attending behaviors, such as eye contact, and verbal communication, such as asking questions or explaining the art. Such implicit microskills are used to build an attuned therapeutic alliance by utilizing unbiased listening and attending to body language communication. Art therapy nonverbal attending skills include the media setup and the handling and provision of nonverbal pragmatic support.

Verbal microskills are enhanced by the use of open, exploratory, and summarizing questions. Art therapy directives are a form of verbal microskills. The request to draw, paint, and create can be posed as a closed or open-ended question or an encouraging or curious statement. Additional art therapy microskills include verbal exploration and interpretation of feelings and meanings associated with the imagery, the art making process, and the explicit narrative.

ATR-N microskills may be component, process, technique, or content based. They are based in the CREATE principles. For example, in Chapter 3 we build upon information from relational neuroscience to suggest that therapeutic movement is a critical art therapy component. In Chapter 4 we increase our understanding of the therapeutic process by discussing the effects of media exchanges on attachment-based interactions. In Chapters 5 and 6 we suggest several ATR-N techniques that can support co-regulation and expressive communication.

The timing of interventions can also be guided by ATR-N considerations. For example, in Chapter 6, which focuses on autobiographical memory, we suggest that the traditional intake timeline directive can be used as an ongoing measure of therapeutic change. We also interpret the timeline according to attachment theory constructs. Thus, as stated earlier, at the end of each chapter we review how an ATR-N approach and each CREATE principle may be used to strengthen the art therapist's therapeutic skills.

BOOK ORGANIZATION AND METHODOLOGY

Six ATR-N CREATE principles organize the book's content. Each chapter focuses on one principle and some principles span more than one chapter. Relational Resonating is emphasized as a major point of distinction; conceptually all the CREATE ATR-N principles are informed by relational therapeutic factors, primarily attunement to, acceptance of, and empathic interest in self and others (Frank & Frank, 1993; Lambert, Shapiro, & Bergin, 1986). As stated, most of the chapters are similarly structured, linking the ATR-N practices with the didactics of IPNB, relevant neuroscience, and clinical skills. Information from neurobiological research is reviewed and integrated with art experientials, thereby shedding light on relational neuroscience applications. A sequence of ATR-N practices, meaning directives, and specific media facilitate creative exploration of the ATR-N skills. In each chapter, we present the ATR-N experiential directives prior to the neuroscience information, as we first like to engage our group members in active learning through art making. Then the relational neuroscience is provided to serve as a scientific context in which personal experience and clinical skills learning can be situated. Readers may find that the information becomes more advanced as they progress. This is because the last three chapters focus on the complexities of Transformative Integrating and Empathizing and Compassion. We also build upon the reader's progressive acquisition of and familiarity with the material. Throughout the chapters, all the CREATE principles are interwoven in the clinical skills section, designed to integrate the information presented with applied clinical ideas and skills.

For those looking to use this material to accompany coursework in ATR-N or the biological basis of behavior and psychology, the chapters' layout can structure the learning. It is suggested that the art practices include personal written work and additional reading. This is similar to MBSR and MBCT approaches, in which teachers, students, or clients continue working outside of the face-to-face group setting. For those interested, the authors offer additional resources on their websites, such as sample course syllabi and assignments (www.noahhasscohen.com).

Chapter 2 presents an introductory review of the relational neuroscience with a focus on interpersonal meaning making and affect regulation. It also introduces our methodological approach. Focusing on regions associated with affect expression and regulation, the primary purpose is to review the main brain structures and their IPNB-related functions. The experientials involve creating paintings of brain maps and reworking two-dimensional brain maps into three-dimensional models. Additionally, we demonstrate how art making assists in building awareness and communication of emotions, as well as in the development of the capacity for personal meaning making. This work also invites investigation of the participants' cultural reactions to the exploration of human neuroanatomical structures and functions. Sensory experiences, visual processing, and group discussion infuse the didactic information with salient meaning.

Focusing on motion, Chapter 3 explores the principle of Creative Embodiment. Distinguishing ATR-N interventions, the inclusion of therapeutic motion, enacted movements as well as symbolically represented motions, and the incorporation of multi-modal interventions can create therapeutic change. We ask participants to create, move around, and manipulate a body-sized representation of their space as well as utilizing this work to connect with others. These activities are intended to result in active matching of one's inner state with art expressions, thereby reducing defensive avoidance strategies associated with stressful or traumatic experiences. In a secure environment motion, particularly when repeated, can help solidify implicit learning and consolidation of new memories. Multi modal expressive choices, as well as moving toward or away from another person, object, or experience, support a felt sense of safety and freedom. As discussed in the chapter's relational neuroscience section, this interface can contribute to a calming of fear responses, increased motivation, and social contagiousness. Symbolized motions can be manifested in art shapes and colors and can be internally experienced as generating movement toward change. Within this action-oriented context, interpersonal space is renegotiated, a sense of self is redefined, and relationships are reshaped. The psychological intersection of motor movements, emotions, and cognitions is often metaphorically revealed.

Chapters 4 through 6 explore the principle of Relational Resonating. Chapter 4 introduces attachment theory as a core ATR-N paradigm and describes the related phenomenon of neuroplasticity. We describe how offering and exploring art media sets the stage for significant relationships to develop and reveal themselves. The concrete and symbolic display of the media can relay personal attachment histories, reveal vulnerabilities to stress responses, and, ideally, support a sense of competence. Working together and representing attachment-based imagery can be powerful gateways to attuned attachment experiences. The acquisition of secure affective experiences with consistent sensory expression can create a new self-representation. The chapter also reviews how attachment styles, which are experience dependent, affect development and changes in the social brain throughout the life span. In Chapter 4, the attachment-based art therapy experientials are the interpersonal media presentations, the family attachment map, and fabric-based attachment albums. While these experientials were designed for use with adults, they can be adapted for children as well.

Illustrating the reciprocal and dynamic qualities of emotive communication, Chapter 5 focuses on the co-regulation and co-creation of relational affect. Co-regulation and co-consciousness refer to attuned communication rather than mere information delivery. We use ATR-N experiential practices to demonstrate that similar to caregiver-infant right-to-right-hemisphere, joint mentalizing and interactions continue to be at the core of interpersonal affect regulation throughout the lifepan. In fact the right brain is used from infancy through adulthood for nonverbal emotional processing and communications. Experientials shed light on how right-to-right-hemisphere brain communication functions within art therapy practices. For example, the pleasures of non-judgmental and therapeutic art making can further support regulatory self-functions. This is because the more we engage in positive interactions, the more efficiently our regulatory neuronal circuitry functions. The chapter's relational neurobiology section describes the lateralized functions of the hemispheres and the neurobiology of positive and negative emotions and affect regulation. All advance the unique relevance of ATR-N practices for affect regulation.

Relationally attuned therapeutic experiences can help create new coherent autobiographical memories and contribute to neuroplasticity. Thus, Chapter 6 focuses on the lifelong role of autobiographical memory. The chapter introduces the self, social, and directive functions of autobiographical memories. The art directives include developing and exploring several autobiographical timelines and making transparent childhood memory cutouts. The purpose is to provide for the formation of a contextualized sense of past, present, and future. We explain how the art directives can update the autobiographical social self and illustrate how art therapists might work with clients to reconsolidate old to new memories while increasing tolerance for episodic emotional memories. In the relational neuroscience section, we discuss research that demonstrates the overlapping neurobiology of autobiographical memory functions and theory of mind. These studies provide further support for the psychological interface of the three autobiographical functions and attachment theory.

Chapters 7 and 8 explore the principle of Expressive Communicating. Chapter 7 focuses on accessing implicit-unconscious emotions, and supporting positive emotions and creative experiences. Inspired by surrealistic art, the ATR-N experiential practices incorporate chance, random, sensory, and playful-based techniques. The purpose is to encourage process artwork, making the implicit explicit. Various regions and neurocircuitry thought to be associated with the unconscious are reviewed in the relational neurobiology section.

Chapter 8 focuses on art mediated interpersonal touch and space (AMITS), describing how physical contact with sensory-rich and unstructured clays can deepen and diversify an inner sense of the self. Stimulated by touch and space, affective and implicit self-awareness may shift to become more explicitly and consciously available for exploration. When the act of AMITS is amplified and used as a means for expression, increased communication occurs. Chapter 8 also focuses on the reparative role of interpersonal touch and space. In this context, we describe different types of interpersonal touch. The interpersonal neurobiology section includes a review of the rich connections between the thalamus, the limbic system, and the cortical brain structures and explores the function of the hormone oxytocin. These descriptions enhance our appreciation of affect regulation by unfolding the complexities of experienced, expressed, and symbolized interpersonal touch.

Chapters 9 and 10 focus on the principle of Adaptive Responding. Chapter 9 focuses on short- and long-term stress and fear responses. The review of the information and art making is linked to the spectrum of stress responses, namely fight, flight, freeze, and turn to others. Art-making offers opportunities to examine bodily reactions, safely express disturbing experiences, reveal related cognitions and emotions, and examine upsetting behaviors. It also supports identifying resources and accessing needed resiliency. Drawing stress responses and constructing a three-dimensional adaptation container provide the opportunity to represent, engage, and practice with safe social relationships. The accompanying discussion of relational neurobiology emphasizes the various states and contexts for coping that arise when an individual faces stressors. Consequently, awareness of coping is increased and practiced through verbal and nonverbal, conscious and unconscious neural pathways. Chapter 10, subtitled "Secure Remembrance," describes an ATR-N model for working with complex trauma. The challenge that complex trauma presents is that symptoms are more difficult to resolve and have a tendency to cycle and reoccur. As such, treatment requires paying deliberate attention to safeness, stabilization, and adaptability. Secure Remembrance is a model with five therapeutic factors: Safety, Relationship, Remembrance, Reconnection and Resiliency (SR-5). Establishing perceived and actual personal safety, engaging in contextual memory processing, and supporting social connection correspond with Herman's (1997) Tri-Phasic traumatology approach. Exploration and development of relationships as well as the practice and application of relapse prevention social strategies make up the other two literature-informed factors. All factors are rooted in the efficacy of nonspecific therapeutic factors, mainly trust, optimism, appreciation of beauty, hope, and resiliency. A sequence of five experiential activities and multiple directives illustrate the five factors. This SR-5 model incorporates directives from two of our previously published ATR-N models (Hass-Cohen & Clyde Findlay, 2009; Hass-Cohen et al., 2014) that include these factors. Altogether, this chapter illustrates treatment methods for developing resiliency; adaptation, coping, and living with extremes of internal duress and stress.

Chapters 11 and 12 explore the principle of Transformative Integrating. Chapter 11 focuses on mentalizing, which refers to the ability to understand and know one's own mental state as well as the mental states of others. Mentalizing recruits implicit and explicit functions and, as stated earlier, is dependent on cognitive abilities and on attachment-based mind states and styles. Several art therapy experiences assist in understanding this complex process. They include constructing paper homes, furnishing their interiors with thoughts and beliefs, bringing the homes together into a community with other artists' structures, making a family environmental map, and discussing written weekly at-home reflections. Such imaginative activities promote mentalizing by allowing our participants to perceive and mentalize others' behavior as purposeful and intentional. Directed sharing of the art augments each group member's internal awareness and facilitates a group component to the transformative integration.

Chapter 12 discusses mindful awareness and describes our approach to art therapy practices that focus on paying attention to and accepting the here-and-now of our experiences. In this chapter, we discuss both formal and informal ways in which the art therapist may promote insight and mindfulness. Several art therapy experiences promote these skills, including collage selection, mindful media awareness, a body silhouette experiential, and mandala making. Informal mindful breathing, formal mindful walking, and a body scan meditation are integrated throughout the experientials. This chapter underscores the integrated brain functions associated with mindfulness practices and the CREATE principle of Transformative Integrating. Unique to this chapter is the emphasis on therapist self-care, which mindfulness practices are particularly well-suited to support.

Chapters 13 and 14 focus on the principle of Empathizing and Compassion. Chapter 13 focuses on the intersubjective experience of empathy and compassionate relating. Empathy results from the integration of right- and left-hemisphere functions with bottom-up arousal and top-down influences. The development of empathy builds upon the capacity for affect regulation and evolves toward acceptance of the self and others in the present moment. At the intersection of attuned attachment and the excitation of emotionally aroused learning, empathic experiences in the art therapy clinic propel the therapist and the client toward change, hope, happiness, and love. To celebrate this possibility, we describe, in Chapter 13, how building an art altar and making a group hand silhouette mural involve mirror neuron systems, which ultimately contribute to mindful empathy, insight, kindness, compassion, and joy.

Chapter 14 serves as an epilogue and concludes with the idea that empathizing leads to the loving of art and art therapy. The full empathic response must include the motivation to relieve suffering and a compassionate response. As fully engaged art therapists expand their efforts beyond a mere cognitive understanding of others' affective states, they become hypersensitive to the messages carried in the art. We suggest that this empathizing response facilitates therapeutic goals and embodies the art therapist's love for art, art therapy, and a deep connection with fellow art therapists.

SUMMARY

Our hope is that this book will serve as a knowledgeable and pragmatic guide to navigating the oceanic waters of arts psychotherapy and neuroscience. Throughout this book, we strive to demonstrate the relational context as the most important component of art therapy–based work, whether between group members and leader, or therapist and client.

Our featured artists made art for self-expression, and engaged in reflective writing and art making. Depending on the activity, we refer to them as participants, group members, artists, or individuals. With the exception of some client work, they are art therapy students and colleagues. In the studio, they pursued art therapy responses and dialogues that captured our attention for endless hours as all of us examined the inconceivable amount of research that contributed to this book. In keeping with the ATR-N concepts, our group is asked to be thoughtful about how to present art media to another person, to anticipate how an individual may approach the provided materials, and to experience how this initial interaction may arouse attachment-based reactions. Throughout the book, we also refer to Noah's and Joanna's responses as "ours" and our contributors' art and responses as "theirs." These first-person claims are not intended to take away from the scientific endeavors in this account. In fact, quite the opposite is true in our phenomenological approach. We insist that this self-laboratory is necessarily part and parcel of our efforts to not only harvest the findings of clinical neuroscience for art therapy, but also interact compassionately with the emerging material.

The ATR-N experiential practices are used to clarify didactic information, increase both inter- and intrapersonal expressivity, develop clinical skills, and promote professional growth. These isomorphic experiences allow for the felt learning to integrate and consolidate. We believe that applying salient relational neuroscience research to the theory and practice of visual- and sensory-based therapies continues a new way of thinking about art therapy and that art making provides an understanding of complex brain information. Our hope in introducing this model is to inspire a dialogue about the integration of complex neurobiological information into art therapy practices.

One distinctive feature of the CREATE ATR-N approach is that it reformulates the issues central to many art therapy approaches in a nonpolemic way. It teaches us that irrespective of the particular art therapy approach (Rubin, 2012), therapy can also be explored via an understanding of the fundamental structures and functions of the interpersonal mind, meaning the relational nervous system, relationships, and experiences. From a neurobiological perspective, sensory, perceptual, emotional, cognitive processing, and memory coding and retrieval are all mind states and functions that support the generation of imagery. Imagery incorporates all senses: visual, kinesthetic, tactile, auditory, and olfactory. In other words, mind states can be manifested as fleeting, sensory, media-based, or clear cognitive visualizations. This imagery, which can be named or narrated by putting words to nonverbal images, contributes to integrated subcortical and cortical functions. An interpersonal neurobiological approach conceives art therapy and imagery as interchangeable concepts. Imagery allows inner experiences to be consciously expressed and is a source of creativity. Hence, at the basis of creative power are the imagination and the image.

Imagery exists at the intersection of mind and body. What we see and what we imagine produce psychophysiological and behavioral responses (Doidge, 2007). The internal activation of mental images is similar to the processes involved in perceiving external imagery from the environment (Dadds, Bovbjerg, Redd, & Cutmore, 1997). This formulation of neural equivalency helps art therapists understand that the symbolic encounter with art making can be experienced as real and is then generalized to life-affirming changes. Furthermore, this neural equivalency can fire up the therapeutic relationship and result in an exchange of mind states and the development of integrated and stable selfhood.

Relational neuroscience provides an atheoretical foundation from which art therapists of any theoretical orientation can approach the interpersonal and felt aspects of art therapy. It utilizes experimental and clinical research as well as evidence-supported practices to demonstrate how brain functions and structures are directly impacted by relational experiences; experiences and information can change the landscape of people's lives as well as their brain. Understanding the relational neurological communications facilitates therapists' development and clients' change processes. We describe how ATR-N practices provide an excellent fit for facilitating relational mind-body exchanges and the unique set of skills that art therapists trained in the CREATE approach possess.

CHAPTER 2

Review of Neurobiology and Meaning Making

The making of art acts as a force of integration and interconnectedness of all the brain systems, creating a greater awareness and understanding of the whole experience. In the creating of art about my mind-brain, the concepts of its structure, function, and psychosocial interaction were more deeply embedded in my memory. The visual experience expanded my understanding of the content, the processes involved, and my own personal emotional connections. The schematic drawing (content and process) engaged the higher thinking skills of my neocortex; the movement of painting (process and emotion) accessed the areas of the brain stem and cerebellum; and the use of color (emotion) connected with my limbic system. Lisa Cerrina

THIS CHAPTER PROVIDES AN OVERVIEW of the main brain structures and functions involved in emotional expression, interpersonal affect regulation, and personal meaning making. Studio experientials, such as copying, drawing, painting, and sculpting visual maps of the brain, expose the reader to using art expressions for learning relational neuroscience, while at the same time stimulating novel reactions and meaning making. Our experiential practices, illustrate how we use the arts to learn the basics of neuroanatomy, the foundation for understanding the ATR-N approach. The creating participants also explore their reaction to this information and consider what kind of implications the approach might have for clinical practice. For example, drawing a brain map greatly facilitates our initial understanding of brain structure and function while at the same time providing insights into the critical role of emotional expressions and regulation throughout the life span. Thus, as stated in Chapter 1, these methods are gateways to acquiring clinical neuroscience knowledge and ATR-N principles and practices. This chapter begins this meaning-making journey. It is in the space between the nonverbal art making and the verbalization of its meaning that the interpersonal self emerges. Aptly named an "intersubjective artistic matrix" (Gerber et al., 2012, p. 41), this interpersonal matrix is the source of meaning-making. Such meaning making informs every square inch of this personal, clinical, professional, and theoretical epistemological map. What we know, how we know what we know, and how this knowledge changes are core epistemological concepts (Hass-Cohen, 1992). This kind of processing and meaning making is anchored in past memories and informed future actions but is influenced as much, if not more so, by what is happening right now (Bateson, 1972). The dreams and truths of the members of our creative milieu are mediated by art making. As these processes converge coherently, interpersonal meaning making emerges. For this to occur, a combined explicit and implicit appraisal, regulation, and integration of emotions, perceptions, thoughts, and behaviors is necessary.

The appraisal of basic emotions, perceptual sensory inputs and developmental experiences occurs in a bottom-up fashion, from lower brain circuitry to the mid-central and then higher brain regions (Panksepp, 1998; Panksepp, & Biven, 2012; Perry, 2006). A schematic formulation of the brain includes three regions: the reptilian-lower brain, the limbic-central brain, and the neocortex, representing higher brain regions (Kalat, 2012). Survival responses are carried by the reptilian brain, and emotions are transmitted from the limbic system, the seat of emotion, to the neocortex, the seat of cognitions (MacLean, 1990). The neocortex is composed of left and right hemispheres. The right engages the nonverbal, social-emotional self, and the left rules over language, motor, and cognitive functions. Consequently, incoming messages link to cortical appraisal, motivation, and interpretation. Horizontal and vertical brain circuitry connects the right and left hemispheres, and the three brain regions contribute to emotional processing and affect regulation (Carlson, 2013). This same sequence also represents the developmental sequence of the brain that emerges from neonatal beginnings to young adulthood when it completes its organization (Eliot, 1999; Giedd, 2004; Kalat 2012).

Affect regulation represents the ability to cope with what arises from reptilian and central areas of the brain (Schore, 2003). In other words, one is able to handle the emotional impact of difficult events without affect dysregulation or external, behavioral collapse. Inhibiting controlling and accepting emotional expression requires integration of sensory information processing and cognitive brain functions (Siegel, 2006). Without it, poorly modulated emotional responses contribute to a diminished capacity for reasoning and meaning making. The expression of such emotion and its regulation also motivates social engagement. Furthermore, they contribute to improvements in mood, cognitive functioning, and learning capacity (Panksepp, 2010). Affect regulation is also directly associated with tolerating, minimizing, and developing resiliency to stress (Siegel, 2012).

Meaning making involves the cognitive and emotional interpretation of facial expressions, nonverbal gestures, and sensory stimuli (Frith, 2009). Due to its sensorial qualities the process of art making, further augments mental models that contribute to deep and personal understanding of the material. Active learning uses verbal, visual, auditory, and kinesthetic strategies to support creativity, build brain capacity, and provide a transformative environment that lends itself to changing the brain and to personal and social meaning making (Diamond, Krech, & Rosenzweig, 2009; Kays et al., 2012). For example meaning emerges as neuroanatomy didactics are brought to life with color infused visual and maps and sculptures.

> *After the group discussion, I made a conscious shift toward thinking of the drawing as "my mind-brain," but it was not until I began to add color that an emotional connection began to emerge. I became less conscious of the more intentional intellectual thought process. The prompt to start with a favorite color provided a safe beginning. I immediately became immersed in the activity (movement) of the painting process, which felt very creative and relaxing, even within the highly defined structure of the previously established schematic drawing. I began with the intention of keeping the three areas of my mind-brain separate, but as color "accidentally" began to run together in places, I did not try to prevent it. Awareness began to emerge as an appreciation for how each area has evolved over time, adding a new layer of functioning to the brain, increasing its complexity, and developing into an interdependent system.* Lisa Cerrina

Each experiential in this chapter mixes the neuroscience and media exploration. Sensory experiences, visual processing, didactic learning, and group discussion assist in the integration. This endows the academic information with emotive, meaningful experiences. In addition, the experientials invite a cultural beliefs and values exploration about the mind-brain quandary. Pertinent questions include discovering what differentiates mind from brain as well as discovering how talking about our bodies, ourselves may present additional personal challenges. Written reflections and verbal discussion further reveal insights that sculpting and painting play a role in connecting emotions with bodily sensations, feelings, and thoughts. Subsequent to such intricate integration, group members also report feeling more socially connected.

EXPERIENTIAL PRACTICES AND DIRECTIVES

Experience I: Brain Maps

For this experiential, the group finds the art therapy tables bedecked with a variety of schematic brain maps. Also on display are anatomical plastic brain models, and sometimes films or social media clips that vividly depict brain function. A variety of illustrated neuroanatomy textbooks provide a visual and tactile reference for individual and group discussion (Carter, 2010; Carter, Aldridge, Page, & Parker, 2009).

We start by discussing a brain map that depicts three major functional brain regions, which correspond to survival needs, emotional protective functions, and complex cognitive abilities. The survival-based region named the "reptilian brain" is located in the lower areas of the brain, connected to the brain stem (Kalat, 2012). Responsible for genetic and instinctual memory, it includes the brain stem, midbrain, and cerebellum, and is innervated by the spinal cord. Evolutionarily referred to as the "mammalian brain," the brain's emotional seat is located within the central and midbrain area (MacLean, 1990). Composed of a system of structures, it is commonly referred to as the "limbic system." Limbic regions transmit emotions and sensations to the neocortex, also known as the cerebrum. The limbic system is directly connected to the brain's right hemisphere. The right hemisphere is biased toward nonverbal and avoidance responses, whereas the left hemisphere is approach-oriented and has a predisposition toward language (Schore, 2003). Complex cognition is conducted by the neocortex. The neocortex receives emotional and sensory information from the limbic system and sends top-down signals to dampen emotional reactivity and direct action (Carlson, 2013).

While most illustrated brain models are oversimplified, they are useful for psychoeducational purposes. For example, they are instrumental in helping people understand why emotions are prevalent in our experiences; there are strong connections between the limbic system and the right hemisphere, which make it easy for emotions to take over. Dominant over human function, the emotional area of the brain lies in its center. At times we role-play how drawing a brain map can help make these connections evident. We ask each group member to: "First, quickly sketch a lateral-side view of the brain." This assists in processing the information, and helps prepare therapists to be able to explain it to another person. Drafting sketches without looking at textbook figures assists us in ingraining the brain structure information into memory. Such a quick drawing from short-term memory allows the artist to capture the main features (Figure 2.1).

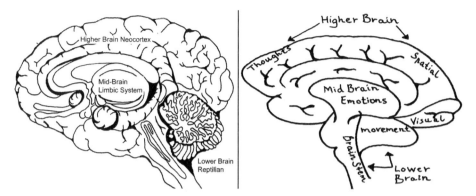

Figure 2.1 *Emotions in the Center.* Illustrated are the lower, mid, and higher brain (on left). Quick illustration of the lateral brain with three parts (on right). Adapted from Lisa Cerrina.

Next, we ask our participants to: "Draw an accurate version of your brain map." Using large, wet-media heavy paper, they then draft, trace, and/or enlarge their drawings to the larger-than-life size of a human head. Adding complexity, some artists, attracted to the process of copying the exact intricate neuroanatomical landscapes may transpose and use several traced schemas. We finalize the directions by asking them to: "Add symbolic color to your pencil brain map, using paint" (Figure 2.2).

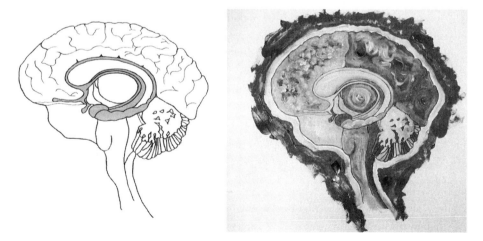

Figure 2.2 *The Brain* (left) and *My Brain* (right). The right brain is adorned with green around the figure. Green also appears in the stem. The center of the brain is light blue, whereas the rest of the regions contain several red, purple, and pink hues. Jessica Plotin.

When I had first drawn the image of the three brains, I was very detached and had no emotional connection to what I was doing. It was strictly an exercise in accurately capturing an anatomical image of the brain. During the painting and coloring process, I discovered my personal relationship with the drawing. As it became "My Brain," it became infused with personal emotion. I started with the color green, which is a color already infused with personal meaning and emotion. It has been my favorite color since childhood and always connects me to a sense of calmness, peace, and contentment. I began to experiment with different shades and I began to enjoy the sensual feeling of thick paint on my brush. I put white and green together on my brush and created thick swirls in a myriad of green shades. Thus began my emotional relationship with "My Brain." Jessica Plotin

For her brain drawing, Jessica drew a lateral-side view of the brain's three systems (Figure 2.2). Influenced by Carter's (2010) beautiful illustrations, her images radiate color. Then she took the opportunity to paint and delineate the neocortex lobes, by endowing each of them with color. Questions arose as to whether to use body-like colors or more symbolic colors. Group members discussed the symbolism behind their color choice, and the thoughts, feelings, and emotions aroused by painting.

In small groups, questions arise such as: What are emotions? Are they limited to specific brain areas? The basic emotions associated with limbic function and nonverbal communication are joy, anger, fear, disgust, and surprise (Panksepp, 2010). As a final step in the process, we offer the participants the opportunity to construct a group mural. Our group participants are asked to: "Find other paintings that resonate with yours and pin them close to each other to make a group mural." This process embodies personal and interpersonal meaning making (Figure 2.3).

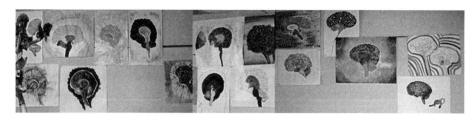

Figure 2.3 *The Mind-Brain Mural.* The multicolored brains are often distinguished by a predominant color; from left to right on the upper part of the mural, the neocortices are painted in pink, red, purples, and blues with contrastingly colored central brains. On the lower part of the mural the neocortices are mixed in color, with one that is a bright yellow.

I was so focused on the painting of my mind-brain that I had paid little attention to the surrounding area. Relating to the empty space, someone asked the question, "And what would be here?" I was very grateful for the inquiry and I began to look at the image as a whole and how I viewed my mind-brain in relationship to its surroundings and vice versa. I began to think more philosophically and emotionally and it was at this point that I felt the process become even more personalized and I became more fully engaged. It was no longer simply a representation of my mind-brain in isolation. It became my mind-brain, my surroundings, and their interrelated energy in time and space. As I looked at all of the art together on the wall, I felt a sense of awe and celebration. I was grateful for the experience, both personally and collectively, and I had a sense that I was not the only one who was feeling this way. Lisa Cerrina

Many of the artists aptly named their brain maps *My Brain*, elaborating on the transformation from didactic learning to personalized meaning making. They reflected on mind-body relationships and on what it means for them and for their personal and professional development.

The human brain has evolved to allow individuals to interact thoughtfully with their surroundings and create meaning. This connection is highlighted in creative expression and even more so in an art directive that encourages one to consider the relationship between various parts of oneself. The neocortex provides hope for humankind to no longer be subject to primitive impulses, but rather to be active participants in our response patterns to the world that surrounds us. As an art therapist, it is important to know what it is that is operating behind a current psychological phenomenon in a client and what that phenomenon might become. The neocortex speaks of human potential in areas of motivation, desire, rational choice, perception, and reaction. It importantly gives hope to act beyond seen activity into a realm of unseen processing that is involved in the activities of the mind. Robin Shanon

Experience II: Modeling the Brain

On our tables, we provide two-dimensional schemas of the limbic system and a selection of polymer clays. An anatomical brain model is also centrally positioned in the middle of the milieu. We ask the group to: "Make a model of the limbic system." Each individual usually gravitates to a specific clay, attempting to make a personal three-dimensional representation (Figure 2.4).

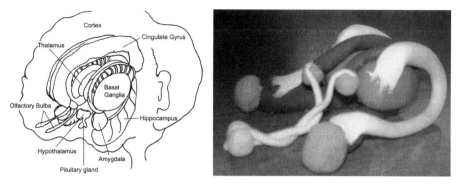

Figure 2.4 *The Limbic System* (left). It includes the basal ganglia, amygdala, thalamus, hippocampus, hypothalamus, and the anterior cingulate cortex. Within the limbic system, the thalamus and the hypothalamus make up the diencephalon, which is situated at the upper end of the brain stem, between the cerebrum and the brain stem. Both are online at birth and sensitive to environmental experiences. The basal ganglia forms part of the motor system. It includes several parts that are not depicted in the image. The pituitary gland is just outside of the limbic system. The cingulate gyrus is on the border between the limbic system and the cortex (on left). Polymer limbic system sculpture (right). The hippocampus is pink, whereas the amygdala is red, which makes it easier to see. Autumn Cade.

> *The fear I felt about my piece was that it wouldn't mold into what I had pictured in my mind that it should look like. The only way that I felt safe was that I felt I was in a protected space in which to bare my soul, that place being with my peers. Over the past few months I feel safe and comfortable enough to be able to share a piece of myself with my cohorts.* Autumn Cade

It can be challenging to construct a cohesive mental image of the limbic system from two-dimensional brain maps or even from the more accurate plastic brain model. Drawing or sculpting an anatomical model that has small soft tissue details and floating parts can be a complex task. Manipulating the clay to reproduce these tissues, organizing the brain structures, and creating a duplicate of each limbic structure sometimes results in clumsy caricatures that can leave individuals feeling frustrated and perhaps anxious. Self-regulation and seeking expressive solutions to these dilemmas thus become a significant part of the meaning-based process (Hass-Cohen, 2008a).

Modeling the brain presents a good opportunity to discuss how rapidly fear, joy, and interest can dominate behavior and possibly reinforce the learning of the art therapist's microskills. In this case, the art therapists are learning what kind of reaction they and their clients may have. These firsthand experiences can clarify what is asked of the therapist in order to support soothing the client's emotional arousal.

As I pondered emotions of love and passion, it is probable that my limbic system was activated and then passed onto my neocortex, wherein I meditated on the greater revelation and significance of such heart-felt emotions. This connection allowed me to feel empowered and free to both feel and express myself in a thoughtfully considered manner. Robin Shanon

Other meaning making discussions may revolve around each person's comfort level with the process of exploring the insides of his or her brain. One's personal history or familial or ethnic culture may not always support the exploration of one's mind or physical brain. In the social context of the clinic or studio, some people may have an intensified emotional reaction to viewing and meta-touching their inside self and brain. Some individuals may find this process unsettling, which can give rise to a gestalt of shared and novel exchanges.

In my family it was a taboo to talk about our insides. We just knew what was right and/or wrong and how we were supposed to behave. It was quite peculiar to think that as I fumbled with the clay, trying to make my limbic system in clay, that this internal part of me was responsible for my emotional reactions. I felt somehow like I was betraying a rule of not questioning too closely. This experience made me aware that I would need to continue a process of personal discovery as well as be super sensitive to explaining the role of neurobiology to my clients. Linda Ross

Emotions that are psychologically and socially remembered and interpreted emerge as mental representations and cognitive schemas (Gross & Barrett, 2011). Although these novel experiences may lead to either negative or positive emotions, their impact on memory and learning are noteworthy for self-realization and growth.

RELATIONAL NEUROSCIENCE: THE NERVOUS SYSTEM OVERVIEW

From an evolutionary perspective, the three main brain regions are the primitive-reptilian lower brain, the emotional-limbic system, which is the central brain, and the higher brain, the neocortex. These developed one on top of the other. The neocortex, the new brain, is the most recently evolved (MacLean, 1990; Figure 2.5).

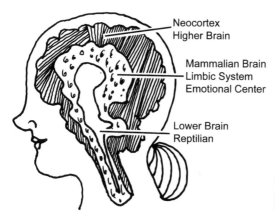

Figure 2.5 *The Triune Brain:* The neocortex, mammalian, and reptilian brain.

In other brain schemas, the lower brain regions are associated with reflexive responses to pain, disgust, and calmness. The central (i.e., intermediate) brain regions are linked to basic emotions such as fear, anger, joy, affection, and interest (Ekman, 1999). Last, the high-forward brain reflects social emotions such as guilt, contempt, envy, humor, and sympathy (Panksepp, 2010). Conceptually, it is more likely that the aforementioned emotions are mental constructs orchestrated by the higher regions. However, lower and middle brain areas give rise to emotional expression and representation (Gross & Barrett, 2011).

The Reptilian, Lower Brain: Motor-Sensory Inputs and Responses

Located at the base of the skull and emerging from the spinal column, the reptilian brain is the oldest and smallest region in the evolving human brain. Resembling the brain of present-day reptiles, which developed millions of years ago, the reptilian brain regulates breathing, heartbeat, consciousness, and the sleep cycle (Kalat, 2012). It is also part of the fight, freeze, or flight response that may accompany fear-based emotions. Furthermore, the reptilian brain is likely concerned with fundamental needs such as survival, physical maintenance, hoarding, dominance, preening, and mating. The basic emotions of attraction and bonding, hate, fear, lust, and contentment emanate from this primal brain. Responsible for heart rate and rhythm, its function can be metaphorically explained as similar to that of the heart (Linden, 2008).

The use of reptilian-based art imagery reflects the importance of this area. Ancient civilizations were fascinated by this primitive part of the brain, and many early civilizations regarded reptiles as power symbols (Cirlot, 1990). For example, the Egyptians depicted the spitting cobra as a symbol of sovereignty, deity, and divine royalty (Eason, 2008). Reptilian imagery is also an archetypal image of life and vitality; in contemporary times, spiraling forms similar to coiling cobras are used as symbols for human DNA. Perhaps this spiral represents not only genetic DNA coding but also movement.

The human brain emerges from the spinal cord, which conducts sensations, or nerve impulses, to and from the brain stem (Kalat, 2012). Fine touch, crude touch, vibration, pain, temperature, and itching are nerve impulse interpretations that have traveled up through the brain stem to higher regions of the brain. These impulses do not cognitively exist until conscious processing occurs. In the higher brain, neural impulses functionally translate into words, feelings, emotions, and so on. In the unconscious brain stem, no such translation is needed. The brain stem connects to the neocortex and spinal cord by the motor (corticospinal) tract. Also acting as a messenger, the brain stem transmits information from the brain back to the body. The brain stem has four parts: the medulla, reticular activating system (RAS), pons, and midbrain. Associated with the functions of the brain stem is also the basal-lower area of the thalamus, which is the brain's sensory gateway (Figure 2.6).

Within the brain stem, the medulla contains the cardiac, respiratory, vomiting, and vasomotor centers. The medulla is also responsible for autonomic involuntary functions, such as breathing, heart rate, and blood pressure. Stemming from the medulla is the RAS, which is a center of arousal and

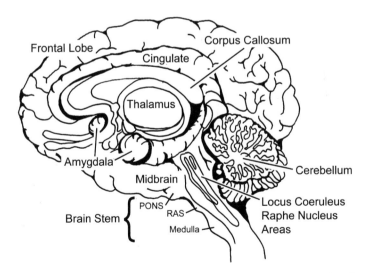

Figure 2.6 *Brain Stem.* The medulla, reticular activating system (RAS), pons, and midbrain. The locus coeruleus produces norepinephrine, and the raphe nucleus produces serotonin. Also shown are the frontal lobe, cingulate, amygdala, cerebellum, thalamus, and the corpus callosum, which connects the right and left hemispheres.

motivation. The RAS connects to the neocortex via the thalamus and RAS activity manifests in the pattern of brain waves (EEG) involved in sleep patterns and wakeful consciousness. The RAS spots novel stimuli, thereby promoting an arousal state that assists in staying awake and responding to danger. Conversely, soft and repetitive sounds, such as mindful breathing, support RAS relaxation. The midbrain portion of the brain stem is associated with vision, hearing, motor control, sleep/wake, arousal, and temperature regulation. Located near the center of the brain, the midbrain connects to the medulla and the cerebellum via a bridge of white matter called the pons. The pons is connected to neurotransmitter-producing nuclei, such as the locus coeruleus, which produces norepinephrine, as well as to the raphe nucleus, which produces serotonin and connects to motor, touch, and pain tracts. The pons also interfaces with afferent and efferent facial nerves, which allow facial expressions to be created and felt (Carlson, 2013).

The cerebellum, also located in the primal brain, helps control complex motor movements and procedural learning and integrates information from sensory receptors in the brain's major extremities, the brain stem, and the neocortex. Skilled or expected automatic movements are supported, and visuospatial signals are analyzed as they correspond to one's own movements as well as the movements of others (Jackson, Meltzoff, & Decety, 2006). Originally associated only with motor functions, the cerebellum is now noted for its cognitive functions as the number of neurons in the prefrontal cortex (PFC) is correlated with the number of neurons in the cerebellum (Herculano-Houzel, 2010). The cerebellum is small, constituting about 10% of our total brain volume, yet it contains more than 50% of the neurons within the central nervous system. In fact, it has many more neurons than the PFC, highlighting its importance in human function (Kalat, 2012; Table 2.1).

Table 2.1 Reptilian Brain Structures

Spinal cord	connects the central nervous system to the peripheral nervous system
Brainstem	controls basic involuntary body functions
Cerebellum	controls complex motor movements and procedural learning
Medulla (oblongata)	regulates autonomic, involuntary functions such as breathing, heart rate, and blood pressure
Midbrain	controls vision, hearing, motor control, sleep/wake, arousal, and temperature regulation
Pons	bridges the cerebrum, the medulla, the midbrain, and the cerebellum, as well as tracts that carry sensory signals to and from the thalamus
Reticular Activating System (RAS)	controls arousal, motivation, and calm based on stimuli detection; is connected to the neocortex via the thalamus

The Limbic System-Central Brain: Generating Emotion

Just above the brain stem and beneath the neocortex lies the limbic system, a collection of individual structures located in the central areas of the brain. Limbic means borders, which is an appropriate name, given that this area is adjacent to the higher and lower brain areas.

The limbic system borders and interacts with the neocortex, which processes the emotions generated by the limbic system and the sensations transmitted by lower areas such as the brain stem. The cingulate gyrus, specifically the front area, the anterior cingulate cortex, defines this uppermost limbic-cortex border. Portions of the brain stem and lower areas of the neocortex are also surrounded by the cingulate. Its frontal part, the anterior cingulate, plays an important role in mediating anxiety. The limbic system structures include the basal ganglia, caudate nucleus, amygdala, thalamus, hippocampus, and hypothalamus (Figure 2.7).

The limbic structures support the maintenance of survival-based behaviors, form basic emotions, as well as process and hold short- and long-term memory. The limbic area generates basic emotions, such as anger and joy. Rudimentary emotions such as these are automatically revealed in facial expressions (Ekman, 1999; Hass-Cohen & Carr, 2008).

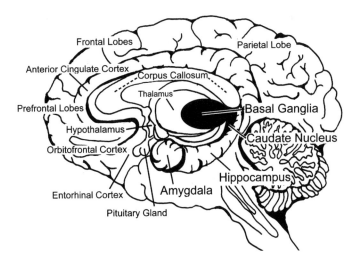

Figure 2.7 *Limbic System and Related Brain Structures.* These include the basal ganglia, caudate nucleus, amygdala, thalamus, hippocampus, hypothalamus, and the anterior cingulate cortex. The anterior cingulate cortex is the front part of the cingulate and is involved in regulating anxiety. The entorhinal cortex, a brain structure separating the neocortex from the hippocampus, sends information to the hippocampus. Also shown are the master hormonal gland, the pituitary, which is located just outside of the limbic system; the orbitofrontal cortex, involved in processing of novel information; the corpus callosum; and the cingulate cortex.

While emotions are generated in this area, they are not cognitively processed there, as consciousness occurs elsewhere (Carter, 2010).

The brain's sensory center, the thalamus, is involved in most of the brain's processes and most likely plays an important part in higher cognitive functions (Carr, 2008b; Hass-Cohen & Loya, 2008; Sherman, 2012). Shaped like two large eggs, it is a sensory gateway that relays almost all sensory and motor information (Kalat, 2012). Sensory processing is key to the activation of the fear response due to the thalamic-amygdala connections. The amygdala comprises a pair of almond-shaped structures that are activated by situations or stimuli that provoke a fear or stress response. Amygdala reactions shape implicit processing of emotion, especially fear, and assist in forming memories (Coan, Schaefer, & Davidson, 2006; LeDoux, 2003b). The amygdala receives messages from the senses via the thalamus as well as from higher cortical regions. In the fear response, messages from the thalamus (known as the low or quick road) bypass the neocortex and stimulate the amygdala to urgently alert the body to perceived threat (LeDoux, 2000, 2003a). The response-biased amygdala converts sensory input to motor output, which in turn excites actions. Linkages between the emotion and motor areas in the brain are provided by the basal ganglia. Part of the motor system, the basal ganglia provide feedback to the neocortex, modulate voluntary motor movements, and support flexible emotional functioning (Kalat, 2012).

Messages from the neocortex, which confirm or negate the amygdala fear response, happen more slowly in a process known as the slow pathway. In this case, based on a conscious evaluation, the neocortex subsequently transmits a signal to the hypothalamus to stop the autonomic nervous system arousal response. The purpose of this signal is to inhibit both the amygdala and bodily arousal, thereby halting the fear response (LeDoux, 2003a, 2003b).

Direct signals from the olfactory lobes are also transmitted to the amygdala. The olfactory lobes receive odors and transmit them directly to the amygdala, bypassing the thalamus. Despite being situated outside of the limbic center, they are involved in the fear circuitry, possibly because they are associated with implicit memories, which are stored in the hippocampus. The amygdala mostly responds to stimuli that evoke unconscious, conditioned fearful memories (LeDoux, 2007; Knight, Nguyen, & Bandettini, 2005). More precisely, it seems that it is the right side of the amygdala that is tuned to implicit stimuli, whereas the left side responds to language-based cues (Costafreda, Brammer, David, & Fu, 2008).

The hippocampus is a stress-sensitive, seahorse-shaped structure that is involved in implicit memory storage and explicit memory formation (Burgess, Maguire, & O'Keefe, 2002). It holds short-term implicit memory for about two years before those memories are embedded in long-term memory.

This neurocircuitry assists in hippocampal consolidation of learning and memory. Spatial learning and navigation also involve the hippocampus, which has been the focus of brain plasticity research. Studies have shown, for example, that the size of the hippocampus in London taxi drivers and Australian aborigines is larger than average (Maguire et al., 2000). This change is likely due to their daily navigation, which relies heavily on spatial memory. More recently, the hippocampus has also been implicated in decision-making processes (Euston, Gruber, & McNaughton, 2012). Most importantly, in 1998 it was discovered that adult neurons can regenerate in the hippocampus (Bremner, 2006). This was an inspiring discovery as reduction in hippocampal volume is associated with uncontrollable stress experiences and memories and with difficulty in recalling traumatic events (King-West & Hass-Cohen, 2008; Woon, Sood, & Hedges, 2010).

While fear processing is essential for human survival, repeated experiences of fearful trauma, such as child abuse negatively affect memory and increase vulnerability to fear and depression (Perry & Hambrick, 2006; Rothschild, 2000). Some people with depression and PTSD have enlarged amygdalas, suggesting that an overactive amygdala may contribute to inhibited hippocampal function (Teicher, Tomoda, & Anderson, 2006). The hippocampus may also appear smaller. The literature suggests that poor affect regulation contributes to heightened activation of the fear, threat, and memory circuitry (Lanius, Lanius, Fisher, & Ogden, 2006). Furthermore, when a research study's participants were asked to reappraise their emotions, amygdala activation tended to increase (Hughes, Crowell, Uyeji, & Coan, 2012).

An important emotional center, the hypothalamus controls the autonomic nervous system and engages the stress response. It contributes to feelings of exhilaration, anger, and unhappiness, directly influencing behaviors. When the hypothalamus is damaged, abnormalities in motivational behaviors, such as drinking, eating, sex, affect regulation, and fighting, may occur (Kalat, 2012). Located near the base of the brain, just in front of and below the thalamus, the hypothalamus transmits information to the pituitary gland. This master gland excretes hormones, which are sent to the adrenal cortex, a structure that sits atop the kidneys. Located just outside the limbic system, the double pear-shaped pituitary gland is part of the endocrine stress response: the hypothalamus-pituitary-adrenal (HPA) endocrine axis (Sapolsky, 2004). The HPA function is the software that bridges the central nervous system (CNS) and the stress response.

As part of the limbic system, the reward system is highly implicated in stress responses, as well as substance use, abuse, pleasure, and dependence. The reward circuitry is associated with the neurotransmitter dopamine (DA), which is produced by the nucleus accumbens (Carr, 2008a). The nucleus

Table 2.2 Limbic and Other Mid-Brain Structures

Amygdala	acts as a gateway to emotion, especially fear; experiences implicit memory
Basal ganglia	provides emotion-motor interface and includes the caudate nucleus, globus pallidus, and the putamen
Hippocampus	controls spatial navigation, learning, and short- and long-term conscious memory
Hypothalamus	bridges the nervous system and endocrine functioning
Thalamus	conducts sensory relay between the body/brainstem and cortical/subcortical areas
Nucleus accumbens	part of the limbic system and the reward pleasure system

accumbens is part of the striatum or basal ganglia, located in the limbic area. Serving as a neurobiological feedback loop, the reward system can strengthen the connection between cues and rewarding outcomes (Vanni-Mercier, Mauguiere, Isnard, & Dreher, 2009, Table 2.2).

Important to the reward system function is the locus coeruleus, a tiny brain structure. Located close to the limbic boundaries within the RAS and the pons, the locus coeruleus responds to arousing or stressful stimuli by sending bursts of a neurochemical, norepinephrine (NE), throughout the brain. When NE is released, it helps facilitate and reinforce the consolidation of new memories and the reconsolidation of old memories. Originally it was thought that memory formation was a stable process. However, research now shows that the consolidation of memory is a labile process, meaning that even old and established memories are susceptible to change (Schwabe, Nader & Preussner, 2014; a review).

These limbic structures and limbic adjacent systems work together, conveying the sensation of emotions from the body and the cerebrum to the neocortex (Kalat, 2012). The limbic system informs higher cortical processing via the cingulate cortex. Divided into the anterior cingulate cortex (ACC) and the posterior cingulate, the cingulate cortex (CC) integrates sensory, memory, and executive functions. It is also centrally involved in maternal care, nursing, and play (Insel, 2003). Meshing subcortical and cortical functions, the CC is involved in sensory, emotional, and memory functions. It contributes to the ability to attune and to focus. The ACC, together with the neocortex regions, specifically the prefrontal lobes and the orbitofrontal cortex, restrains inappropriate limbic-aspired action, prompts effective decision making, and coordinates activity between the neocortex and lower brain–mediated responses (Carlson, 2013).

The Higher Brain: Affect Regulation and Meaning Making

The neocortex controls higher-order thinking, reason, and speech (Goldberg, 2009). It also processes emotions and sensory information. Frontal neocortex regions, responsible for our highest level of functioning, can be the most vulnerable to traumatic brain injury. Most susceptible to brain damage are the two protruding poles in the frontal lobe area and in the posterior occipital lobe. Graphically, the neocortex looks like wrinkled, soft gray matter with ridges and indentations. When a person experiences a concussion, the soft brain matter hits the skull, usually with temporary effects, but sometimes resulting in long-term damage (Corrigan, Selassie, & Orman, 2010).

The neocortex's intricate surface includes bumps (gyri), grooves (sulci), and deep grooves (fissures, Figure 2.8). These forms are gray matter, composed of cell bodies, dendrites, and synapses of neurons without myelinated

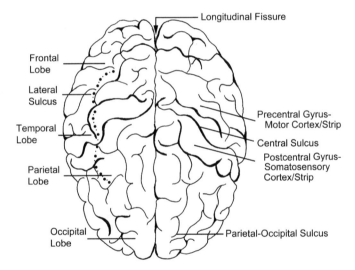

Figure 2.8 *Schema of a Dorsal View of The Neocortex with Selective Sulci and Gyri.* These divide the brain into lobes and connecting processing areas. The longitudinal fissure divides and connects the two hemispheres. The lateral sulcus divides and connects the frontal lobe and parietal lobe (above) from the temporal lobe (below). It is usually longer in the left hemisphere. The precentral gyrus is associated with the motor cortex, which includes the premotor cortex, as well as several subcortical brain regions. The motor strip functions to plan and execute movements and is connected to the spinal cord and neurons that control the muscles. The central sulcus separates the parietal lobe from the frontal lobe and the primary motor cortex from the somatosensory cortex. The postcentral gyrus, associated with the somatosensory cortex or strip, is an end point receiving area for tactile sensory information from the skin and joints. Touch, pain, pressure, and temperature sensation are transmitted to this region. The parietal-occipital sulcus runs deep into the end of the corpus callosum. It separates the parietal and occipital lobes as well as two regions associated with creativity: The cuneus, which is involved in basic visual processing, and the precuneus, which is involved with episodic memories, visuospatial processing, and reflections upon the self (not shown) (Buckner, Andrews, & Schacter 2008; Carlson 2013; Kalat, 2012).

fibers or axons. This is in contrast to white matter, which is composed of neurons with myelinated axons (Kalat, 2012; Christian, 2008, p. 63). Connections between gray matter neurons create a pattern in the gyri and sulci. All human brains have similar gyri and sulci patterns. A two-dimensional dorsal view represents the most traditional schema.

However, because life experiences, especially learning and education, result in diversely shaped connections, every person has unique brain topography (Cozolino, 2010). For example, the more connections there are, the heavier and more resilient the brain (Kalat, 2012). Studying and learning are among the strongest contributors to unique differences and to such increased connectivity

To organize this information and maximize ease of use, we guide our group to first notice the longitudinal fissure, which is the cleft between the hemispheres, and the central sulcus, which divides the frontal and posterior lobes. Also highlighted is the dotted line representing the sylvian lateral fissure, a prominent structure of the human brain. This lateral sulcus divides the frontal and parietal lobes from the temporal lobe below (Figure 2.9).

Anterior (before) and posterior (after) to the central sulcus are two important gyri, the postcentral gyrus and the precentral gyrus. The postcentral gyrus, involved in somatic sensation, lies immediately behind the central sul-

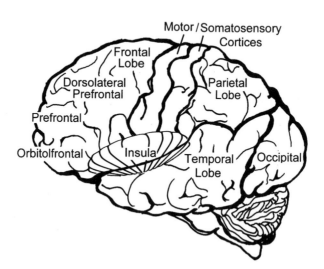

Figure 2.9 *Lateral View of the Central Sulci and the Cortical Lobes.* The temporal lobe, prefrontal lobe, frontal lobe, sensory motor cortex, parietal lobe, and insula with sulci and gyri. The insula is interior to the surface lateral sulci. The frontal lobe includes top-side (dorsolateral), prefrontal areas. The orbitofrontal cortex, also part of the frontal lobe, is located above the eyes and behind the forehead.

cus, also known as the somatosensory cortex or strip. Laid out like a map inside our heads, the somatosensory strip processes sensory information. It contains specific areas that represent each of our body parts and is responsible for receiving sensory input from each of these body parts in order to send this information to other areas of the brain for processing. We have reviewed the somatosensory cortex previously (Hass-Cohen & Carr, 2008, pp. 34–35), and do so again in Chapter 5 when we discuss the sense of touch. Lying in front of the central sulcus is the precentral gyrus, known as the primary motor cortex or strip, which controls voluntary movement. This motor cortex, which lies in front of the central sulcus, is discussed in greater detail in Chapter 3. Like the somatosensory cortex, the primary motor cortex contains specific regions dedicated to regulating movements for each part of the body (Kalat, 2012).

The brain is divided into parallel hemispheres. Neural pathways in each hemisphere work in a contralateral (cross-sides) fashion to control the opposite side of the body. Each hemisphere has somewhat different processing specializations that are interconnected via neural pathways called commissures. Connecting the right and left hemispheres, and flanked by the cingulate cortex, is the corpus callosum, the largest commissure (Figure 2.7). The corpus callosum becomes operational during middle childhood, potentiating the left hemisphere's eventual dominance over the right hemisphere (Eliot, 1999). When the right and left hemispheres connect, children efficiently learn how to read, write, and speak with more adept vocabularies. The corpus callosum is larger in women, suggesting stronger hemispheric connections (Sullivan, Rosenbloom, Desmond, & Pfefferbaum, 2001).

In the brain, bottom-up, and back-to-front processing complements such right-to-left connectivity. Bottom-up interfaces of mid-brain to high-brain pathways contribute to the integration of sensory information, memories, and executive functioning. The cingulate cortex above the corpus callosum connects subcortical to cortical tracts, adding sensory inputs to cortical processing. Located between the higher cortical areas and limbic structures, the cingulate cortex plays an instrumental role in affect regulation by bridging body and limbic information with cortical processing. Strong connections between the limbic system and the right hemisphere associate with left cognitive processing that includes information coming from the back of the brain; visual and auditory streams bring information forward to the frontal lobes (Carter, 2010).

The neocortex is responsible for sophisticated social-cognitive functions. Frontal lobes, the largest lobes in the neocortex, are situated at the front of the brain and lead us in action. Separated posteriorly from the parietal lobe by the central sulcus and from the temporal lobe inferiorly by the lateral sulcus, the

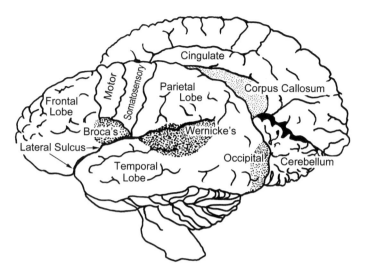

Figure 2.10 *The Neocortical Lobes.* The occipital, parietal, temporal, and frontal lobes, and the insular cortex are shown. The insular cortex is located within the sulcus that separates the temporal lobe and inferior parietal cortex. Dotted areas in Broca's area represent language and motor processing. Dots in Wernicke's area represent auditory association and language comprehension areas. Dots near the occipital lobe represent the beginning of informational association areas that take information across the cortex to the frontal lobes. The corpus callosum is shown as a bridge between the left and right hemispheres.

frontal lobes are responsible for cognitive, language, and motor functions. The lateral side of the left frontal area primarily controls speech output and motor functions on the right side of the body, while the right side of the frontal area assumes the same functions on the left side of the body (Figure 2.10).

Located in the frontal lobes are prefrontal regions (PFC) which are part of the motor-efferent system in the brain. These areas send messages throughout the central nervous system, leading it to action. Contained within this region are the precentral gyrus, the motor strip, and Broca's area, which is responsible for speech production (Kalat, 2012). Also connected to the brain stem and the cerebellum is the motor strip. The cerebellum feeds motor and basic body reactions to the frontal regions. Located in the frontal lobes behind the forehead, the PFC is responsible for the highest level of cognitive functioning: planning, organization, sequencing, categorizing, abstraction, and problem solving. Collectively, these are executive functions. The PFC directs the anticipation of impactful events, helps configure and reconfigure perceptions, maintains attention, regulates affect, and coordinates behavior. This primary executive area is responsible for integrating perceptual, volitional, cognitive, motor, and emotional processes.

The temporal lobes, which occupy areas that are located roughly above our ears, are responsible on the left for verbal memory, language comprehension, and word retrieval, while the right temporal lobe handles visual and nonverbal memory and nonverbal sound comprehension. Temporal lobe functions are multifaceted, integrating complex sensory, verbal, auditory, and emotional functions. They contain the primary auditory cortex, as well as a language comprehension section called Wernicke's area (Figure 2.10).

The parietal lobe exists behind the frontal lobe and demarcates the foremost part of the posterior part of the brain. Arithmetic, reading, verbal intelligence, and right-body tactile functions are controlled by the left parietal, while the right parietal is responsible for visual-perceptual and spatial construction, perceptual intelligence, and left-body tactile functions. Moreover, the right parietal processes external sensory cues and facilitates awareness, creating an understanding of one's own body within a given environment (Vuilleumier, 2005).

Located in the posterior portion of the brain, the occipital lobe processes visual information. It organizes visual input received by the primary visual cortex and passes it forward for further processing. Hidden deep in the cerebrum between the lips of the lateral sulcus is the smallest lobe of the brain, the insular lobe. The insula conveys sensory information about bodily states to the cortex. It is responsible for taste, hearing, and visceral sensations. The insula also transmits bodily sensations, such as disgust, to the cortex. It processes interoceptive stimuli and tracks ongoing bodily conditions. Additionally, the insula helps mediate extreme emotions, awareness, and expressions of bodily states, such as pain. Implicated in a multitude of social emotions, embarrassment, guilt, and envy, insula function contributes to theory of mind and empathy (Table 2.3).

Table 2.3 Main Cortical Structures

Frontal lobe	responsible for executive function, the frontal lobe includes the PFC and the motor strip; handles motor processing
Prefrontal cortex	controls the highest cognitive and regulatory functions
Orbito-frontal cortex	responsible for autobiographical memories
Motor strip	regulates movements for each part of our body
Somatosensory strip	receives and relays sensory input from body parts
Parietal lobes	handles visual-perceptual and spatial processing
Temporal lobes	responsible for memory and complex visual, auditory, linguistic, emotional, and motivational functions
Occipital lobe	receives, processes, and forwards visual stimuli as the action of seeing
Insular lobe	bridges brain-body functions

CREATE PRINCIPLES AND CLINICAL APPLICATIONS:
AN OVERVIEW

This chapter provided an introduction to the basic brain structures and functions associated with interpersonal neurobiology. For the ATR-N activities the participants engaged in a quick drawing, copying, and coloring of the brain map. They also modeled and sculpted a three-dimensional brain model and constructed murals, as well as shared and discussed related personal and mutual experiences that might eventually be applied to clinical work. Also provided is an introduction to integrated and transformative learning, covering the process through which experiential learning contributes to psychological change. In the quest to understand the complexity of interpersonal neurobiology, our participants work on realizing and becoming aware of changes in their belief systems. Furthermore, balancing artistic expression with affect regulation induces interpersonal change and develops the self of the art therapist. Such transformation is facilitated through consciously directed learning that includes perceiving, receiving, analyzing, and understanding the symbolic contents of one's art. It also has the potential to challenge and change the person's worldview of self and other.

In the following sections, we suggest how the information and experientials presented in this chapter manifest the CREATE principles. Most of the chapters in this book follow this convention. Connections to the CREATE ATR-N principles are outlined below as well as implications for art therapy microskills that can be used for the purposes of clinical work, teaching, or the development of research protocols.

The Creative Embodiment principle is activated through mural making, which stimulates movement and discussion. Supporting a range of therapeutic movements, the art therapist's space facilitates growth and development for clients. Movement and motor system pathways strengthen beneficial links between emotion and cognition. The creative process is enhanced with newfound understanding and freedom from constricting affect.

The active co-creation and co-ownership of a wall mural increases as well as supports interpersonal bonding and Relational Resonating. Although this chapter is mostly devoted to drawing and learning about the didactics of clinical neuroscience, the initial gathering and discussion represent group foundations for social interaction, contributing to the emerging of therapeutic Relational Resonating. Similar to art therapy based psychoeducation groups, this step is where learning becomes socially enhanced, thereby supporting meaning making.

With regards to the Expressive Communicating principle, it is the unique versatility of paints and painting that allows clients to creatively express, reflect, and contain a broad spectrum of emotions. Associated with the use of paint, color invites communication of the basic core emotions, including surprise, fear, anger, disgust, joy, and sadness. Emergent qualities of color and movement in painting can inspire personal insights, placing emotion processing at the center of art therapy. Since color is linked to personal and symbolic meanings, its use consequently increases optimal levels of excitation and motivation. At home or in the clinic or studio setting, the discussion of images displayed on the wall supports the communication and sharing of emotions and meaning making.

Liquid paint and color application, as well as the request to form a brain model from polymer clays, can contribute to a stressful experience. The media's fluidity, variable controllability, and possible negative personal connotations can challenge and stimulate the need for Adaptive Responding. At the same time, the sensory qualities of the media can also be attractive and may provide clients with rewarding experiences. The juxtaposition of stress and excitation can elicit clients' expression of conflicting feelings and increase tolerance levels for affect. It may also bring forth a subjective experience of control as the individual adapts to the novel and fluctuating demands of art making.

The CREATE principle of Transformative Integrating is represented through the art making process. Adding color to the pencil drawings of the brain integrates cognitive and emotive learning while consolidating a more expressive understanding of the self. As they acquire color and paint, the visual maps' creative transformation contributes to a sense of pleasure and well-being. The same process can be used when providing clients with psychoeducation services. They will benefit from this activity, as drawing and painting information will assist them in better absorbing and owning it.

Finally, the principle of Empathizing and Compassion is represented as the capacity to tolerate emotional frustration, such as that associated with making the limbic model or any other complicated three-dimensional clay structure. As clients experience and learn new information, the therapist can guide them toward self-empathy rather than self-judgment. Deliberately monitoring and shifting thoughts, feelings, and perceptions as well as adopting kindness-based values is linked to the transformation of the self-other dialectic. This self-other dialectic not only may encourage deeper self-awareness, but the resulting empathic attention may also serve as a springboard from which to nurture and relieve suffering. Within a group setting, self-awareness can deepen social connectivity as we can better join with others. Empathic associations, or empathic attention, provide a gateway to compassion as well as kindness and nurture the desire to alleviate the afflictions of others.

CHAPTER 3

Creative Embodiment: In Motion

It is believed that motor information related to motor actions is stored in the cerebellum and can be retrieved as needed. Perhaps emotions and memories associated with particular movements are also easily recalled when that motor information is elicited from the cerebellum. If so, then creation in action has therapeutic uses in fostering general art therapy practices such as safety, calmness, and hope. When painting, I created a scene that reminded me of a pleasurable experience. The act of creating required movement. When moving is done simultaneously with thinking or feeling, it might have a more profound impact than thinking or feeling alone. In addition, next time I look at the artwork, my brain will remember the movement involved in its creation, and the positive memories will be elicited again. When I enter the space I created for art making, I will immediately be engaged in orienting me to that space, and the freedom and well-being I felt last time I worked there will hopefully be felt again when I move or even anticipate movement in my space. Tamara Cates

EXPRESSIVE THERAPIES SUCH AS ART, drama, and play therapy utilize concrete fine motor movements and large actions; rhythmic or not, they are also symbolized in scribbles, loops, and reiterative lines and symbolic images. This chapter focuses on the first CREATE principle, Creative Embodiment, and it describes how the art therapist's skills and space support actual and symbolic therapeutic movements. The space in which art therapy occurs can range from a spacious area with dedicated tables and closets to a small office space that was quickly converted into an art studio. Utilizing movement, no matter how large or small the art therapy space, lends significant clinical benefits. The motor dimensions of art making directly contribute developmental, emotional, and symbolic values to the Interpersonal Neurobiology (IPNB) therapeutic context.

Developmentally directed movement, such as kneading clay, provides opportunities to hone gross and fine motor skills, as well as visuospatial skills that affect social function (Kramer, 1986). Drawing bold gestures on large canvases assists in warming up and releasing emotions (Kwiatkowska, 1978). Motor-based activities can also increase cognitive function, such as understanding the differentiation between left and right (Kramer & Erickson, 2007). These activate, motivate, excite, and release emotions, and, when successful, can symbolize the potential for change. Rhythmic movements whether walking, dancing, playing percussion instruments such as drums or even moving speak directly to lower brain functions of the motor system that are responsible for survival responses. When repeated with the support of a caring therapist these kind of multimodal interventions have the capacity to soothe and lull and perhaps recalibrate the functions of the motor system and cranial nerves involved in instinctual fear based and defensive reactivity (Perry & Hambrick, 2006; Porges, 2011, 2013).

Emotions such as fear and happiness, when compassionately processed as metaphors, can additionally generate motion and propel people into action. A studio art therapy experience in which the group members create and infuse with color a body-sized drawing, My Space, first demonstrates this chapter's principle. Then the artists engage in an interpersonal space exploration, Group Space.

Day-to-day therapist-client actions and interactions are therapeutic. Such motions, which can be taken for granted, include covering the workspace with protective paper, putting the crayons and paints where they can be easily accessed, and reaching out for the crayons. Picking up the brush, dipping it in the paint, creating, and then cleaning brushes and putting away all the materials are other examples. We propose that such simple beginning and ending gestures provide emotional and cognitive motion-based outlets (Hass-Cohen, 2008a). Our hands and bodies perform hundreds of simple and complicated automatic movements daily, to which we usually do not pay much conscious attention. These automatic motions initiated by the art therapist allow for several noteworthy therapeutic gateways: Communicating interest, conveying respect, showing appreciation of the client's difficulties in beginning to create art, helping to abandon judgment, and providing attuned acceptance. Moving from nonverbal knowledge to explicit verbalized meaning making can be challenging yet it can effectively consolidate therapeutic gains. As examples, our artists' accompanying narratives, reflections, and processing of a group mural facilitate this explicit process (Manders & Chilton, 2013).

The study of mirror neurons (MN) and their functions provide additional important insights to the connections between movement, cognition and intersubjectivity. MNs, located near the motor strip play a critical role in intersubjective functions of familiar motions and motor-based goals (Rizzo-latti, Fadiga, Gallese, & Fogassi, 1996). This is an intersubjective function, as without the observer's internal knowledge of the observed action, he or she cannot understand their purpose (Gallese, 2010). Thus, embodied simulation theory shows that "people reuse their own mental states or processes represented in bodily format to functionally attribute them to themselves" (Ammaniti & Gallese, 2014, p.16).

The explicit conveyance of interest, attuned acceptance, and trust (Frank & Frank, 2004; Lambert, 1986) are significant ATR-N therapeutic skills. The effective therapist skillfully communicates these factors nonverbally. For example, even a simple act of moving the media so that it is within the client's reach (Hass-Cohen, 2008a) may begin the needed process of reducing defensive and avoidant states and initiating adaptive action systems (Ogden, Minton, & Pain, 2006). Approaching the media, scratching the page with a pencil, and loading a brush with paint are concrete actions that transform into symbolic meaning while breaking the barrier of entry to a new dimension of expression. In addition to carrying specific content, the created image may also allegorically convey the actions that contributed to its creation. The goal is to generalize these successful tangible and emblematic motions to daily function. As children and adults alike experience a sense of control in the studio, they also gain a positive cognitive belief in themselves and bolstered confidence to take control and ownership outside of the studio (Moon, 2001). Repeated moving occurs in space. As the studio environment and context are negotiated this movement becomes safe and relational. Sharing media, being careful not to bump into each other's creative space, watching others' creative endeavors is an embodied opportunity to engage in safe and supportive relationships.

Important to this work is a review of the neuroscience of the motor system and its relevance for IPNB approaches and Art Therapy Relational Neuroscience (ATR-N) interventions. Due to neuronal isomorphism between the motor system, specifically the cerebellum and the prefrontal cortex (Baizer, 2014), motor activity also most likely increases cognitive, emotive and social function. Sensory-motor based work, involving touch and music go hand in hand with motor activation and are considered critical for recovery and development of trauma resiliency (Perry, 2006). Such repetitive movement must include positive, nurturing interactions with trustworthy others. Therefore the nature of art making, which is rooted in a deep respect for the artist's need for space, safely supports a tentative negotiation of the pace, quality, and quantity of potential lifelong attuned relationships and friendships. What has been advocated for traumatized children (Malchiodi & Crenshaw, 2013; Perry & Hambrick, 2006) is most likely effective for a variety of clinical problems. This is partially because art making, listening to music, and dancing are activities that can be generalized and used in clinical milieus and in day-to-day practices. Different from cognitive focused work, ATR-N interventions have the potential to modulate lower motor systems' over-arousal and put motion to therapeutic use.

EXPERIENTIAL PRACTICES AND DIRECTIVES

Experience I: My Space

Creating the creative environment, an essential part of the experiential process, is the first step in transforming the creative work space into an interpersonal environment. This step sets the course for our work together. Because this is one of our first group art therapy experiences, our walls, although soon to be festooned with art expressions, are typically bare and uninspiring. Thus, inviting relational and personal creativity, each group member first covers his or her work table with colorful butcher paper. As red, blue, yellow, green, black, and white paper lay out on the body-sized tables, the ordinary studio transforms into a vibrant working space. We encourage the large body sized paper in order to physically, emotionally and symbolically stimulate embodied movement. Setting a protected, safe and socially respected base for creation, each tabletop is completely wrapped in paper, which is securely taped. There is also enough space between the tables to allow for easy interaction and maneuvering without getting in each other's way, enabling artists to approach the space from any angle or point of view; close yet far enough apart, the group space is set for action. With individual spaces now nested within the interpersonal setting, the group is invited to: "Explore your space, the tabletop, using your choice of either acrylic or tempera paint or soft pastels." It is suggested that everyone use the whole canvas, thus filling it up. They may either use their own paints or feel free to use the community table media.

Group members are also encouraged to share their art materials with one another, which fosters movement within the clinic or expressive arts studio and influences creative motivation. To maintain an environment conducive to intrapersonal and social reflection, we ask the artists to avoid verbal social exchanges (Badenoch, 2008). This inner attention enables the focus to be on the tactile and kinesthetic experiences as well as on any emotions or thoughts triggered by the process and by others. Such an inward focus provides the opportunity for individuals to center themselves, synchronizing inner states with outer states. Such measures create a space for the group members to reflect on their sense of being present in the ATR-N space, thus allowing each person to become actively aware of the potential of here-and-now processes for change and social learning.

Coined as My Space by many of our cohorts, the work involves the creation of a self-space. In this open-ended realm, each individual paints something personal and meaningful, while the media's fluidity on an expansive canvas allows felt, unrestricted, kinesthetic movements to emerge. These movements concretize as art forms that outwardly reveal the individual internal space. As a result, the process transforms the space and canvas into symbolic self-spaces. Kazuko's painted rhythmic curves, which represent movement, along with her written reflection, offer a wonderful example of this experience (Figure 3.1).

> *I did not feel that my space was intended to mean my working space. Rather, I felt that my space, for this work, should represent my whole self: body, mind, and spirit. Therefore, I thought of the paper as my physical body and the art represented my mind and spirit. I felt that my spirit would be a feminine color and shape. Therefore, I chose a pink pastel and drew a curve. I enjoyed the physical sensation of drawing curved lines. I felt that I was conveying my energy with each stroke of the pastel, so the curved lines represented my flow of energy. I drew several curves with the pink because I had a huge amount of energy. Moreover, I added several oil pastels and acrylics over the pink*

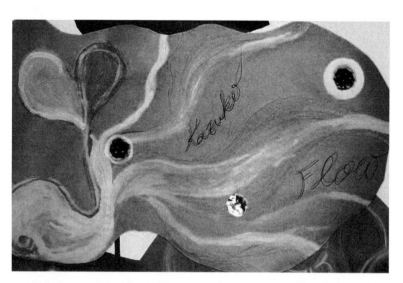

Figure 3.1 *My Flowing Energy.* On a soft yellow foundation, a light pink form spreads from a bulb in the lower left corner up into a deeper pink heart and diffused pink tendrils. At the top, the base, and in two distinct spots, hot red-pink contrasts with the yellow. Kazuko Numata.

pastel curved lines. These different media represented my different characteristics: kind, curious, genuine, dependable, and easygoing. I then added a heart symbol to symbolize a generator of my spirit that is connected with the source, which could be called God. Therefore, my energy will never be exhausted. Next, I cut the paper into a curved shape. As I already mentioned, the paper represented my physical body, so it was curved as a female body. Kazuko Numata

Integral to embodying supportive movement and espousing therapeutic universality is creating communality (Riley, 2001; Yalom & Leszcz, 2005). One way in which we do this is by viewing a critically acclaimed documentary, *The Living Museum*. The film's director, Jessica Yu (1999), showcases art produced by patients at the Creedmoor Psychiatric Center, the largest state psychiatric care institution in New York City. Inspired by artists such as Hans Prinzhorn, André Breton, and Jean Dubuffet, the Living Museum was founded and created by Bolek Greczynki and Janos Marton. Serving as a psychiatric refuge, the therapeutic focus is on raw process expression and art brut, rather than on technical skill. The film culminates with the patients' external exhibit, validating the residents' artistic abilities and the group expressive arts approach. We project a 20-minute segment of the film onto a large wall while the artist-participants start working at their table spaces, thus bringing us directly inside the Living Museum, and embodying the patients' work. Another reason we choose to have the group watch and respond to this video is that it provides a glimpse of the interface of client art, therapeutic art, and fine art. Seeing the film can clarify the therapeutic value of art making for the novice as well as the seasoned art therapy participant. It is also hoped that through the process of participatory identification with the art made by the Creedmoor patients, the viewers can eventually become more accepting of their own art.

While the film is being shown, some participants watch to its end, while others start painting right away, occasionally looking up or listening to the film.

I chose to create my space as a reflection of my new experience as an artist in the program. From the beginning, I wasn't sure what I wanted my space to look like or what meaning it should have in the end, so I just started to draw. I opened my brand-new NuPastels and chose one of my favorite colors, a pale blue, and began to draw a small circle in the center of the paper. As I became enthralled with the process of creating my space, I added more vibrant colors and created swirling patterns from the small center circle like curving pathways. I

tore strips of purple and yellow paper, curled them around my fingers, and attached them around the circle. In the process of creating my space, the art came alive to me. The marks on the paper became symbols that were meaningful to me. I thought about the artists in the video we had just watched, and I realized that this drawing was symbolic of myself as an artist. Just as the small circle seemed to be bursting through the space, my identity as an artist is changing and emerging through my experience. I was inspired by one artist from the film, Helen, a woman with severe depression who drew straight lines with a ruler to create patterns of color. Using her technique, I created lines with black charcoal and white chalk pastel to create gradient lines representing the "bars of judgment" that can hold back my true self as an artist from emerging. I then smeared the lines away from the center, symbolizing the "bars of judgment" being erased (Figure 3.2).
Rachel Tate

Here, Rachel reflects on what she experienced at the "bursting" interface of motor movements, emotions, and cognitions. Using motion-based language, she describes first looking at the empty space and the blank paper and how, at the same time that she is feeling uncertain about how to move, she begins action by drawing. The neuroscience information reviewed in the next

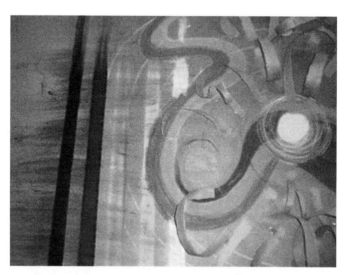

Figure 3.2 *Bursting Through: Emergence and Freedom.* The process of creating my own space helped me to rethink how I see myself as an artist. Softening from black through to light gray and white, vertical lines cross the paper. A wide mid blue line is flanked below by lavender and above by red, flowing from a pale green circle. A thick vibrant red line also lies to the lower right of this circle. Lavender and yellow paper ribbons also curve out from this central point. Rachel Tate.

section suggests that this kind of thoughtful pre-activity is of tremendous significance. The pre-activity activates the motor and cognitive areas of the brain, suggesting the connectivity of motion, emotion, and cognition. These amalgams are revealed in symbolized motions that are contained in the interpersonal creative space. Patty reported a similar experience, where moving her arm became physically and symbolically soothing:

> *After taking that deep breath, I started to draw. I drew circle after circle of different sizes. As I began to use more colors, I mixed and blended them with my fingers and the palm of my hand. Doing this, I realized, gives me a sense of control over what the colors will be and what the final image will look like. The simple circular motion my arm was moving in was soothing in itself, and at this point I knew what I wanted to draw.* Patty Russell

The group members have also reported that standing up or moving around in order to make the art stimulates greater self-awareness and generates the safety to expand and experiment, which allows for the release of emotions, pain, or painful feelings. Robin Vance wrote about how making art while dancing invites the creation of new self-memories and supports positive memories along with the natural forgetting of difficult memories (Vance & Wahlin, 2008). Frequent movement around the tables while creating large-scale drawings permits glimpses of each other's space, giving rise to a natural borrowing or sharing of imagery.

To support the expression of the individual range of experiences, we sometimes suggest selecting one of the following directives: "Paint your own space (My Space), paint your name (My Name), or paint your reaction to the film (My Reaction)."

> *I chose to draw my name. I stood there in front of my table trying to decide what I was going to create. I had no idea where to start, what materials to use, or what the product would look like. I finally decided to choose a medium and begin. I figured that if I just stood there I would never decide what to do and that I would find direction after I began. I picked up pastels and started making random marks in the center of the paper. I used various colors to make random marks that overlapped one another. Eventually, I realized that what I created looked like a wall. It suddenly came to me what I wanted to create in regards to my name. I wrote my Chinese name on the left side and my English name on the right. I did this because I feel as though I do not fully fit into the American society that I was born into. Typically,*

Caucasian Americans do not think of me as American due to my obvious Asian characteristics. On the other hand, Chinese people do not see me as fully Chinese. I am a "toe gee," an American-born Chinese who has lost much of what is considered Chinese. Hence, I am an American-born Chinese, an ABC. I found a picture of a naked woman covering her face with her arm. When I saw this image, I related to the woman in the fact that I, too, felt vulnerable and exposed. I cut out the image and placed it in the center, where I had drawn the wall. Once this directive was completed, the group was asked to title our pieces. Since I rarely title my pieces, I found it difficult to decide on a title. I thought over what I wanted to name my piece until it came to me: Somewhere in Between. *My title,* Somewhere in Between, *reflects these feelings of not fully belonging anywhere (Figure 3.3).* Maggie Fong

As participants discuss their experiences and art, some may mention how they have become inspired to envision their dedicated space for their art making at home. Thus, claiming and owning one's creative space becomes symbolic and can be generalized into taking action outside of the clinical studio.

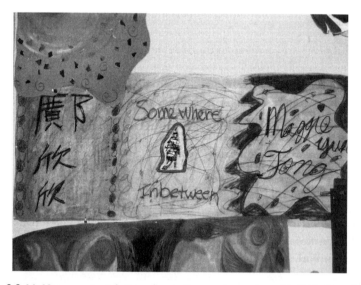

Figure 3.3 My Name experiential: *Somewhere in Between.* A central panel is divided into three sections with lavender on the left behind Chinese letters, pale blue in the center under the collaged image, and pale gray blue surrounded by red brown on the right, under the artist's name. A bright golden yellow sun-like shape sits to the upper left of the image. On the lower left, a rectangle of marbled multicolored swirls lies next to the central panel. Maggie Fong.

Experience II: Group Space

Once finished working, group members share their work's narratives and create a group mural. To begin this process, we walk about in the creative milieu and hand each person a pair of scissors with large silver blades. With scissors in hand, the artists are asked to: "Release your art piece from its binding to the table and hang the cutouts in a large group mural." Some members choose to cut around the boundaries of My Space as it is, but others may cut out areas that they wish to discard around the edges, or divide the art into multiple images. This is a pivotal point in the process, as the meaning of the art can be changed by active release, elimination, and restructuring, contributing to a sense of control and mastery. As such, purposeful motions and actions empower self-agency.

We are inspired in this art directive by Henri Matisse's paper cutouts (http://www.henri-matisse.net/cut_outs.html). Following surgery and a cancer diagnosis, Matisse used a wheelchair for the last 14 years of his life. In the video *Painting with Scissors*, Matisse's studio assistants would paint sheets of white paper with gouache paint. They would hold the paper and Matisse would then cut out elements from the vivid handmade color stock and place them in often life-sized compositions that were tacked onto a white wall, which served as the background. As he does this, he playfully reflects on the cutouts and moves them around in his hands as if they were a three dimensional object. Watching a movie of him and his assistants working together is a transformative experience, as it becomes a shared "we" experience.

Some of our artists take eagerly to this task, allowing themselves to reinvent their art by boldly cutting out and then pasting their table cover or mural. Some will change the orientation of their art from horizontal to vertical or vice versa as they place their images on the wall, adding to the collective mural. Studio participants often seem to revel in the interplay between their consciously painted imagery and the chance effects created by the scissor cuttings. This kind of playfulness has been associated with therapeutic relational benefits (Jernberg & Booth, 1999). Symbolically this is a way of processing multiple possibilities for representations of the intersubjective self. If we are successful in attuning to ourselves and to our clients, it is as if each time we decide to make a change, we experience an internal shifting. In essence, creating and reflecting on the multiple possibilities for the construction of selfhood.

> *Even if I did not verbally share what I was feeling, that art piece was a witness to what I felt and to what my chaotic and overwhelming thoughts were all about. Having been able to leave behind [some of*

the original artwork] and alter my art piece gave me the freedom to transform its meaning. I left behind all unwanted thoughts and feelings on the table while I allowed my wishful thoughts [to] hang on the wall. I felt safe enough to allow others to see my art piece. Ilene Lopez

Others experience an expansion of self-sense and emotional relief as they release their art from its binding and hang it on the wall, seeing it as a whole from a new vantage point.

I followed the directive to cut our pieces off the table in any manner that we saw appropriate. I liked my piece just the way it was. Therefore, I left it intact as a whole. Our last directive was to hang our pieces up on the wall so that they were next to other peoples' pieces. Maggie Fong

I moved forward and toward finding a connection within the group. I did not feel as alone or feel that I was going to be judged by (my) art piece. I felt better and more energized with each movement, but I suppose I placed into action the reward circuitry. One of the simplest transformations was when (after I released it from the table) I placed my art piece vertically instead of horizontally (on the wall) as I had originally intended to do. It gave a sense of feelings coming in and exploding under the pressure of containment and then the release of what was left. Ilene Lopez

The group unconsciously negotiates the space, develops relationships, and supports ownership and confidence. Periodically, within this action-filled context, the group stands back and reflects on the richness of the diverse images and emotional responses. Studio participants may find echoing themes and shared symbols such as hearts, stars, and sky in each other's work. Once tacked up, they may discuss adding to the wall and spatial changes. Some want their art to touch other pieces, while others layer one space over the other to reflect their overlapping interests and strong relationships. Movement prevails throughout, stimulating social and individual synergy. This kind of work is again reminiscent of Matisse's work, specifically the *Swimming Pool*, which he constructed in 1952. Positioned just above the level of his head, his assistants taped a broad band of what looks like butcher paper all around the room on which he taped ultramarine blue forms of swimmers, and sea creatures. The room, which was paved in tiles, became a pool where anticipated movement, pleasure, joy, and interactions could be sensorially embodied. This kind of environment is a wonderful coming together of movement and expression at the most elementary level of human existence.

RELATIONAL NEUROSCIENCE: THE MOTOR SYSTEM

Over the eons, the human body has become engineered for immediate, adaptive, accurate, and relevant motion-based responses to stimuli. Managing motion has played an important role in building evolutionary linkages between surviving and enhancing life. Living beings that don't move also don't have a brain; thus brain circuitry is specifically designed to generate motion and behaviors in response to the environment (Ratey & Hagermaan, 2010). The motor system is involved in maintaining body balance as well as initiating, producing, controlling, and coordinating both simple and complex movements (Kalat, 2012). The ATR-N principle of Creative Embodiment is based on research suggesting that motor system pathways facilitate and strengthen beneficial links between movement, emotion, cognition, and social interaction (Baizer, 2014; Ratey, 2008). For example, an unexpected movement, such as tripping, can initiate a startle response that triggers self-protection movements (Kalat, 2012). Such a response also activates the brain's reward circuitry, stimulating adrenaline and dopamine as it brings forth both a realization of fear and a sense of reward or pleasure (Sapolsky, 2004). So, the initial fright and moving away from others can turn into an agile dance, accompanied by relief and laughter at the realization that the danger has passed and that social life can continue. We contend that utilizing expressive art motions can provide similar relief and support.

The motor system is intricately interwoven with the central nervous system (CNS). The CNS consists of the brain and spinal cord, and is intricately linked to the peripheral nervous system (PNS; Carlson, 2013). Through the CNS, messages travel to and from the body's muscles, organs, and brain. The PNS consists of two branches, the somatic and autonomic nervous systems. The somatic nervous system informs voluntary movements by using efferent (outgoing) neurons to carry instructions from the brain to the body. The somatic nervous system also includes afferent (incoming) neurons that conduct visual, tactile, auditory, kinesthetic, proprioceptive, and other sensory information from the body to the brain. Afferent neurons compose the sensory portion of the somatic and autonomic systems that give feedback to the brain, allowing motor system actions to be refined both consciously and unconsciously. That is, the incoming somatic sensory information allows the brain to compare planned or habitual actions with actual feedback about

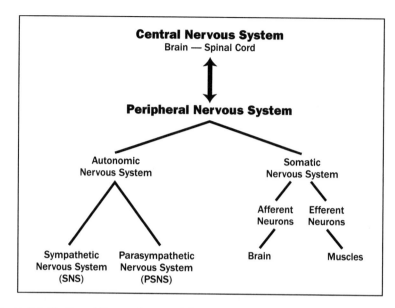

Figure 3.4 *The Central Nervous System and the Peripheral Nervous System.* The CNS includes the brain and spinal cord. The spinal cord connects the PNS with its somatic and autonomic nervous system branches in the body. The spinal cord and PNS simultaneously transmit motor information down to the body and sensory information up to the brain. The somatic/sensory nervous system conveys incoming or afferent sensory messages to the brain and carries outgoing or efferent messages to the major voluntary muscle groups. The autonomic nervous system (ANS) contains the sympathetic (SNS) and parasympathetic (PSNS) nervous systems. The SNS is excitatory, quickly initiating action, while the PSNS ("para" meaning "over") helps restore normal function by counterbalancing or inhibiting the SNS.

actions as they happen. Furthermore, parts of the motor system continuously correct movements to increase performance accuracy (for an extended discussion, see Carr, 2008b; Christian, 2008; Kravits, 2008b; Figure 3.4).

The motor system consists of primarily efferent neurons whose role is to transmit information from the CNS to the PNS (Kalat, 2012). The motor system also includes the automatic nervous system (ANS), which very rapidly initiates responses to fear, stress, and exciting stimuli. The efferent and afferent neurons of the motor system communicate through the spinal cord to the brain and body with various body responses over which we have little to no conscious control. This allows further feedback of feelings, emotions, and gut instincts.

The motor system can be imagined as a tree, with branches that extend to the tree's crown, adorning cognition with affect and motion, which emerge from its trunk and roots. Thus the impacts of motion on emotion and cognition are reflected in the motor system organization. For ease of comprehension, we describe the motor system as three distinct structural levels, but in

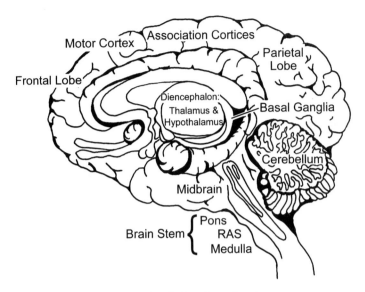

Figure 3.5 *Brain Areas that are Associated with Motor System Functions.*

reality these subsystems and their functions are interdependent and integrated with one another. So schematically, the motor system has three levels. They are: (1) the higher level, which includes the cortical association areas (the parietal lobe, temporal lobe, and dedicated areas of the frontal lobe); (2) the middle level, which includes the motor cortex and subcortical structures (the thalamus, hypothalamus, and cerebellum); and (3) the lower-level spinal cord and brain stem (Kalat, 2012; Figure 3.5).

Normal motor development relies upon establishing specific connections between the muscles and pyramidal neurons. The structural hierarchy also includes the pyramidal motor neuronal system, which connects lower- and higher-level systems and controls voluntary movement. The pyramidal motor neuronal system connects the executive center in the frontal lobe with the spinal cord and the muscles. The neocortex and the spinal cord are also connected by pyramidal neurons. When successful, these connections allow pyramidal cells to act as part of the circuitry responsible for vision-guided motor function (Salimi, Friel, & Martin, 2008). The prefrontal cortex (PFC) receives input from all brain areas involved in processing sensory modalities. Within the PFC, pyramidal cells have been implicated in cognition processes involving sensory and visual inputs (Elston, 2003). Horizontal pathways also connect the system's different levels, protecting us from consequences resulting from immediate damage to one of the three vertical links. This complex organization enables the different levels of the hierarchy to influence each other (Table 3.1).

Table 3.1 Motor System Structures and Functions

UPPER HIGHER LEVEL

Association cortices include the parietal, temporal, and frontal lobes along with most of the cerebral surface of the human brain. They are largely responsible for the complex processing that occurs between the arrival of input in the primary sensory cortices and the generation of behavior. The parietal association cortex is especially important for attending to complex stimuli in the external and internal environment. The temporal association cortex is especially important for identifying the nature of such stimuli. The frontal association cortex is especially important for orchestrating and planning appropriate behavioral responses to the stimuli.

Basal ganglia: Extrapyramidal subcortical nuclei are probably involved in the selection of actions. The basal ganglia include other structures that assist in its activities: the caudate nucleus, putamen, and globus pallidus, along with the substantia nigra, the red nucleus, and the sub-thalamic nucleus. All are synaptically connected to one another as well as to the thalamus, brainstem, cerebellum, and the pyramidal system.

MIDDLE LEVEL

Motor cortex: initiates movement. This area includes the primary motor cortex, pre-motor cortex, and the supplementary motor area in the frontal lobe.

Diencephalon: area includes the thalamus and the hypothalamus. The thalamus acts as a gateway to the sensory system, receiving sensory information and forwarding it to areas of the motor system. The hypothalamus controls body temperature, hunger, thirst, fatigue, sleep, circadian cycles, survival or stress responses, and links the nervous and endocrine systems.

Cerebellum: facilitates the coordination of voluntary muscle movements, equilibrium, and tone, accompanied by an analysis of the timing of visual signals that correspond to one's own/others' movements. The cerebellum informs the brainstem, which is involved in involuntary bodily functions and movements as well as sustaining memory processes that enable fine motor skills.

LOWER LEVEL

Brainstem: The brainstem includes the pons, the reticular activating system (RAS), and the medulla oblongata. It is generally responsible for autonomic involuntary functions such as respiration, heart rate, blood pressure, etc.

Spinal cord: The spinal cord, a long, thin, tubular bundle of nervous tissue and support cells, extends from the medulla oblongata in the brainstem to the pelvis. Two of the spinal cord's three main functions are the conduction of motor information to the muscles, and transmission of sensory information up the brainstem to the thalamus for distribution to cortical and subcortical brain areas for further processing.

PYRAMIDAL MOTOR NEURONAL SYSTEM

Motor neurons descend from the motor strip in the frontal cortex to the lower brainstem areas (the midbrain, the pons, and the medulla oblongata) and on to the spinal cord. These long neuronal fibers terminate at different points along the spinal cord, where efferent nerves of the peripheral nervous system carry motor impulses to voluntary muscles. In conjunction, afferent sensory feedback into the cerebellum details fine motor aspects of these particular movements. Each discrete movement (for instance, picking up an object) triggers afferent nerves to send the cerebellum very specific information about each position during the movement sequence so that the cerebellum can send messages that fine-tune the muscle movements, adjust balance and redirect actions to accomplish the task.

Adapted from Carlson (2013)

The upper level contains association cortices, where auditory, spatial, visual, proprioceptive, kinesthetic, touch, and sensory inputs are processed. The association areas are responsible for the highest level of information processing in the brain, deciphering incoming information and connecting afferent sensory inputs with efferent outputs in order to construct and sequence motor responses in a timely manner. These processes occur simultaneously while the individual considers a myriad of possible behavioral responses and making decisions about which behaviors to execute, and when (Chakravarthy, Joseph, & Bapi, 2010; Stocco, Lebiere, & Anderson, 2010). The upper level is where the sensory information generated by art making is assembled, and where concrete movements become meaningful and symbolic: "The commonly held view that sensory and motor computations in the cortex are separate and hierarchical in organization needs to be reconsidered and interpreted in relation to the fact that all sensory pathways also carry copies of motor instructions so that sensorimotor processing is unified throughout all levels of thalamocortical functions" (Sherman & Guillery, 2011, p. 1075).

The association pathways receive information from the middle level, which is composed of the motor cortex, thalamus, basal ganglia, and cerebellum. These structures transmit incoming sensory information to the association pathways. This higher-level circuitry translates the information, resulting in more accurate movements. Their efforts are concerned with tactics aimed at avoiding collisions with objects and people. Comparisons of the desired versus actual results allow for corrections in movements as they occur.

It is partially due to the cerebellum's function that the motor system is associated with both emotional and cognitive function (Strick, Dum, & Fiez, 2009). The cerebellum, appropriately named the little brain, is involved in the coordination of voluntary and involuntary movements (Kalat, 2012), hand movement and language (Baizer, 2014), and the direction of emotions (Turner et al., 2007). Furthermore, it analyzes the timing of visual signals that correspond to one's own movements and those of others by balancing the excitation and inhibition of impulses. The cerebellum helps control complex motor movements, procedural learning, and muscle contraction sequences to create appropriate actions. Utilizing sensory input from the thalamus, the cerebellum works by balancing its own excitatory output with the inhibitory output from the basal ganglia to refine movement and increase coordination.

Historically, it was thought that both the cerebellum and the basal ganglia chiefly functioned as contributors to motor control. However, it is now known that these bodies have additional roles (Bostan, Dum, & Strick, 2010). The basal ganglia assist in emotion regulation (Ochsner & Gross, 2007), while the cerebellum is involved in language and memories of fine motor sequences, among its diverse neurobiological duties. "The range of tasks associated with cerebellar activation is remarkable and includes tasks designed to assess attention, executive control, language, working memory, learning, pain, emotion, and addiction. . . . [Data], along with the revelations about cerebro-cerebellar circuitry, provide a new framework for exploring the contribution of the cerebellum to diverse aspects of behavior" (Strick et al., 2009, p. 413). This newer conceptualization of cerebrum function suggests that expressive art making movements may facilitate linkages to these functions.

The lower level of the motor system is responsible for transmitting information to the middle level and receiving commands from the higher level. For example, when one picks up a paintbrush, the motor cortex receives this information and, in turn, sends the appropriate messages to the hand. The hand's muscles adjust and balance fine motor actions, allowing one to fulfill the action and load the brush with paint, thus allowing art making to become an executed reality.

> *Creating art provides us with new information about ourselves as well as a means of communicating thoughts and feelings that otherwise might have not been available to us through verbal communication. It is the movement of creating, the action of it, that begins this therapeutic process.* Lisa Cerrina

Movement seems to be critical to the process of ATR-N change and learning. Taking a variety of forms, movement occurs in standing and using an easel, practicing painting, and scribbling motions before creating art, or dancing, or moving toward the finished product (Cane, 1983; Kwiatkowska, 1978). Other embodied work includes play therapy and drama therapy. These therapeutic and playful therapies can stir the imaginative self in such a way as to not only experience pleasure but also anticipate successful outcomes (Jernberg & Booth, 1999; Lahad, 1993). Understanding the neurobiology of motion affirms ATR-N principles and has the added advantage of relieving art therapists from any polarized discussion on art versus therapy (Hass-Cohen, 2007; Kramer, 1971; Riley, 1999).

Younger clients may benefit developmentally from the inclusion of therapeutic motion, since it also supports the development of coordination skills. More specifically, children with neurodevelopmental deficits such as autism, nonverbal learning disorders, and attention-deficit/hyperactivity disorder (Allen & Courchesne, 2003; Schmahmann, Weilburg, & Sherman, 2007) may benefit, as motion can help to organize, coordinate, and navigate space. Such advantages have been linked to improved communication, enhanced social skills, and higher cognitive functions such as the ability to shift attention (Akshomooff & Courchesne, 1992). Children with a history of developmental abuse benefit from repeated therapeutic movement as it can help calm their flight or fight defensive responses to attempted relational interventions (Crenshaw & Mordock, 2005). Furthermore, movement is associated with catecholamine release by the reward system, that can balance the release of stress neurotransmitters and hormones, again increasing both pleasure and cognitive and regulated parasympathetic functions (Hass-Cohen et al., 2014).

From an IPNB perspective, perceived danger can inspire action and evoke movement. Survival needs have primed the nervous and visual systems to quickly detect motion, respond with action, and seek safety (Siegel, 2012). Two main visual processing streams forward environmental visual cues from the occipital lobe to the frontal lobe (Kalat, 2012). The dorsal or "where-how" stream is hypervigilant about motion in space and can stimulate a fear response.

The neurocircuitry of the "where-how" dorsal stream involves areas in the brain that are sensitive to actual, perceived, and implied movements, whether in the environment or in imagery. The cerebellum has direct linkages to the dorsal lateral PFC, the executive center of the brain (Herculano-Houzel, 2010, Figure 3.6). Therefore, art therapists should exercise caution and specificity when presenting clients with imagery that contains movement (Hass-Cohen & Loya, 2008). People also tend to resolve fears by moving away from or toward the stressors that cause them (Sapolsky, 2004). Motion is then triggered by limbic-based emotions, such as actual and

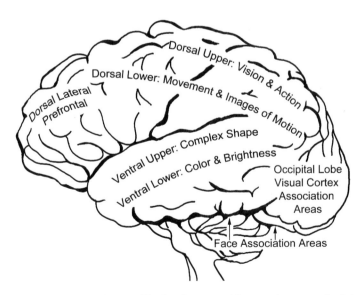

Figure 3.6 *Visual Processing Streams.* The dorsal upper and lower pathways are the "where-how" stream. The ventral pathways are the "what" streams responsible for the recognition of objects by their physical attributes which also include auditory inputs.

remembered fear. This knowledge guides the art therapist in initiating enactments of approach or avoidance that stimulate motion. Creating a sense of physical and emotional safety involves providing a supportive and adequately sized environment:

> *A sense of safety was set up early on and it was important to have a defined, ample space in which to create. We had the freedom to use the space to release and explore in a supportive environment in a manner of our choice.* Jessica Plotin

Understanding the Creative Embodiment principle is important when working with clients who have post-traumatic stress disorder (PTSD). Individuals diagnosed with PTSD often use avoidant strategies such as dissociation, thus inhibiting the recovery process (Cozolino, 2010; Porges, 2011). Vance and Wahlin (2008) suggested that dancing while making art increases memory functions and decreases pain, and Talwar (2007) explicated that dance and movement can support conscious processing of traumatic memories. It is likely that these actions stimulate the pleasure associated with catecholamine release by the reward system, which is discussed in later chapters. Furthermore, Talwar structures the art space in such a way that clients walk back and forth between the media table and the paper, which is taped on a wall. She holds that this assists in establishing proprioception. In other words, clients can gain a felt sense of the relative position of neighboring parts of the body and of the intensity of effort. In summary, engaging in nonverbal action provides a safe outlet for self-expression, as well as a sense of physical control (Hass-Cohen, 2006a). In addition, the neurotransmitters released during movement can calm the body while increasing energy, supporting clients' willingness to process traumas and relieving emotional and physical pain. As researchers continue to investigate the specific roles of each component of the motor system (Coffman, Dum, & Strick, 2011; Stocco et al., 2010), support for the importance of Creative Embodiment as a therapeutic factor in art therapy grows.

CREATE PRINCIPLES AND CLINICAL APPLICATIONS

In this chapter, the principle of Creative Embodiment is illustrated through experiential practices and directives. In particular, the larger art format and the creation of a group mural promote movement and enhance the ATR-N therapeutic advantages of motion. As an example, the motor system can become coordinated with the planning and with cognitive, emotive and social systems. This enables the integration of actions, emotions, and thoughts, promoting increased motivation and reduced inactivity. Motion, especially when repeated, can help clients solidify implicit learning and the consolidation of new memories. Motion can be embodied concretely, as in movement, or symbolically accessed. It is also an opportunity to joyfully interact.

In the same manner, relational interactions are encouraged between group members through experiential movement, sharing, and reflection. Associated with Relational Resonating, these ATR-N microskills allow for clients' growing awareness of others as well as their own relation to using interpersonal space. Group members attune to each other through rhythmic lines and shapes, motion-based imagery, words, and motions. In addition to the advantages of personal sharing, the sequencing of individual and group directives supports the creating participants' active awareness of others' art processes. Moreover, conveyance of interest in others' art through these discussions is motivating and rewarding, which enhances clinical change. Consequently, active co-creation and co-ownership of the wall mural increases interpersonal bonding and reduces isolation.

Experiencing the movement associated with painting a large surface with color and forms provides access to primary emotions such as joy or fear, feelings of self-doubt, and/or anxiety or self and interpersonal judgments. Expressive Communicating of emotions is released via the My Space experience. Once aroused states are reflected upon, the creators may be able to access subjective meaning making. For example, releasing the art from the table is an emotionally transformative moment in which what was created and expressed can be further communicated and changed. Realization of such impact through mutual discussion can provide the client group members with shared emotional moments of bonding, ownership, and pride.

Adaptive Responding takes place as the group members respond to moving around the art space and shifting toward mural making. In other words, movement assists in adapting to the demands of art making and the emotive reactions that arise. Moving both away and toward the art facilitates solutions that can balance emotional arousal and stress responses to novel situations. Supporting the capacity to tolerate emotional frustration and defensiveness, overall adaptation to concurrent stressors can be achieved in various ways. Navigating available space results in increased sensory motor experiences, possible emotional frustration, cognitive defensiveness, and the ambiguity of art expression, which are all means toward such adaptation. Experienced in exploration of fear-based impulses, these results are generated by the request to change the art, and turning to creative action for resolution of the fear response. The therapeutic request to change the image can be experienced as demanding by the creator. Such skillful ATR-N interventions provide clients with the opportunity to experience coping and adaptation. When feeling safe, clients identify and explore fear-based impulses, such as avoidance and withdrawal, thereby regulating any ambiguity in their art and life.

Transformative Integrating is demonstrated by the sequencing of the experientials. ATR-N microskills include the creative sequence of painting, expressing, cutting out the My Space art, reconsidering, and displaying the art. When therapeutically applied, creative sequencing of art directives assists clients in new meaning making. Such changes contribute to saliency, which transforms experiences and assists with achieving personal goals. Moreover, adding motion to the art making contributes to the integration of cognition, emotions, and sensory processes. This process mirrors the integrative process of creating, reframing, and witnessing oneself therapeutically. Viewing the *Living Museum* art in our relational space, moving about both during and after the art making, and shifting from personal art making to collective mural work in the Group Space experience supports many aspects of integration. Releasing the art from the personal context activates its interpersonal function. Furthermore, the creative transformation of the art in shape and orientation contributes to a sense of pleasure and well-being. Similarly, the integration of feelings, thoughts, and actions through the display and discussion of the art can promote flexibility. Flexible responses support balanced affective and cognitive function.

The progression from working individually to collectively, creating a mural, also enables an integration of personal- and group-meaning making. This unified sense of belonging aligns the group members' affective states, increases group bonding, and integrated cohesiveness. A feeling of membership in such a setting can increase relational security associated with integrated neurobiological functioning. Such integration is represented by the synchronization of the PFC, limbic system, sensory system, and motor system, which contributes to a sense of well-being and facilitates cognitive function. Viewing *The Living Museum* video showcases the CREATE principle of Empathizing and Compassion. Working as a group, watching the film, and seeing others' art collectively gives rise to empathic resonance with both the film participants (the psychiatric patients) and with present group members. Prosocial responses, such as helping each other and seeing oneself as part of the helping profession, are ignited by recognizing each individual's professional identity formation. Discussing and viewing art made in the presence of the film and each other supports a deepening connectedness and compassion as one witnesses and participates in the unfolding experiential. Looking at each person's My Space image supports the recognition that social loaning of imagery through the mimicking and mirroring of each other's actions, gesturing intentions, and symbols is a relational exchange. Within the arts psychotherapy clinic or art studio, in therapy groups or individual work, such repeated sharing experiences support the building of connected and empathic responses across a diverse group of people.

CHAPTER 4

Relational Resonating: Attachment and Neuroplasticity

I can see my growth as an artist, who is learning to become more in tune with her feelings towards making art, and more understanding of the feelings that can appear because of the art. From my mind's perspective, I believe that this semester, more than any other semester, has expanded my mind the most, in many ways. . . . Learning about neuroscience and how the brain works has also opened my eyes and my mind to new perspectives on life. Everything I have learned and participated in from this creative milieu has helped me understand what it might feel like to be the client, and has given me perspective on how I can foster that relationship and help it to grow. Autumn Cade

ATTUNED THERAPEUTIC RELATIONSHIPS AND COMMU-nication promotes stable internal and flexible psychobiological states and interpersonal interactions. Such social exchanges and their ensuing mental representations have the potential to activate and mend attachment ruptures, stabilize affect regulation, update autobiographical memories, and contribute to earned attachment. Specifically collaborative and coherent art therapy relationships can increase experiences of positive affect and help disengage from negative feelings. Clients' abilities to access and share autobiographical memories will be influenced by their attachment style and history. Those with secure relational histories can use past positive memories for comfort, while those with less secure models or chronic trauma histories may experience difficulty evoking coherent past narratives.

This chapter is dedicated to the CREATE principle of Relational Resonating. It describes the multiple interpersonal dimensions of offering and sharing media, touching others' art, functioning together, and representing attachment-based imagery. As in Chapter 3, we contend that sharing art with others as well as making art in the presence of others most contributes to therapeutic change. Here we describe how interpersonal exchanges and representations can mend attachment ruptures and change relational schemas or attachment-based internal working models. Thus, such art therapy exchanges can contribute to the development of regulated and adaptive mind states and an earned secure attachment style.

Over the lifetime, aversive experiences such as early childhood developmental trauma, may negatively impact the maturation of critical linkages in the brain related to the development of secure internal working memories of attachment (Perry, 2001). However, positive experiences, such as those within attuned relationships, can still transform relational insecurity to earned security (Hesse, 1999). Because internal working memories of attachment are for the most part implicit, the development of contingent verbal and nonverbal expression supports security and coherency. As ATR-N practices easily engage emotive-implicit and cognitive-explicit functions and non-verbal right-to-right hemispheric communication they are particularly suitable to achieve these ends. We have operationalized Relational Resonating to mean co-creation, co-consciousness, co-regulation and co-meaning making. Relational Resonating witnesses a fluid, stable alignment with oneself and with another person, giving rise to self and relational compassion. Such mindful awareness entails a non-judgmental acceptance of others and supports secure attachment experiences. Propelled by the additional support of non-verbal communication, the experience of a mindful, attuned presence in the client-therapist relationship is a foundation for self-regulation via contingent communication. In recalling, projecting, and altering the images of the self and others in the past, present, and future, the directive function of memory can then be used to envision future relationships, promoting representations of secure and caring attachment experiences. Sharing with others, being heard, and having one's experience empathically felt reinforces emotional regulation. Throughout this book, we describe several sequences of ATR-N directives, media, and processes that promote Relational Resonating.

The capacity to change one's sense of relational security and gain stable, regulated emotional states is a reflection of the brain's propensity for neuroplasticitity and change (Cozolino, 2013). Interpersonal neurobiology (IPNB) approaches suggest that individuals' attachment styles are experience dependent and can change throughout one's life span (Siegel, 2012). This understanding of the neuroscience of attachment and brain plasticity is central to the CREATE principle of Relational Resonating. Both negative and positive experiences can change brain structures and function. Persistent abuse and neglect, or, conversely, love, mindful awareness, and empathic attunement, shape the social brain (Badenoch, 2008). In this chapter, we review the neuroscience of such dynamic plasticity across the life span, with a focus on the influence of early caregiver interactions on adult attachment styles. Additional information on the neurobiology of attachment is covered in upcoming chapters.

Attachment theory is a paradigm for understanding interpersonal psychosocial interactions (Wallin, 2007). Attachment strategies and styles form a system of proximity-seeking behaviors. Generated by parent-child interactions, these interactional patterns develop an internal working model (IWM), which is maintained across the life span (Bowlby, 1988; Main, 2000; Siegel, 2012; Sroufe, 2000). IWMs represent internalized repetitive and meaningful expectations. They are internal representations of other's mental states. The capacity for sensing and mentalizing another's state of mind begins with the development of object constancy during the first two years of life (Piaget & Inhelder, 1973), and then evolves as theory of mind (ToM; Frith & Frith, 2003; Premack & Woodruff, 1978). IWMs components include (a) memories of attachment related experiences, (b) beliefs about relationships, (c) attitudes about social interactions, (d) expectations about ourselves and others, and (e) learned confidence or lack of in being able to successfully connect with others.

Thus, IWMs develop in an interpersonal context and are represented by successful mentalizing (Allen, Fonagy, & Bateman, 2008; Fonagy & Target; 1997). Originally conceptualized as a cognitive capacity ToM is now understood as a social emotional ability. For example, lacking the ability to read social skills, children on the autism spectrum do not seem to follow age expected milestones and have difficulties with ToM. Relational stressors trigger the reenactment of these mental representations (Cozolino, 2010). The need for interventions will depend upon whether secure or insecure attachment styles are evoked. The exchange of intimate feelings and partnership relationships can augment or alter child attachment strategies or adult IWMs. Therapist relationships or friendships may also help attain a more flexible and resilient earned security.

For the experiential practices, we begin with an introduction to the personal and relational aspects of the art therapist's art media. It is at this stage that the participants begin to earn relational competency as they engage with the material (McNiff, 1992). This also presents an opportunity to practice affect regulation (Moon, 2001). As potential negative and disturbing feelings toward the media are processed via the art, the new images become what McNiff has called an "antitoxin" (1992, p. 3). Acting as antidotes to deregulating emotions and feelings, antitoxins lead the way to earned emotional stability. In this regard, from the first art therapy encounter, direct engagement with the media and the creative arts can become a regulatory experience (Malchiodi & Crenshaw, 2013).

From an ATR-N Relational Resonating perspective, the creative experience is also broadened from intrapersonal (i.e., what is stirred within the person) to interpersonal awareness (i.e., what is stirred between the therapist and the client and the group). Art therapy embraces the relational context in the artistic products and in the creative process (Moon, 2008). We teach that even the layout of the media on the therapist's table and the introduction of the various media to the client help access Relational Resonating. These are critical art therapy microskills.

In this chapter, the attachment-based art therapy experientials are the Interpersonal Media presentations, the Family Attachment Map, and the Fabric-Based Attachment Albums (Clyde Findlay, Lathan, & Hass-Cohen, 2008). Although they can be adapted for children, the experientials mostly focus on adult experiences. These practices serve to foster an empathic understanding of secure and insecure attachment-based styles. Personal engagement furthers the development of interpersonal flexibility needed for successful sensory-based relational interactions. Throughout the didactics, experientials, and personal reflections, the art therapist may become aware of his or her own attachment style. Our experiences are augmented by ongoing, written reflections where the individual creators are invited to journal about what they have learned and their experiences of felt or perceived relational safety.

ATTACHMENT THEORY

Attachment styles are blueprints for relating to others (Cassidy & Shaver, 2010). Secure IWMs emerge from early childhood repetitive and meaningful expectations of attuned attention from a formative caregiver. The capacity to cognitively mentalize social actions (Baron-Cohen, Leslie, & Frith, 1985), is linked with affect regulation, attachment history and social empathy (Hughes, & Leekam, 2004; Mikulincer et al., 2011).

For adults intimate lifelong partner experiences converge into complex, feeling-based working models. Parents' attachment styles are the strongest predictors of their children's attachment classifications (Hesse, 1999; van IJzendoorn, 1995). Both child and adult attachment styles describe states of mind activated in the face of attachment-related stress. These states do not represent absolute brain functions or expressions of unchanging traits or personalities (Siegel, 1999). The main adult attachment styles are secure and insecure. Insecure is further divided into three categories: preoccupied, dismissive, and disorganized (Hesse & Main, 2000). Each adult category corresponds to a child attachment style. Insecure-resistant and anxious correlate with the adult preoccupied style, and insecure-avoidant with the adult dismissive style. For children, the disorganized category does not stand alone; it is part of avoidant or resistant attachment. This is because child styles are still in flux (Hesse & Main, 2000; Main & Goldwyn, 1998; Figure 4.1).

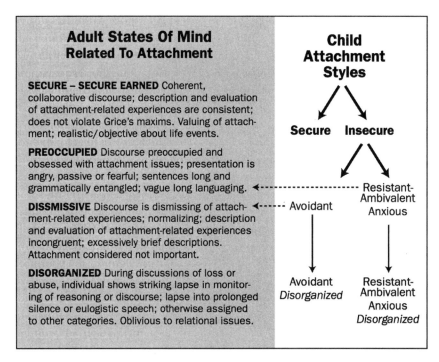

Figure 4.1 *Review of Child and Adult Attachment Styles.*

Adults with an insecure-preoccupied attachment style are prone to feeling underappreciated, seek to gain proximity by pleasing others, and become very anxious about close relationships. Adult preoccupied attachment styles, however, are concordant with a resistant-ambivalent-anxious attachment style in children. Arising from irregular caregiver attention, very anxious children expend considerable effort to ensure adequate attention when stressed.

Similarly, adults with a dismissive IWM are also anxious about relationships. In contrast to children, adults are more prone to anticipate rejection by rejecting others first. Adults with dismissive models find trust difficult and often see others as a threat to stability and control. Paralleling children with an avoidant attachment style, both consistently refrain from seeking comfort in times of stress. These adults have learned as children that reassurance is unavailable and that consequently a sense of sustained control is not possible (Henry & Wang, 1999).

Infants who exhibit a disorganized attachment response typically have caregivers who exhibit frightening, intrusive, or unpredictable behavior. Examples include cases of child abuse, child neglect, and domestic violence. However, abuse and neglect are not the only causes of disorganized infant attachment responses. In other instances, the caregiver experiences the infant's needs, expressed through crying or dependent behaviors, as internally triggering, intrusive, frightening, and disorganizing. The parental figure may then unconsciously respond with angry grimaces and snarls at the infant. These caregivers likely experienced extreme relational confusion in their own childhood relationships; they may have been frightened by a caregiver, and developed a disorganized internal working model (Hesse & Main, 2000).

Adults or children with a disorganized interactive style may exhibit a confused fight-or-flight or proximity-seeking response. In other words, they will not know whether to run away, fight, or come closer. Thus their usual insecure response to relational stress, either anxious, avoidant, preoccupied, or dismissive, becomes unstable and disorganized. Unsafe contexts leading to intense or prolonged flight, fight, or freeze responses predispose a person with an insecure attachment style to engage in survival reactions rather than social solutions. Some extreme psychopathologies, such as borderline and narcissistic personality disorders, have been linked to critical attachment inabilities to regulate emotion, resulting in a lack of successful social experiences (Wallin, 2007). In contrast, positive attachment-based experiences allow for the possibility of changes in attachment classification from insecure to earned secure (Schore, 2003).

Earned secure attachment categories represent interactional processes that can interrupt familial patterns associated with insecure attachment (Badenoch, 2008). As an example, even under stressful conditions, the parenting skills of people with suboptimal attachment histories who currently have an earned secure style remain sensitive and nurturing. When an adult with an insecure attachment style forms an ongoing intimate relationship with a person grounded in a secure IWM, such as a therapist, mate, close friend, or an adult sibling, the insecurely attached person may become more flexible and resilient, and develop an earned secure style of relating. For married couples, this change takes about seven years (Hesse, 1999). The capacity for affect regulation allows for tolerance of distress and continued function of the prefrontal cortex (PFC; Christian, 2008). Rather than distress shutting down higher thinking, regulation evokes meaning making (Briere & Scott, 2012). Thus, even with difficult childhood experiences, the mind is capable of achieving an integrated and coherent perspective that permits parenting behavior to be sensitive and empathic. Over time, as the earned secure attachment state of mind develops, the individual begins to mentalize, anticipate and even provide for positive relational interactions and resiliency.

MENTALIZING

Mentalizing represents an integrative framework for psychotherapy (Connors, 2011). Many approaches including psychodynamic, cognitive behavioral, systemic approaches and social ecological approaches embrace the value of understanding human relationships on such a micro and macro levels.

Successful or unsuccessful mentalizing is the reflective ability to understand and contingently respond to others (Fonagy & Target, 1997). Directed by IWMs, successful or unsuccessful mentalizing happens and develops throughout the life span. The capacity for reflective mentalization has been correlated with IWM. In other words, whether our attachment needs are met, and whether our strategies to achieve these needs are successful, is directly correlated with successful mentalization. For example, about 87 percent of children who were classified as securely attached to either mother or father at 12 months were successful at the TOM task, as expected at age 5. In contrast, those who were classified as insecurely attached at age 12 months were slower at developing ToM. They were only successful at a 50 percent rate at age of 5 years (Fonagy & Target).

Fundamentally interpersonal, mentalizing is a function that supports engaging in relationships with others, listening to others and being receptive to how others think and feel, as it enhances how one thinks and feels. Adaptive and maladaptive mentalizing of these states form the foundations of mental health (Bateman & Fonagy, 2011). Thus, the social emotional representation of one's own and others' minds is a form of imaginative mental activity, namely, perceiving and interpreting human behavior in terms of intentional mental states. These imaginative states include needs, desires, feelings, beliefs, goals, purposes, and reasons that guide dyadic and familial interactions (Asen & Fonagy, 2012). Consequently, family conflicts can arise when family members misunderstand each other's needs, desires, feelings, and intentions. Therapeutic interventions that help parents and children to better understand each other's minds can therefore improve closeness, problem solving skills, and individual child social and emotional development (Wallin, 2007). Within a therapeutic relationship the experience of being thought about makes people feel safe enough to reflect upon and participate in their interpersonal environment (Asen & Fonagy, 2012). Across therapeutic modalities, the study of mentalizing suggests that successful social mentalizing is tied to secure attachment, which is key to coherent intersubjectivity, and therefore to successfully partaking in learning and social contexts.

EXPERIENTIAL PRACTICES AND DIRECTIVES

Experience I: Interpersonal Media

For an artist, thinking about how to present media for someone other than oneself represents a paradigm change from the intrapersonal to the interpersonal. As those with prior fine arts education evolve into art therapists, there is a need to shift from relating to the media as fine arts tools to acknowledging and utilizing their relational role. For example, touching another's art materials is typically taboo in the fine arts, which may arouse attachment-related stress for the artists. We attempt to assist group participants in developing a flexible balance between personal artistic and clinical art therapy expressions (McNiff, 1992; Moon, 2001). This distinction facilitates an understanding of the relationship between the client, the therapist, and the art productions, and aids in the development of art therapy microskills.

In preparation for this experience, the group is asked to bring a personalized toolbox with a wide range of structured and unstructured art media. As the participants come into the creative space, they are asked to: "Organize the media selection on your individual tables, providing your materials to someone other than yourself, such as a client". Then, one table at a time, participants move around the milieu exploring the variety of media displays, discovering the different containers, and the wide range of possible setups (Figure 4.2).

We set up the relational context by asking group members to offer their supplies, touch each other's art materials, and move in and out of each other's spaces. Together, we explore the variety of relationships offered by the different displays. For example, we ask participants to reflect upon questions such as, "How would the touch and intimacy offered by new pastels differ from the context of well-used and smudgy pastels? Would new pastels suggest special care? Would they invite tentativeness and worry about waste? Would

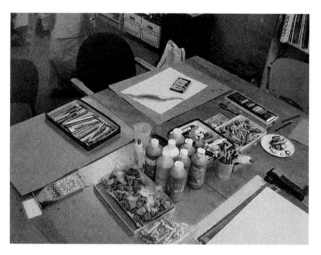

Figure 4.2 *The Art Therapy Media Setup.* A combination of new and used media are set up for easy access. The media are set up in this way to provide access for several participants.

previously used pastels suggest intimate closeness and nurturance or be experienced as overly personal?" Latent relational patterns of interaction, especially when the artist participants are new to each other, are often stirred.

> *I am uncertain as to how others will feel when they look at my table, for surely my items do not bring them the same comfort as they do me. I peer at their tables, which contain identical materials, but different all the same. Different in the way they are arranged, in their newness and their wear. I begin to wonder how others will feel, with me looking at their things, touching them, using them. This table, covered in my art supplies, is now my space. A little window into me. While some items are too new to be special, others are part of stories, memories that can never be detangled from the physical object. Those are the items I want to share the most. I feel a kinship with the strangers who examine the tin containers holding my colored pencils, which I received for my birthday many years ago. The original pencils have long since been replaced, but the tins, which I've carted around since high school, have become part of me, like a child's blankey or the lingering scent of your mother's perfume. A shrug settles in my shoulders as someone examines the oil pastels on my table. These are not part of me. They are foreign, messy objects that I have not liked since childhood. They are new, purchased solely for this work. They are not me, but they are here, misrepresenting me. I think about this, and consider that, since the moment I walked through that door, the me I knew before is changing. I now must make room for the "art therapist" me, a me that is comfortable using whatever media the client would like, a me that not only does not mind getting oil pastels all over my fingers, but also understands why that might be calming, useful, perhaps even necessary. I examine my space. It is my own personal blueprint.* Emily Skelton

As the group wanders around the room, individuals may remark on their peers' choices, directly touch their supplies, while taking in attempted non-verbal and verbal contributions. For most, these experiences trigger internal attachment models. Exploring the art therapy media may feel familiar and comfortable for some, while others may feel less at ease. Individuals with secure IWMs may feel nurtured by these experiences and feel safe to engage with social commentary. In the face of attachment-related stress, securely attached adults may be better able to tolerate anxiety because their IWMs allow them to feel connected, protected, and understood (Main, 2000; Siegel, 2012). These individuals also tend to experience less stress and exhibit more resilience when exposed to stressors. Providing support for the examination of such art psychotherapy interactions, our Israeli colleagues Sharon Snir and Dafna Regev have researched the relationships between the reaction to different art materials and attachment strategies. Subsequently they developed an art-based instrument to qualify and quantify these interactions (Snir & Regev, 2013a, 2013b).

Individuals who are more prone to relational insecurity may find exposure to art psychotherapy interactions more challenging and may need to self-regulate. For example, they may respond with dismissive remarks, withdraw, or become preoccupied with rearranging their media. Some may manage this stress with an air of indifference, placing their materials on the table randomly, as if to suggest the lack of importance of the experience. Other reactions may include hesitation, seeking guidance on the correct position for material placement, doubting their own preferences, and exhibiting a desire to follow the lead of others. These experientials allow art therapists to gain empathy for the internal attachment states of their future clients.

> *Prior to this experience, I had no understanding that wet media, paints, and clay could be considered emotionally unsafe. However, following the media-based directives, I was able to understand why, in many instances, structured and concrete media are deemed safer media over paints and clay. The term "containment" came alive for me in this course and I realized that we as therapists are not only called upon to contain safety for our clients within the interpersonal holding environment, but also to provide containment through the art. Although we want to explore deep-rooted emotions, feelings, fears, and presenting problems through our clients' artwork, we are responsible for slowly revealing these things through a process. This experience allowed me to understand the impact different media have on an individual and realize the repercussions using certain media may attain.* Jennifer Klein

In the art therapy clinic or therapeutic studio, the development of significant relationships can interface with attachment-based reactions. Relationships may become personally meaningful and expressed in the working interactions. Symbolic representations of personhood, personal history, and self-perceptions of competence may emerge in personal reflections and group discussions. More specifically, in such a social lab and creative environment, strides can be made toward secure attachment experiences; The interaction between the group members and the studio facilitators directly contributes to earning relational confidence.

For example, in her reflections, one person confided that she had been

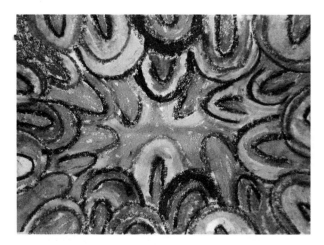

Figure 4.3 *Touching Not Touching.* An abstract representation of a cohesive group. Anonymous

able to dramatically reassess her own parenting. Joanna asked to share her discoveries by reading her poetic reflection aloud. Supportive group witnessing and sharing can support the development of IWM coherency and contingency. Similarly, the facilitator's IWM is exposed. In preparation for this kind of meeting, one artist once made a pastel image of what she would expect (Figure 4.3).

> *As I was contemplating the upcoming experiential, I reminded myself how the initial experience of personal art therapy making can invite closeness and attachment bonding and how it also requires safety—expressed here in the directionality and coming together of the colorful half rounds drawn above, each protected by two to three layers of lines evoking the individuals in the group. As I looked at the image above a few years later, I was reminded of aboriginal drawings of women—represented as half circles gathering as a community. I was pleased with the association because it represents the kind of nonverbal, visual-based intimacy that the dialogue around media can promote: the small groups that we often fall into are often primarily female gendered and the evolving, secure, and contained self is represented in the encapsulated half rounds.* Noah Hass-Cohen

Experience II: The Family Attachment Map

For the Family Attachment Map (FAM), we ask that the group members explore and represent their family relationships. The activity demonstrates how personal histories shape IWMs. One way to call upon these family rela-

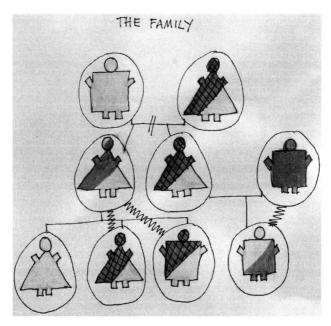

Figure 4.4 *Art Therapy Genogram.* The use of color and design indicates the type of relationships. For example, the hatched areas indicate the transmission of neglect through three generations. The female participant who created the genogram is depicted as a combination of neglect and loving.

tionships is to invite individuals to chart attachment-based episodic memories (Figure 4.4). Holding, attending to, and tolerating the emotional manifestation of the past in the present is required, in addition to examining attachment style. Completing a FAM also requires the employment of cognitive skills such as selecting, categorizing, planning, and meaning making. We ask everyone to, "Create a visual family map of all the important people in your life, including children, parents, and grandparents." Each person is encouraged to go as far back in time as they desire so that their map records significant personal relationships and family events, such as divorces, deaths, and migrations. To facilitate the art making, they thus first create an art-based or visual genogram.

To assist in organizing the genogram, we often suggest creating a series of traditional questions (McGoldrick, Gerson, & Petry, 2008). Traditional genogram questions focus on understanding the structural organization of the family, major family life-cycle events, and patterns of closeness and conflict. We have added such questions below. We suggest asking these and any other questions for different periods of each individual's life. For example, the first five years, five to 10 years, 10 to 18 years, and so on (Table 4.1).

Table 4.1 Genogram Questions

1. How many generations would you like to present?
2. How many siblings did you have?
3. What was your birth order?
4. Did either parent pass away while you were growing up?
5. Were you adopted or raised by someone other than your parents?
6. Did you live in foster care for any length of time
7. Were your parents ever divorced?
8. Were they divorced more than once?
9. With whom did you live?
10. Did you have stepparents?
11. What was your relationship with them like?
12. Did either parent have a relationship with or live with a person to whom they were not married?
13. What was your relationship with them like?
14. What significant events occurred (e.g., moving, hospitalizations, experiencing the death of someone) and how old were you at the time?
15. Would you consider either parent to be emotionally, physically, or sexually abusive? Were you ever subjected to racist remarks or prejudice?
16. What was your weight and body build?
17. Was it a problem?
18. What other questions should we ask or talk about?

For the next FAM experiential, we suggest that the group members use collage material or copy family photos to: "Show what it was like growing up in your family." The premade and photocopied images assist in depicting attachment-based relationships. Additional colors and symbols are used to describe details of their family life story, such as communication style, types of connections between people, and emotional background. Attachment-based questions examine perceived security of the family base, including feeling comforted, loved, and supported (Bluck & Habermas, 2000). This narrative supports the development of a secure life-story schema, which can be used repeatedly. A list of possible attachment-based FAM questions focus on mapping the emotional salient quality of the family system (Table 4.2).

Representing and reflecting upon one's own and other's mental states in this narrative supports mentalization (Asen & Fonagy, 2012) and memory reconsolidation. FAM-based questions are intended to lead individuals to represent their episodic memories of their family relationships and put them together as a meaningful amalgam (Figure 4.5).

Table 4.2 Family Attachment Map Questions

1. How would you show your emotional interactions with each parent and sibling as an infant/toddler? When in primary school/secondary school? As a teen? As an adult?

2. Were there any conflicts with any of the people in the above question? How were they managed? And how would you show that?

3. What were some of the exact words used in your communications with each in the above two questions? Write those in or cut them out from collages.

4. With whom were you the closest and why? How would you show that?

5. With whom were you the most distant and why? How would you show that?

6. Were you treated with respect, dignity, and love? If not, why? How would you show that?

7. Did you ever feel rejected as a child? Choose an image to show that.

8. Did anyone feel psychologically intrusive as you were growing up (e.g., head games, double messages, your feelings used against you)? What would that look like?

9. How did your parents discipline you? And under what circumstances? If you wish, choose an image to represent it.

10. What were your responsibilities as a child (chores, taking care of siblings)? If you wish, choose an image to represent it.

11. Were you ever left alone for periods of time? Choose an image to represent these feelings.

12. Were you ever frightened? What caused it? How did you and others respond to your fright? Choose an image to represent these feelings?

13. How would you characterize the emotional atmosphere of your home—warm, tense, edgy, quiet, calm? Choose an image or colors to represent these feelings.

14. How and from whom did you receive recognition? Show it with marks.

15. What were holidays like? Birthdays? How were gifts given in your childhood? Were strings attached? What did the gifts look like to you?

16. How did your parents communicate with each other? Was there conflict? Choose colors to show what that might that look like (e.g., passive, aggressive, violent, yelling, hitting, threatening). Under what circumstances? What did you do when conflict occurred? What does conflict look like?

17. How did your parents demonstrate love to each other, your siblings, you, and others? Under what circumstances? Were there favorites? How did that manifest?

18. Did you feel loved? Make a symbol for your feelings.

19. What was your experience of leaving home? Were you relieved, sad, anxious, excited? Choose images that show this.

20. In relation to losses, abuse, or other traumatic events you may have experienced, how did you feel at the time and how have your feelings changed over time? Choose different colors and marks to show this.

21. Have there been changes in your relationships with your parents since your childhood? Add images or colors that show this.

22. Why did your parents behave as they did in your childhood? Add your understanding through symbols or images.

Adapted from Baranowsky, Gentry, & Shultz (2011), Asen & Fonagy (2012), George, Kaplan, & Main (1996), and Hesse (1999).

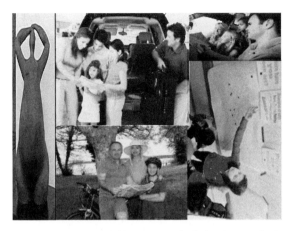

Figure 4.5 *My Family Trying to Find Itself.* A photograph of a female statue looks out over three photographs in the center and top right. The photographs show parents and kids using a map as if looking for directions. A young girl points to a notice on the lower right. The young girl is me. I often felt I needed to provide my family with directions. Louise Smith

> *Oh my goodness, this so represents the different fathers and mothers that I have in my head—those that are close and far apart and how I felt so close and so far from my siblings. Now I am thinking that this is the map that I use every day when we are stranded and don't know what way to go, and when my children are in the driving seat and hence just pose for the world. I must say that I like this so much better than the dry genogram drawing. And I admit that most of the time I feel like that little girl in my mind navigating this world. Which required that I stay distant and dismissing? Can I change that through the eyes of my here-and-now figure? Can I come to this thing called earned security? That is the challenge, isn't it?* Louise Smith

When the map comes to a finish, we invite our participants to create an oil or polymer clay-based figure, representing the self, and to place it in front of or to the side of the picture. Thus each person is brought directly into the picture of their past relationships. These tasks, ordering and representing one's family history and then connecting to the representation today, can potentially evoke strong feelings. The variety of attachment-related representations can touch deep limbic reactions, thereby stimulating distressing experiences. Conversely, we contend that representing these experiences in shape and form recruits higher cortical functions that provide the opportunity to practice affect regulation. In addition, the request to connect current behavioral patterns with past difficult or affirmative familial experiences can allow strong emotional responses to be understood and contained (Baranowsky et

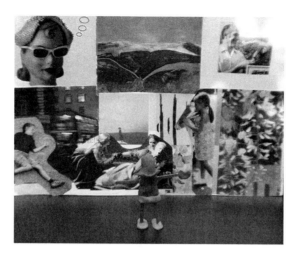

Figure 4.6 *Family Attachment Map with Three-Dimensional Self-Clay Figure.* A blue oil-based clay figure with outstretched arms faces a family collage. The top left corner shows an adult woman and the top right an adult man, between which there is a colorful landscape. In the lower left a boy leaps and in the lower right a girl carries flowers. The central image between the children is one of a dramatic family scene. It depicts the kind of support that was extended in our family. Anna Louisa Kingston

al., 2011). Furthermore, moving to a three-dimensional format promotes a symbolic reengagement with attachment figures and strategies. This symbolic act can support moving toward an earned secure attachment as the individual is called upon to express and regulate emotions and consider different ways of interacting with others, with current family and with their family of origin (Figure 4.6).

> *I found making my family environmental map helped me crystalize the dynamics in my family of origin as the collage images distilled what I wanted to express. The images obliged me to describe my family in a simplistic form yet revealed a great deal about our interaction, roles, and emotions. Modeling and then placing my plasticine sculpture of myself in front of the collage was liberating. I decided to make my arms outstretched as if to say, "Here I am today; I see this environment for what it was in the past," but I can step back from it and calmly observe it.* Anna Louisa Kingston

As we come together to talk about the work, the group members are invited to place their family environmental maps around them. Some prop up their maps against the walls, while others lay them out on cleared tables. The discussion and reflections on the familial IWMs require mentalizing. Engaging with such metacognitions can form a bridge between a triggering memory and a defensive response. In other words, as the group members reflect, they can move toward a new way of knowing themselves. The group reflections are later storied in individualized formats.

Experience III: Fabric-Based Attachment Albums

In order to integrate attachment theory and strategies with personal development and clinical applications, participants are asked to represent their significant relationships as either recipients of caring or providers of support and loving. To start the work, we ask that the participants first respond implicitly in imagery or verbally to any of the following words: *mother, father,* or *parental figure (grandparent, sister, brother, guardian)*. We discuss that though some are more common labels, their meanings are far from universal. The next directive is to: "Create a cloth album illustrating the four principal adult attachment styles or child attachment strategies." Alternatively, they can choose to use the five-page album to: "Fully illustrate one style with one or more significant others." These choices invite the creator to imagine their young self's blueprints and/or the adult living expression of early relationship modeling. The use of fabrics brings forward a kinesthetic understanding of the styles, meaning the felt experience of security or insecurity (Clyde Findlay et al., 2008). Through the proposed attachment album activity, we access the personalized experience of each artist, each individual's constructed relational story (Table 4.3).

Table 4.3 Fabric-Based Attachment Albums

1. Choose one or more significant-other relationships that you want to explore
2. Decide if you will be exploring the album as a child or as an adult.
3. Illustrate the related four principal adult attachment styles or child attachment strategies with one or more significant others.
4. If you like, you may choose to fully explore just one style.
5. Decide on the fabrics and media that you will use for the album.
6. Make an album with at least five pages. A book format is needed. One must be able to turn pages in space. There are no size limitations.
7. Use one page for each of the four attachment categories or to explore one style. The last page is a visual reflection.
8. Make an image for each attachment style. The last reflection page is also an image.
9. Underneath each image or across from it give a title for the attachment style of the image.
10. Add a three- to five-page written tale explaining how each image goes with each attachment style and a personal reflection.
11. Discuss how you may directly, or in a modified fashion, use attachment albums with clients.

Adapted from Clyde Findlay, Lathan, & Hass-Cohen (2008).

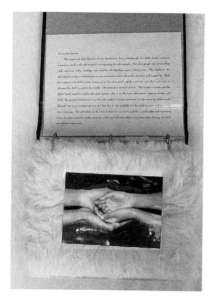
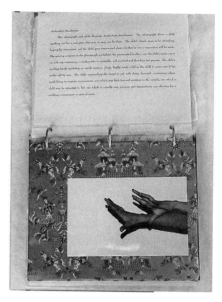
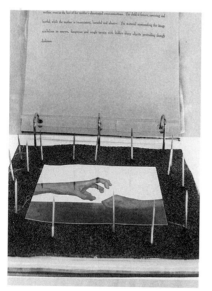
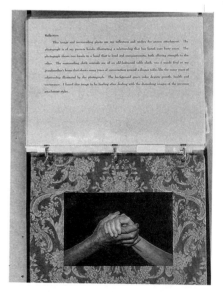

Figure 4.7 *Attachment Album.* Top row left to right: secure representation followed by an ambivalent representation. The secure image is adult hands supportively cupping a younger pair of hands glued onto a soft furry fabric. The ambivalent image is two sets of hands echoing each other in a repulsing gesture glued to a fabric with a repetitive motif. Bottom row left to right: disorganized attachment representation followed by an earned attachment image. The latter is a reflection on the process of making the albums. The disorganized image shows a vulnerable closed hand being menaced by a clawing adult hand mounted on dark sandpaper pierced through with three-inch nails. The reflective image shows supportive older male and female hands holding each other, set upon a richly textured fabric.
Jessica Tress Masterson

Sewing, gluing, and fastening parallels symbolized earned secure attachment processes. For the creator, carefully stitching a cuddly blanket fabric can mimic and express the warmth of a child's secure attachment. Salvaging a torn rag can represent mending the disorienting effects of an adult's disorganized attachment style. Sharing these vested textured albums furthers the development of a coherent autobiographical narrative. In this way, album making and sharing can be reparative as the work may promote the creator's affective tolerance for his or her personal narrative.

Creating attachment albums may often evoke strong metaphors. One example is Jessica's use of a combination of graphic black-and-white photographs. She expresses closeness with her placement of hands set upon backgrounds of textured fabric. The multi-dimensionality of her imagery projects a powerful and vivid representation of IWMs. Disorganized attachment is illustrated by a large, menacing hand reaching over a withdrawn, curled-up hand, mounted on rough black sandpaper pierced with dangerous three-inch nails. In contrast, the image of open and receptive pairing of hands, supportively cupped together as in a secure attachment, is embedded in warm and fuzzy fabric (Figure 4.7).

Sharing the albums requires a dedicated and well-defined structure and time frame. The size of the full group determines how much time each member can have for sharing. Sometimes if the group is very large it is necessary to dedicate two meetings to sharing. Group cohesion will further influence the degree of cross-talk, reactions, peer feedback, and discussion. The secure adult may feel connected and protected, which consolidates learning. Others with more preoccupied, anxious or dismissive, or avoidant patterns may, with guidance, learn to experience art making as comforting and safe. For those experiencing dissonance, the relationally based autobiographical images can provide the opportunity to close some gaps and coherently narrate childhood memories. The attachment album experience can be a profound opportunity for group members to reach back in time in order to repair the present and prepare for the future.

RELATIONAL NEUROSCIENCE: ATTACHMENT-BASED NEUROPLASTICITY ACROSS THE LIFE SPAN

While genetics account for the basic layout of the brain, experience sculpts our neurons into orderly processing networks (Eliot, 1999). Thinking, learning, and behavior alter the brain's physical structure, connectivity, and function (Kalat, 2012). Brain-scanning technology continues to give dramatic insights into the functioning and development of the brain and the impact of early childhood experiences on the development of brain structures, networks, and tasks (Perry, 2002a, 2002b).

The human brain triples in size during the first year of life alone. Throughout the first two years of life, the brain cells and neural pathway linkages begin to develop (Eliot, 1999). While the brain changes throughout the life span, it grows to full size by the time a child is ready for kindergarten. Interestingly, connections that are seldom or never used weaken, whereas those that are frequently used are reinforced and grow. In fact, shaping of the cortex goes through a reiterative process until age 25, when it organizes, disorganizes, and reorganizes the prefrontal cortex (Drury & Giedd, 2009). Throughout life, new neurons are also formed in the adult brain, usually in the hippocampus, the brain structure involved in learning and memory (Jessberger & Gage, 2008; Kalat, 2012).

The caregiver's warm support and capacity for attunement are key to the developing nervous system and to resiliency. Many early brain linkages are dependent on the emotional and social attachment relationship with the caregiver. Nurturing and attuned caregiver responses support the brain's optimal maturation processes and growth trajectory. The quality of caring relationships contributes to the development of specific attachment styles and the capacity for affect regulation. These early experiences form the foundations for lifelong interpersonal affect regulation skills. Severe and persistent maltreatment can compromise attachment, creating persistent mistrust of interpersonal connections, social isolation, and problems with regulating affect and attuning to others. Depending on when the trauma occurred and which resources were available, the developmental delays and corresponding neurobiological deficits may present as distorted cognition, lack of behavioral controls, poor confidence, and medical problems (Perry, 1997).

Predictable, escapable, or controllable stressors, or situations where some safe caregiver contact was available or was restored, can protect neurobiological development (Champagne & Meaney, 2001; Schore, 2001a). Importantly, deliberate therapeutic development of steady interpersonal abilities can compensate for these deficits and be protective in the long term. Specific interventions should focus on the development of affect regulation, mastery of cognitive abilities, use of affirmative motivation, and growth in self-trust (Cohen, Mannarino, & Deblinger, 2006). This is particularly critical for working with child survivors of prolonged and severe abuse or neglect (Crenshaw & Mordock, 2005).

Infancy: Brain Shaping Through Relationships

From the moment a baby is born, sensory organs begin to relay environmental information to the brain through neural impulses. The newborn's brain develops as a result of potentiated and pruned synaptic connections that respond to sensory inputs (Eliot, 1999). Synaptic pruning eliminates weaker neuronal connections (Hebb, 2002), and strengthening and potentiation of activated neural pathways shape the brain (Kandel, Schwartz, & Jessell, 2001). The sensory and affective nature of the attachment relationship is central to this synaptic thickening and reorganization of neural networks.

At birth, neurons are not mature, and their brain axons are unmyelinated; thus the connections between them are slow (Deoni et al., 2011; Hass-Cohen, 2008a). Developmentally, myelination begins in brain structures that are responsible for primitive functions before progressing to areas responsible for higher functions. Myelin is an insulating white sheath surrounding axons that facilitates electrical communication, hence the name "white matter." Unlike dendritic connectivity and the pruning of synapses, myelination is genetically wired (Eliot, 1999). Myelination of axons occurs sequentially from the back to the front of the brain. It begins in sensory regions, such as the visual cortex, and then progresses into areas involved in motor function and higher cognitive and emotional functioning, related to the parietal, temporal, and frontal lobes' development (Eliot, 1999; Toga, Thompson, & Sowell, 2006).

Myelinated neural pathways transmit communications quickly. This is in contrast with unmyelinated brain matter, aptly named gray matter, which wraps the outer brain areas and serves to protect the myelinated pathways. For most parents, it is easy to see the expression of myelination as a child masters motor tasks such walking and grasping objects. Less obvious but equally important is parental praise, which reinforces emotional and social neuronal pathways through myelination.

The first gene-environment interactions occur in the exchanges between mother and infant (Weaver, 2011). Magnetic resonance imaging reveals that the infant brain is able to alter its shape within the first weeks of life, suggesting a structural bias for adaptation to physical, relational, and mental activity (May & Gaser, 2006). During these formative times, the attachment relationship directly regulates the genome and the way that the genes will encode the proteins (Barry, Kochanska, & Philibert, 2008; Spangler, Johann, Ronai, & Zimmermann, 2009). If there are positive attachment experiences, the potentiality of the genes will be carried out to the fullest (Kochanska, Philibert, & Barry, 2010).

The relationship between the mother and infant also stimulates hormones, such as oxytocin, connecting to opiate and endorphin systems. At 10 or 12 months of age, the genetic systems encode the connections of the brain's highest parts with top areas of the limbic system. These are bottom-up and top-down social-emotional neural pathways. Additionally, the anticipation of secure interactions involves the reward circuitry, which stimulates release of the neurotransmitters dopamine and noradrenaline (Carr, 2008a). Furthermore, the more the infant's social-emotional neural pathways are stimulated, the quicker and more automatic his or her proximity-seeking actions become (Tronick, 2007).

Not all caregivers can provide sufficiently responsive and sensitive care for the baby to be able to form a secure attachment. Infants will modify their nurture-seeking strategies to cope with the emotional capabilities of their specific caregivers. In order to elicit as much comfort and attention from the caregiver as possible, the baby may use an indirect approach, such as extensive crying and, or avoidance. The infant may exhibit hypersensitivity to physical contact, problems with coordination, and a weakened body tone. These stressed behaviors are a function of the autonomic nervous system, which mobilizes arousal through its sympathetic branch. When a prolonged need for adaptation occurs, it can be accompanied by a long-term stress response and the release of cortisol. Neural development is also influenced by the release of cortisol, a stress hormone (Bakermans-Kranenburg & van IJzendoorn, 2007). Stress responses can influence long-term potentiation (LTP), or learning on a synaptic level, as it can strengthen and quicken specific stimulus-response links between nerve cells. For example, LTP can contribute to a conditioned fear response. Cortisol effects both prenatal and postnatal development. Predictable neural network linkages result from LTP consolidation, taking anywhere from hours to years. These processes of learning and forgetting exist on the neural basis that cells that fire together, wire together; cells that do not, die together (Carr, 2008a; Kandel et al., 2001).

Contingent responsiveness to the infants', at first automatic expressive displays, through "mirroring" interactions in secure attachment establishes a cognitive platform from which the infant learns she is understood and thought about, building the foundation of mentalization (Asen & Fonagy, 2012). In contrast stress-based interactions in infancy will influence the nature of an individual's interpersonal interactions throughout the life span and can lead to the tendency to overreact to any stressor, however mild (Schore, 2001b). This can often create an internal mixup where external stressors and internal startle response confuse and disorient the child and later the adult. This type of lower brain reaction that is guided by lower and mid-central brain functions can create a vulnerability to aggressive relational dispositions (Crenshaw & Mordock, 2005; Mikulincer & Shaver, 2010, 2012; Perry, 1997). So while it still holds true that attachment styles are malleable, the quality of the relationship with the primary attachment figure heavily influences the dominant and long-lasting IWMs, social skills, and the ability to cope with stress.

Early Childhood: Language and Higher Brain Development Respond to Caring Systems

Early childhood continues to be a time of tremendous brain growth. As children orient and react to their interpersonal environment, functions of the central nervous system (CNS), peripheral nervous system (PNS), and endocrine system continue to evolve. In particular, areas that filter sensory inputs, such as the thalamus and somatosensory cortices, continue to link with structures responsible for fear, the amyg-dala; meaning making, the hippocampus; and affect regulation, the PFC (LeDoux, 2007).

Infants and young children's brains are still right-hemisphere dominant (Chiron et al., 1997). However, there is an increase in the development of language centers. The brain also experiences an explosion of growth in the frontal lobes, allowing the toddler to employ self-control as well as gain self-awareness (Eliot, 1999). This burgeoning and language development are responsible for the burst of *I, me, my,* or *mine* words and parallels the development of the capacity for ToM (Premack & Woodruff, 1978), which is linked with affect regulation and attachment history. Tested by the ability to cognitively mentalize social actions (Baron-Cohen, Leslie, & Frith, 1985). The capacity for object permanence and for ToM, which develops slower for children on the autistic spectrum and those with intellectual delays, can benefit from social scaffolding (Bruce & Muhammad, 2009). Thus, maturation continues to be embedded in a relational context (Cozolino, 2013; Hughes & Leekam, 2004).

Environmental interactions continue to shape the capacity for relationships throughout the life span, creating specific neural pathways in the brain that are involved in the dynamics of attachment, safety, and stress (Siegel, 2003, 2006). Cumulatively, the child's early experiences influence the quality of his or her ability to connect with others. This includes the development of empathy and the ability to control aggression, which are relationally dependent (Kimonis, Cross, Howard, & Donoghue, 2012).

Smooth flow of information throughout the brain depends largely on the structural integrity and maturity of linked myelinated pathways. Non-optimal relational experiences, such as abuse or neglect, can lead to the underdevelopment of cortical, limbic, and spinal area linkages (Burrus, 2013). Critical periods for these linkages may be missed, and connections between areas of the brain responsible for survival, and for affect regulation, may not be optimally linked. Thus disruptive attachment experiences contribute to interruptions in brain connectivity, which is associated with the persistence of primitive, immature reactivity. Neurobiologically, this is because the interaction of the environment and experience may not provide for optimal gene expression. Again, behaviorally, this may appear as hyperactivity, inattention, aggression, and anger (van der Kolk, 2005).

The young child's specific pattern of response to abuse, such as prolonged dissociation and or hyperarousal, may further contribute to permanent neurobiological changes (Briere & Scott, 2012). The effects of disorganized and fear-based attachment responses can promote a sensitized fear response and severe affect dysregulation, as long-term potentiation in the lateral nucleus of the amygdala is thought to lead to dysregulation (Rodrigues, Schafe, & LeDoux, 2004). These neurobiological changes have been linked to long-term affect regulation problems, anxiety, and mood disorders (Perry, 1997, 2002a, 2002b). Finally, it is the timing of the assault on the brain that will determine the exact damage.

Middle Childhood: Integrating Affective and Cognitive Security

Middle childhood is a time for tremendous cerebral-cortical growth. Growth is particularly impressive in the corpus callosum (CC), a brain structure that connects the left and right hemispheres. During middle childhood, growth rates continue to be highest in associative and linguistic neural networks, sharpening language functions (Thompson et al., 2000).

As the CC develops and myelinates, the two hemispheres connect and interact. There is a shift from right-hemisphere (RH) abstractions, such as sensing and feeling bias, to left-hemisphere (LH) foci: language, reasoning, logical planning (De Bellis, Keshavan, & Shifflett, 2002; Kagan, 2003). As the CC connects RH and LH functions, children's abstract and logical abilities develop, connect, and specialize. Integration of spatial and linguistic capacities supports higher-order cognitive processes, such as fluent reading (DeBoard, Kilian, Naramor, & Brown, 2003).

During this development phase, the increase in hemispheric communication may contribute to the shift from being I-centric to noticing the outside world (Erikson, 1959; Piaget & Inhelder, 1973). Suddenly, the once carefree child is self-conscious and aware of what others will say and think. As children reach puberty, their interest in peers and social interaction increases, as do parental and educational demands.

Meeting the demands of novel psychosocial and environmental tasks puts a heavy burden on the relationally insecure child. Experiences of attachment-based trauma can hinder LH and RH integration, which may contribute to the seemingly unreasonable behavior responses of traumatized children. Such behavioral responses from a child express a distrust of interpersonal relationships; he or she may also have problems with perspective taking and with effectively enlisting others as allies (Cook, Blaustein, Spinazzola, & van der Kolk, 2003). The traumatized child will most likely find it difficult to identify, express, communicate, and adapt his or her emotions (Perry, 2001, 2002a). These inabilities to self-regulate put some of these children at risk for oppositional and conduct disorders (Ford, 2009; Ford et al., 2000; Sroufe, 2000). Child maltreatment usually happens in the caregiving environment, the very setting on which the child relies for safety, stability, and comfort. This contradiction can lead to cognitive dissonance for the child in addition to ensuing emotional dysregulation.

Attachment-based psychotherapies have been shown to be effective for externalizing child problems, as they can assist in increasing the family support base (Gil, 2010; Malchiodi & Crenshaw, 2013; Moretti, Holland, Moore, & McKay, 2004). Praise and positive reinforcement are critical aspects that have the potential to repair attachment-based insecurity and trauma. In addition, it is necessary for the caregivers to both believe the child and tolerate his or her emotional reaction. This support is especially critical when children react with rage. A structured, behaviorally managed, strength-focused program is effective in sustaining these re-parenting efforts (Cohen et al., 2006b). The caregivers must draw upon the child's cognitive abilities and personal strengths in order to assist him or her in acknowledging, recognizing, labeling, and coping with emotional distress (Proulx, 2002a, 2002b; Schore, 2009).

Adolescence: Linkages of the Social Emotional-Based Prefrontal Cortex

Researchers have discovered that the process of myelination increases twofold during adolescence, primarily in the areas of the PFC (Giedd et al., 1999). The PFC is one of the last parts of our brains to mature, and is not fully developed until age 25. Furthermore, although the most rapid growth of the CC occurs at younger ages, as mentioned above, the CC continues to increase in size throughout adolescence (Drury & Giedd, 2009). Overall, until the PFC catches up and the RH and LH are fully connected, the adolescent brain—which is inundated with emotional impulses—lacks the the full capacity to inhibit or regulate such impulses.

As in the toddler years, puberty prompts a gray matter growth spurt in the frontal lobe (Giedd, 2004). The PFC is responsible for complex executive functioning such as motivation, reasoning, judgment, and the inhibition of impulses. Specifically, the dorsolateral PFC is crucial for control of impulses, judgment, and decision-making. The PFC also acts to control and process emotional information sent from the amygdala, the fight-or-flight center of the stress response, which may account for the mercurial tempers of adolescents. While the PFC steadily develops throughout the teenage years and into young adulthood, myelin covers the limbic center more quickly than in the PFC. Studies have also suggested that the brains of females will typically myelinate faster than the brains of males, which may contribute to their faster emotional and cognitive maturation (Strauch, 2003).

In the limbic areas, the main structures that receive a boost in myelin are the hippocampus and the cingulate gyrus (Benes, Turtle, Khan, & Farol, 1994). The hippocampus is the part of the limbic system that plays an important role in long-term memory and spatial navigation. Also part of the limbic system, the cingulate gyrus partially wraps around the CC, which connects the LH and RH. It also connects to our brain stem and spinal cord, which control basic gut reactions and movements. The cingulate gyrus is involved in emotional formation and processing, as well as learning and memory. This increased speed of connection can explain the impulsive emotional reactivity and importance of social evaluation during adolescence (Crone, 2009).

In regard to the social and emotional context of adolescent brain development, adolescents seem to employ different neural strategies for thinking about others' intentions than do adults (Blakemore, 2012; Blakemore, den Ouden, Choudhury, & Frith, 2007). In adolescence, deficits in self-regulatory abilities or an insecure IWM can have a notable impact on daily functioning. When endured in the absence of sustaining adult or peer relationships, insecure attachment strategies contribute to a number of maladaptive behavioral patterns. For example, the adolescent may experience self-regulation disruptions, interpersonal mutuality difficulty, reality disorientation, and or a combination of critical competency deficits. Such disruptions may respectively manifest as eating disorders, conduct disorders, thought disorders, and addiction. As discussed earlier, attachment-based psychotherapies are effective for this age as well (Diamond, Siqueland, & Diamond, 2003).

Adults: Engaged Resiliency

Brain plasticity is considered constant throughout the life span and, in adults, is often most easily illustrated in the effects of learning or recovery from brain injury. Over the past decade, data have indicated that the adult brain is capable of substantial structural and functional reorganization after a stroke (Nudo, 2011). Some limited recovery is known to occur spontaneously, especially within the first month following a stroke. Furthermore, interventions based on the modulation of neuroplasticity mechanisms are used in neurocognitive rehabilitation.

Cognitive training can produce performance gains with both younger and older adults. Practice-oriented studies reveal improvement on specific tasks, such as for working memory (Buschkuehl et al., 2008). It is debated whether increased prefrontal activity, common in adult brains, is due to durable plasticity or age-related changes in functional supply (Lovden, Bacman, Lindenberger, Schaefer, & Schmiedeck, 2010). Nonetheless, increases in gray matter density and volume as a function of learning abstract knowledge and complex motor skills have been confirmed (Draganski et al., 2006).

Mindfulness-based practices have also been seen to alter functional connectivity in the adult brain. Specifically implicated is the auditory cortex and areas associated with attentional and self-referential processes (Kilpatrick et al., 2011). Important for resiliency, gray matter density likely increases (Hölzel et al., 2011; see Chapter 9). The positive effects of enriched lifestyles on adult cognitive changes are a reflection of such brain plasticity (Hertzog, Kramer, Wilson, & Lindenberger, 2009). Cognitive activity can spare the brain some of the negative effects of aging such as depression and stress, and mitigate some of the assault on the brain. Increasing cognitive activity through enriching therapeutic activities helps to increase the density or mass of thick gray matter in the brain. Throughout the life span, a heavier brain, which has a heavier mass of thick gray matter, provides more protection against time's assault (Bishop, 1995; Satz, 1993).

The neuroscience of resiliency requires balancing the nervous system's arousal (sympathetic nervous system [SNS]) and calming (parasympathetic nervous system [PSNS]) functions. The stress response is partially automatic and influenced by rapid transmission of impulses along multiple pathways. What results are complex responses, including flight, fight, freeze, affect regulation, and social engagement (Hass-Cohen, 2008a; Kravits, 2008b; Porges, 2001).

Exaggerated and prolonged stress responses, found in generalized anxiety disorder and post-traumatic stress disorder, have been thought to exemplify an anxious attachment style and allostatic overload. In contrast, benign stressors can trigger a search for pleasure and proximity seeking (i.e., attachment behaviors), thereby promoting the rebalancing of altered physiological and psychological states (Esch & Stefano, 2005). Research on the earned secure attachment style suggests that there can be plasticity in internal representations (Roisman, Padrón, Sroufe, & Egeland, 2002). The adult brain is able to move to more coherent integrated functioning that frees earned secure parents to nurture securely attached children. In other words, the neurobiology of allostasis, control, lack of control (Henry & Wang, 1999; Kravitz, 2008a; Hass-Cohen, 2008b), and affect regulation are involved in the neuroplasticity of attachment-based interactions (Hass-Cohen & Carr, 2008).

Older Adults: Positive Social Influence on Brain Compensation and Maintenance

Aging can bring with it loss of cortical function through a variety of pathological processes (e.g., stroke, dementia). The result may be a loss of cortical modulation of arousal, impulsivity, motor hyperactivity, and aggression. These all represent functions mediated by lower portions of the CNS (brain stem, midbrain). Equally, the progressive effects of mild cognitive impairment and Alzheimer's disease (AD) erode executive functions of decision making, thoughtful action, and memory, primarily located in the PFC, entorhinal cortex, and hippocampus (Small, Herlitz, & Backman, 2004). In midlife, high-density brains with compensatory neural network capacities, brain reserve capacity, and cognitive reserve can slow the onslaught of aging and AD, and compensate for brain injury (Allen, Bruss, & Damasio, 2005; Galbraith, Subrin, & Ross, 2008; Satz, 1993; Staff, Murray, Deary, & Whalley, 2004). Exercise, ongoing learning, stimulating occupations, and lifelong social activities protect and enrich the brain through the increase in gray matter (Allen et al., 2005; Satz, 1993).

Aerobic exercise and cognitive stimulation have been shown to promote neurogenesis, or the production of new neurons (Horner & Gage, 2002; Ratey & Hagerman, 2008). For example, the best predictor of health and well-being in older adults is the level of activity and exercise (Goldberg, 2005). Additionally, a relational context has an impact on the aging brain. Greater social resources, as defined by social networks and social engagement, are associated with reduced cognitive decline in old age (Barnes, de Leon, Wilson, Bienias, & Evans, 2004). Intellectual stimulation through social interaction has been associated with increases in brain volume as well as with cognitive improvements (Ishizaki et al., 2002; Mortimer et al., 2012). Research also suggests that new learning can be successful when embedded in a relational context (Gallegos, 2009). Art therapy outcome research has also suggested that thematic arts programming can be beneficial for increased perceptual and cognitive abilities (Levine-Madori & Alders, 2010).

CREATE PRINCIPLES AND CLINICAL APPLICATIONS

The primary focus of the art therapy experiences in this chapter is the CREATE principle of Relational Resonating. Art therapy interventions provide unique opportunities for the kind of playful and supportive interactions that the developing brain thrives on. When working with clients, expressive practices and coherent communication promote stable internal psychobiological states and fluid interpersonal relationships. Collaborative and attuned therapeutic relationships support these states; they increase experiences of positive affect and help disengage from negative feelings. Relational art therapy directives either can be interactive, as in the media experience, or can focus on interpersonal content, as in the family map and the fabric albums. Specific ATR-N microskills combined with the art therapist's steady and constant attunement can thus generate a new sense of security, which provides the basis for earned attachment. Relational art making is the therapeutic cornerstone that facilitates attachment-based change (Hass-Cohen, 2008b).

In this chapter, the connotations associated with the therapist's or peer's shared media may be attachment-based triggers for clients. The offered media in the Interpersonal Media experience may stir clients' attachment styles. Using the therapist's media may arouse anxiety around what is allowable and what is not: "What will happen if I break your crayon or use too much of it?" Clients may also wonder if they are worthy or unworthy of the therapist's attention. For example, they may ask themselves if they are good enough or loved enough if they receive used crayons. They may also experience an emotional response to a specific brand of crayons, such as Crayola, as it may bring up distressing or, conversely, joyful childhood memories. Furthermore, learning how to display interpersonal interest in others is a critical ATR-N microskill. The experiences of the media table, making attachment-based art, and witnessing others' representations of relational memories and attachment styles all support the development of such a microskill. Likewise, the sharing of the therapist's media supports the taking on of relational risks and of making relational connections.

Additional ATR-N microskill sequences and directives that promote the capacity for relational resonance are (1) the construction of the FAM, which builds the foundation for creating the cloth album; (2) sharing and narrating the art with a trusted group; and (3) reflecting on the process in writing. The FAM allows collection of the information needed for the albums. Then the album making gives rise to nonverbal aspects of each person's internalized attachment style. Inviting clients to use fabric media and create attachment-related objects, such as an album of their significant relationships, provides several opportunities. Examples include explicitly approaching, reflecting upon, naming, and organizing implicit self- and attachment-based mental representations. The verbal communication makes these implicit states explicit, and supports the development of a coherent, autobiographical experience. Clients who share a challenging attachment history may find that the structured, concrete activities of searching for specific images and colors, manipulating materials, planning, and finally gluing their pieces together help them to focus and regulate. The media assist in developing the ability to discriminate between experiencing and knowing (Allen, 1995). An example would be

"I am happy. I feel happy; I know I am happy; and I want to continue to be happy." The therapists can adapt these directives and sequencing. Therefore, therapeutic opportunities exist for affect regulation as the experience involves being listened to, heard, and felt by others and vice versa.

The principle of Creative Embodiment is embedded in the interpersonal media experience. Individuals move to other art media displays and welcome others at their own media tables. Encouraging clients to physically explore the creative space can excite the possibility of forming a new relationship and new acquaintances. The activity is structured and contained, providing an opportunity for success despite a history of unsuccessful social endeavors.

The principle of Expressive Communicating is inherent in a therapeutic exploration of attachment. This chapter also provides for the ability to actively acknowledge and recognize the expression, processing, and communication of attachment-based emotions, such as sadness, guilt, shame, fear, surprise, and joy. It is important to note that attachment experiences and reactions are for the most part unconscious. Such nonverbal phenomena consist of emotions, cognitions, and behaviors that can be difficult to express in words alone. Unique to art therapy, a consistent media display can provide tangible reminders of therapeutic attunement. This constancy invites the anticipation of secure interactions and a sense of being fundamentally connected with other people. Making attachment-related objects, such as the albums, allows attachment experiences to be felt in a regulated manner. It concurrently emphasizes the importance of providing attachment-sensitive media, such as felt and fabric, as these can often evoke attachment experiences.

The opportunity to revisit attachment memories through bilateral processing also permits memory consolidation (Vance & Wahlin, 2008). The execution of the art task requires cortical taming of possible strong limbic emotions and provides for an integrated verbal (LH) and nonverbal (RH) expression (Hass-Cohen, 2008a). This experiential puts fabric, a long-neglected art medium, in the forefront of our thinking. We propose that sensory and felt attachment-based media are useful clinical micro-tools. In group therapy, seeing attachment-based art images provides clients with direct access to others' emotions while communicating many related feelings and thoughts.

Adaptive Responding is encouraged as clients use the media to shift in and out of coping states; whilst actually and symbolically reaching their hands to touch the therapist's media offerings they practice resiliency. The art activities can be adapted to provide clients opportunities to revisit and cope with many reminders of relational stressors or breaches of trust. For example, the request to use the therapist's media can be a relatively benign stressor that can activate anxious or avoidant types of attachment insecurity, providing an opening for safe exploration. The experientials allow for safely engaging in a nonverbal, felt, and sensory discovery of one's past and current attachment strategies and style. Creating the art provides a sense of tangible and symbolic mastery of attachment issues. With guided verbal and nonverbal discovery, this can be generalized to a perceived sense of security and hope for an internal working model that can be altered. For example, the creation of the clay self-interacting with the family map provides for emotional relief and self-regulation through concrete distancing.

Transformative Integrating is promoted throughout the sequence of attachment-based experientials: making, narrating, and reflecting. These activities support an integrated autobiographical narrative via right-to-left hemispheric integration. The RH holds the nonverbal autobiographical memories, and the LH contributes to integrating them into an explicit verbal story. Another example, the Attachment Album art simultaneously represents and integrates implicit/unconscious basic emotions and explicit/conscious relational memories contributing to integrated reconsolidated memories.

Empathizing and Compassion form through the interpersonal media and attachment-based art experiences, and by the witnessing of others' representations of relational memories and attachment styles. They also support the evolving professional empathic presence and the understanding that an empathic therapeutic relationship can build toward an earned-secure attachment status. The therapist's sensitivity to embedded relational transactions is associated with the offering and sharing of art media, and his or her unconditional acceptance of the art product. Thus, the client can process the therapist's compassionate understanding and acceptance, allowing for hope in gaining relational security.

CHAPTER 5

Relational Resonating:
Co-Regulation and Co-Creation

Making my collage alongside my daughter reminded me of doing things together at the kitchen table. Sometimes I was absorbed in figuring out my tree and sometimes I noticed how she was working. I was impressed by the boldness of the way she drew and pasted her images. I realized my process was less clear, and she saw me adding new sheets of paper and starting over. I loved that we seemed to share a private world. I intentionally did not comment on what she was making. We just shared the materials and worked side by side. I felt silently connected in a special way. Joanna Clyde Findlay

IN THIS CHAPTER, WE DISCUSS and illustrate the contributions of visual communication and creative expression to co-regulatory interactions. The premise is that individuals communicate with each other implicitly, without talking or using words, just as much as they do explicitly (Cozolino, 2010; Fonagy, Gergely, Gurist, & Target, 2005; Rothschild, 2000; Schore, 2003). We hold that interpersonal, nonverbal right-to-right hemisphere regulatory communication lies at the heart of Relational Resonating, and the Art Therapy Relational Neuroscience (ATR-N) approach.

Co-regulation's evolutionary purpose supports survival as it assists in the physiological maintenance of homeostasis (Sbarra & Hazan, 2008). The capacity to regulate and self-soothe is furthermore central to successful interpersonal interactions. Without co-regulatory experiences, cognitive and emotional brain resources can also diminish. This is because an attuned attachment relationship relieves some of the burden that independent emotional and behavioral control puts on high-order prefrontal cortex (PFC) function (Hughes, Crowell, Uyeji, & Coan, 2012). Co-regulation represents a dynamic mutual and reiterative process, which systemically supports reparation and personal development and change (Tronick et al., 1998; Tronick & Beeghly, 2011).

Early life mother-child co-regulation fuels the development of self-regulation, contributing to the development of a secure internal working model (IWM). From infancy through young adulthood, sufficient co-regulation experiences build up the individual's capacity for independent self-regulation, attuned relationships, secure attachment, and coping with change and stress (Hughes et al., 2012). Attuned co-regulatory experiences help balance the stress response, as seen, for example, in normal blood pressure and temperature of babies. Similar down regulated arousal was documented in lowered blood pressure levels of partners that have close daily social interaction (Sbarra & Hazan, 2008). Furthermore, the infant-caregiver implicit communication system provides the foundation of a person's meaning making.

Within the therapeutic relationship, co-regulation is an implicit interactional procedure that evolves into co-consciousness (Tronick et al., 1998; Tronick, 2001). Co-consciousness is a shared meaning system that provides the scaffolding for flexible reflectivity (Fonagy et al., 2005) autobiographical coherency and personal stability (Wallin, 2007). These regulated states contribute to developing interpersonally stable personality traits and an earned relational sense of security (Siegel, 2006). Thus, the function of co-regulation across the life span evolves and includes implicit and explicit communication and meaning-making systems (Badenoch, 2008).

From a neurobiological perspective, several brain functions contribute to regulatory processes. The first are brain lateralization functions: Throughout the life span, attuned right-to-right hemispheric (RH) interpersonal communication serves to facilitate several important purposes. These include access to unspoken emotions, support for active affect regulation development, evolving social and emotional information processing, and confidence in decision making. Left hemisphere (LH) functions contribute to these abilities through explicit verbal processing, resulting in integrated function (Mac-Neilage, Rogers, & Vallortigara, 2009).

Additional areas responsible for affect regulation and integrative processes are the connections between the PFC and the amygdala (AMY). The AMY processes and prioritizes emotional cues received from the visual cortex, such as facial expressions (Schupp et al., 2007). Face-to-face experiences develop the capacity for trust and self-soothing (Tronick, 2007). Bidirectional feedback loops between the PFC and the limbic areas, the frontolimbic circuitry, are involved in regulation of emotions (Hughes et al., 2012) and in bonding and caring relationships (Siegel, 2012). Neurobiologically, bonding and secure attachment experiences infuse the frontolimbic circuitry with feel-good neurochemistry, including dopamine (DA), serotonin (5-HT), and oxytocin (OXY; Hughes et al., 2012). Mental states are thus comprised of an amalgam of cognitions, feelings, and emotions.

For the experientials and guided experiences, we suggest a sequence of directives that progressively demonstrate affective co-regulation, co-creation, and co-consciousness. These directives illustrate how the interactions between art psychotherapists and clients may provide immediate access to RH non-verbal communication. The first experiential is called My Right Hemisphere. Each group member first creates a color-based impression of her RH, and then imagines parent-child face-to-face and right-to-right communication. Drawing, erasing, and redrawing techniques are used to track this dialogue. Next, we simulate a parent-child dyad art therapy directive, which involves creating a Tree of Life alongside one another. Such co-creative dyadic occurrences have been associated with attachment experiences (Snir & Hazut, 2012). Playful and deliberate use of colors, forms, tactile media, and images, which are primarily processed by right-brain functions, are obvious RH-based microskills. As stated earlier, LH verbal processing of the artwork can further support regulated integration. Finally, a nonverbal Dual Drawing role-play supports adult in vivo co-creative interactions that contribute to co-consciousness and meaningful communication (Moon, 2008). Our ATR-N directives support the development of specific microskills as they attend to a continuous and dynamic process of mutual influences and affect regulation. Within a safe relationship, the interpersonal art therapy laboratory offers a co-regulatory environment. Co-creating alongside each other and together is an ATR-N skill. When the therapist and client work together, yet with separate purposes in mind, the therapist can maintain an attuned environment. Co-creating as well as engaging in response art within and outside of the session allows for the attachment relationship to develop and supports the capacity to process difficult experiences (Fish, 2012; Franklin, 2010). This kind of attuned co-creation offers the opportunity to experience, practice, and develop emotional regulation. Art therapists have developed similar directives that support parent-child attachment processes (Ball, 1998; Brown, 2008; Choi & Goo, 2012; Hosea, 2006; Isserow, 2008) as well as assess attachment styles (Kaiser, 1996; Kaiser & Deaver, 2009).

AFFECT REGULATION

It is through nonverbal interaction that infants and toddlers internalize regulation strategies, practicing expressing and understanding nonverbal interpersonal cues. The caregiver's gestures, tone of voice, eye contact, touch, and facial expressions indicate the intensity, timing, and physical proximity of his or her nonverbal affect. Attuned back-and-forth implicit communication is the carrier of interpersonal meaning, and the overall effect contributes to synchronized resonances (Chused, 2007; Schore, 2008). Neuroscience research suggests that humans need such exchanges to maintain their social resources (Hughes et al., 2012). The formation of early secure attachments fuels successful adult emotional regulation and teaches how to effectively reach out to others for social and regulatory support (Hughes et al., 2012). Attuned caregiving in the face of stress offers the growing child a supportive model of how to self-soothe and digest overwhelming experiences (Schore, 2003, 2008; Siegel, 2012; Cook, Blaustein, Spinazzola & van der Kolk, 2003).

Insufficient regulatory capacities of physical arousal and emotional states in adults are associated with early on poor caregiver attunement (Siegel & Hartzell, 2003). Children whose parents repeatedly dismiss or reject them may learn to disregard or distrust their emotions, relationships, and even their own bodies. They may dysregulate and disconnect from others if they sense important adults are getting too close or too distant emotionally (Ainsworth, Blehar, & Waters, 1978; Kravits, 2008a). As relationally insecure children grow into adults, an insecure avoidant or anxious IWM expresses as insecure anxious or avoidant attachment styles. When faced with a significant interpersonal stressor, the person may feel numbed or flooded by intense emotions. In order to self-regulate, the relational insecure adult may turn to isolating strategies and will likely avoid, dismiss, or feel deeply ambivalent about close relationships (Hesse, 1999). Cognitive problems with sustaining attention and concentration are also common (Gillath, Giesbrechtb, & Shaver, 2009), which may contribute to reduced rational compensatory coping skills. Overall, insecure, anxious, or avoidant IWM result in inadequate interpersonal strategies, leading to a consistent recycling of excessive dependency and/or disengagement, depression, and anxiety. While difficult, this is an organized pattern of interpersonal interaction. Therefore, it is usually predictable, which makes it easier for the therapist and client to recognize the pattern of insecure behaviors, attitudes, and feelings and work together toward change (Wallin, 2007).

In comparison, disorganized attachment responses can be experienced as chaotic and destabilizing (Cassidy & Shaver, 2010). The pace and intensity of emotions increase under stress, which contribute to feeling like one's emotions are out of control. As a result, the individual may experience a significantly diminished capacity for reasoning, and communication may become incoherent. In other words, a cycle ensues where emotions affect cognitions and vice versa. Repercussions of this course of events are that cognitive and emotional interpretation of verbal communication, facial expressions, gestures, and sensory stimuli becomes skewed. A person with a propensity for negativity, for example, will be even more prone to negative interpretations and to catastrophizing reactions (Lanius, Bluhm, & Frewen, 2011). Because cognitive function is constrained, recognizing and differentiating between one's own feelings and those of others becomes convoluted and confusing. Subsequently, current stressors may be experienced as if one is a helpless and hopeless child. It may also take the person longer than it would take someone with less negative cognitive patterns to return to a functional baseline (Wells et al., 2009).

Chronic or severe dysregulation of affect associated with disorganized attachment experiences have been hypothesized to interfere with the development of neural connections in critical brain areas and contribute to biological-based dysregulation (Schore, 2001b). Analytical, LH capacities may fail, and emotional RH schemas of the world take over, provoking uninhibited helplessness and fury (Kagan, 2007; Teicher, Andersen, Polcari, Anderson, & Navalta, 2002). This dysregulated state can become chronic, which has been associated with borderline personality disorder (BPD) behaviors (Linehan, 1993a). Among other BPD problems, affect dysregulation is the most damaging to interpersonal functioning. BPD is primarily a dysfunction of the emotion regulation system (Shearin & Linehan, 1994), characterized by a pattern of harmful impulsivity and unstable affects, interpersonal relationships, and identity (Wupperman, Neumann, Whitman, & Axelrod, 2009).

The facility for affect regulation requires the integration of sensory, emotional, and cognitive functions. As emotions transfer from the limbic system to the cortex, the right brain, which implicates the nonverbal, social-emotional self, integrates with the left brain, which dominates language, motor, and cognitive functions. The integration of nonverbal RH communication with LH cognitive processing is well served by art therapy practices (Chapman, 2014).

CO-REGULATION

Emotional expression, communication, and regulation are best contextualized as intrapersonal and interpersonal processes across the life span (Hughes et al., 2012). The function of co-regulation shifts from survival and affect regulation to co-conscious meaning making. Mother and infant attuned interactions, such as gazing, cooing, and smiling, present as a cycle of communication. Should the mother withdraw her participation, for example, by persistently freezing her expression, the infant will visibly react in a distressed manner, eventually turning his or her head away, appearing depressed (Tronick, 1989, 2007). These cycles of effective or ineffective connection, disconnection, and repair then generalize into the development of either trust or security or a distorted sense of the self and the other (Tronick & Beeghly, 2011). Patterns of verbal and nonverbal exchanges between infant and mother are also social, meaning-making moments. The moment-to-moment communication may be as follows: the infant pulls the mother's hair; her face expresses irritation; and the infant may defend against potential disconnection by raising both arms in front of his face (Tronick, 2007). The mother may repair by playfully blowing on the infant's face. As the baby lowers his hands, he smiles while eye contact and connection are successfully restored.

Co-regulation is hence understood as a continuous dynamic process, in which each person affects the other, rather than the exchange of discrete information (Fogel & Garvey, 2007). As children grow, parents function to help them manage their emotional arousal (van der Kolk, 2005). In early childhood and toddlerhood, the child is seen to become a more equal partner in parent-child exchanges, sharing in turn taking, initiating communication, and maintaining mutual interaction (Kim & Kochanska, 2012). Nonverbal communication through matching intensity of eye contact, tone of voice, and movement remain central to parent-child interactions. The young child's emotional response to an experience is co-regulated by the parent's affective response (Hughes, 2004). In essence, a child's attention is directed by the quality of the parent's attention. Furthermore, how the caregiver processes experience shapes the child's capacity for reflective thought (Fonagy, Gergely, Jurist, & Target, 2005). Parents who provide appropriate vocabulary for children to use allow for the gradual identification and expression of their inner life, supporting such mentalization (Siegel & Payne Bryson, 2012). Mutual influences emerge as the parent's affective communication is impacted by the moment-to-moment connections with the child (Fonagy et al., 2005; Hughes, 2004).

Parent-child dyadic emotional regulation prepares the child for peer interactions, supports practicing autonomy, and frees resources for cognitive growth (Harrist & Waugh, 2002). While preschool children are expected to manage emotions and impulses more effectively, they can still be quickly overwhelmed by the demands of their environment, thus at times needing extra external soothing and support in order to keep their frustrations well managed (Bath, 2008). Accordingly, an inverse correlation was reported between teacher ratings of preschoolers' behavior problems, such as non-compliance or aggression, and the level of attuned mother-child interactions (Deater-Deckard & Petrill, 2004; Lunkenheimer, 2007). In fact, preschool years are seen as critical to the development of adaptive or maladaptive regulatory abilities (Cole, Teti, & Zahn-Waxler, 2003). What were once evolving nonverbal interactions of parent-infant affect regulation crystallize into dyadic patterns of parent-child interaction (Cozolino, 2013). For example, anxious mothering can look like over controlling and critical parenting, which contributes to the child's internal avoidance and withdrawing behaviors. Distant, inconsistent, or hostile parenting can contribute to fear and unremitting aggressive, under controlled behaviors. In contrast, attuned and flexible parenting promotes security. Secure parenting teaches that the repair of relational dissonance and conflict is possible. This modeling and support helps the child experience quick recovery and develop regulated internal working models and behaviors (Granic, O' Hara, Pepler, & Lewis, 2007).

In middle childhood, parent-child mutuality is also negatively correlated with externalizing behavior problems (Lunkenheimer, 2007). Dyadic joint attention, co-occurring positive affect, responsiveness, and cooperation are pathways toward emotional resiliency. The growing child and the environment are mutually influencing systems that actively organize the self. Over time, back and forward transactions between the child and his or her context develop into regulatory traits. The products of past recurring dyadic interactions can support or constrain future dyadic behavioral patterns.

As the adolescent prefrontal brain regions reorganize, attuned dyadic relationships help the teenager manage overwhelming emotional arousal. This entails acknowledging the young person's distress, supportive silence, and an invitation to reflective problem solving (Bath, 2008). In contrast, transactional coercive parenting can turn into a cycle of mutually reinforcing negative affect and disrupted parent-adolescent relationships (Kim, Conger, Lorenz, & Elder, 2001).

The mutual regulation of early biobehavioral processes extends to an adult dyadic intersubjective state of consciousness (Tronick, 2007). Collaboration with another gives the opportunity to expand into more coherent complex states (Siegel & Payne Bryson, 2012). In fact, throughout the adult life span, the capacity for affect regulation is enhanced in the presence and support of trusted others (Siegel & Hartzell, 2003). Robust adult attachment continues to be co-regulatory. Healthy dyadic reparation, recovery from argument, and the return to previous or new ways of relating are secure attachment functions (Gottman & Driver, 2005). Patterns of adult co-regulation form a complex organizing system that includes dynamic connections, disconnections, and repairs (Tronick & Beeghly, 2011). Even the mere presence of support by a parent, spouse, or significant other decreases the amount of independent resources required for emotional and social self-control and contributes to cognitive and mental functioning (Beckes & Coan, 2011). Under affirming interpersonal conditions, the ability to express and regulate emotions motivates social engagement and increases the ability to tolerate negative social experiences. Furthermore, in the face of duress, learning to rely on others permits co-regulation of affect, reducing the likelihood that threat-based circuitry will be activated, thereby promoting resiliency (Beckes & Coan, 2011). It also contributes to improvements in mood, cognitive functioning, and learning capacity. For example, in groundbreaking interpersonal research, women who held their husband's hands during lab-induced stress showed less activation in fear- and threat-sensitive areas of their brains. In the presence of secure adult attachment figures, women were able to resource affect regulation by literally holding their spouse's hands (Coan et al., 2006). While loss of an attachment figure can trigger biobehavioral dysregulation (Sbarra & Hazan, 2008), regulatory benefit can still be achieved by calling on mental representations of an attachment figure.

Change in therapy has also been linked to the dyadically regulated relationship between client and therapist. In this type of relationship, co-regulation has been linked to co-consciousness and to shared meaning making. Additionally, implicit and explicit shared emotional dyadic states offer opportunities to practice and experience affect regulation. Thus, we hypothesize that art therapy activities offer an ongoing flow of co-interaction, co-creation, and co-consciousness. Affect regulation and change are supported by the nonverbal and verbal communication, collaborative art making, and mutual witnessing of this therapeutic process.

EXPERIENTIAL PRACTICES AND DIRECTIVES

Experience I: My Right Hemisphere

For the first experiential, we invite the participants to embody their RH, the interpersonal brain. Each group member creates a representation of his or her RH function, particularly as it relates to interpersonal communication and affect regulation. In support of the directive, we showcase the artwork of Alex Grey, who vividly illuminates the experience of human relating (http://www.alexgrey.com). His X-ray vision art *Contemplation* depicts vibrant human biological systems, anatomy, and brain.

> *Alex Grey's painting brought the academic images, drawings, and scans of the brain and body that we had studied to life. It made me think about what goes on inside my skin and brain. I wanted to explore my own brain and what it is like to know the origins of my emotions and behavior as located in my different minds or so-called hemispheres.* Louise Smith

We start by asking participants to: "Make a detailed pencil drawing of a right hemisphere." We then ask them, using color, to "transform the image into My Right Hemisphere." Inspiration for this imagery can be found in Carter (2010). In each chapter, she provides an illustration of the brain that

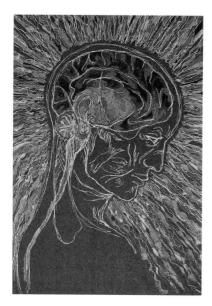

Figure 5.1 *My RH: Mind, Body and Soul.* A dark pink central brain is enveloped by green folds of the neocortex. The entire brain-mind pulses with multicolored energy. Lisa Cerrina

symbolizes its functions. Nonvocal background music or the use of music-therapy instruments can also assist in this shift from a cognitive perspective to an integrated RH focus (Scheiby, 2005; Thaut, 2008). The titles that participants give their own art, such as *What My Right Brain Does for Me and What My Left Brain Does*, will usually spontaneously reflect this idea (Figure 5.1).

As we gather to discuss the group's experience of the activity, there is often a lively debate. Some express a preference for left-brain-related tasks, such as the copying of brain images, which involve high levels of cognition, attention, and control. Further, they may comment on the sense of focus and calm brought upon the creation of the controlled pencil drawing. Others are more oriented toward right-brain-related tasks, such as creating a symbolic representation of the brain, which involves emotion. They may report feeling energized by color, process art, painting, and the rhythms of the music.

The experiential leads to a talk about the expression of RH and LH lateralized functions. The RH function is key to understanding the gestalt of the creative experience. It has a role in the processing of visual, prosodic auditory, and gestural signals as well as the holistic reasoning aspects of language, such as intonation and emotional emphasis. In contrast, left-brain functions support the verbal processing of the art. Calling upon both the RH and the LH allows for functional integration and supports affect regulation. Either the pencil drawings or the adding of color or paint may bring on insecurity and emotional dysregulation. These responses may be related to a fear of artistic failure, fear of judgment, or other personal reasons such as negative memory, requiring affect modulation.

Experience II: Right-to-Right Hemisphere Communication and Co-Creating

In the studio sketching has therapeutic value as it tracks implicit dynamics. So next we ask each group member to sketch the flow of nonverbal exchanges. First is that between a parent and an infant, and then between a parent and a young child. We prompt each person to imagine feeling the physical contact of holding an infant in their arms, the weight and warmth of the baby, gazing face to face, and then say, "Draw the right-to-right interaction of a mother and infant." They may want to explore their own memories of holding or being held. They are invited to conjure up the gentle sense of movement and shifts in posture of mother and child. Some participants feel pressured to literally draw a mother and baby and are reassured that they can simply set an empathic intention to mentalize and explore the experience of the caregiver-infant interaction. As they draw, they search out forms that represent the reciprocal act of communication, including the gestures and facial expressions of parent and infant. In pursuit of attuned representation and mutual regulation, they are encouraged to erase, smudge, draw, and redraw the relationship. Thus mental co-creating occurs. Heavyweight drawing paper is provided with the idea that it can bear the wear and tear of the activity and symbolically support attuned holding. As the images emerge, the pencil or charcoal marks approximate, track, and mirror the represented interactions. While best achieved with wood-based charcoal, using a soft lead-based pencil works as well. Henri Matisse was a master of such techniques, which he used for drawing faces of the women he loved.

Using the left hand to smudge the pencil marks may bring forward unexpected imagery and deliberately engage the RH, which controls the left side of the body. In general, the right cerebral hemisphere controls the left side of the body, and the left cerebral hemisphere controls the right side. However, a person's hand dominance may not be an indication of cognitive function location. In 95% of right-handed individuals, the left side of the brain is dominant for language. Even in 60–70% of left-handed individuals, the left side of the brain is used for language (Knecht et al., 2000). Participants experiment with what feels right, familiar, or different for them. Sometimes both hands are used. Giving right-to-right hemisphere communication art a title activates the LH, bringing it cognitively online and allowing for integration of the nonverbal and verbal aspects of the work (McNamee, 2003; Figure 5.2).

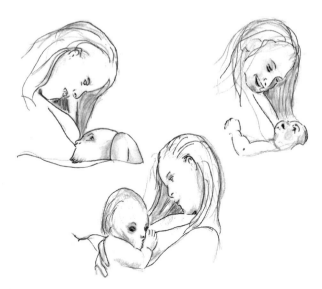

Figure 5.2 *RH-to-RH Mother-Infant Gazing.* Gazing supports the development of affect regulation and growth in infants. In this drawing, the mother intuits the regulatory need of the suckling infant, which is to move toward and away from her. Joanna Clyde Findlay

Sketching, erasing, and rubbing out the drawing, followed by a resketch of the mentalized image, leaves energetic tracks that can remind us of gazing, touching, holding, and the good feelings that can be associated with such co-created embracing. These positive feeling states are thought to be mediated by oxytocin (OXY). OXY is a hormone that is thought to be released during breast-feeding, hugging, touching, and orgasm. In the brain, OXY is a neurotransmitter that is involved in social bonding and in the formation of attuned trust between people (Kosfeld, Heinrichs, Zak, Fischbacher, & Fehr, 2005).

> *The smudging and erasing brought forward images of what an attuned relationship might be. I found the request to sketch the communication between a parent and small child really difficult. It reminded me of my relationship with my mother. I am not sure that she felt comfortable holding me for too long. As we erased, smudged, and redrew more of what we thought, the exchanges made me feel more attuned to the activity and perhaps to myself. It opened possibilities to understand mothering. I started to think about communication more like a loop or a swirl of lines. I guess it helped me understand that the connections between parents and children are always altering.* Lisa Kandros

RH-to-RH communication is involved in mother-infant gazing; it supports the development of affect regulation and growth in infants (Schore, 2008). The RH has, so to speak, an emotional lens, and it is the holder of autobiographical memory. The inclusion of faces and facial expression in the images as well as the use of the left hand intentionally calls on RH functions. The RH stores the mental working models of attachment and is informed by visceral bodily states. It is functionally dominant during the late prenatal stages and the first two years of life. In infancy, RH-to-RH, face-to-face communication is engaged by what has been named proto-conversations (Trevarthen, 2006). Proto-conversations involve attuned vocalizations such as cooing and "umm," hand gestures, strokes, and movements of the arms and head. Proto-conversations and facial expression act conjunctly and support the development of secure attachment and effective affect regulation (Hughes et al., 2012; Schore, 2001a; Tronick & Beeghly, 2011).

Between mother and infant, there is a dyadic verbal and nonverbal interworking of contingent communication where their psychobiological systems are co-regulating (Kravits, 2008a; Tronick, 2001; Tronick & Beeghly, 2011; Tronick et al., 1998). The infant can be observed maintaining the mother's gaze during nursing, then breaking the eye contact, turning away in order to self-regulate. As discussed earlier, should the mother turn away or develop a still face, difficulties with emotional regulation may result in depression. The mother may talk to the infant and the infant will reengage. The marking traces left during sketching can be seen as mental and executed correspondences of proto-conversational gestures. These are symbolic of self-regulation cycles.

Similarly, we ask for a drawing of a parent–young child interaction: "Draw yourself together with your very young child, or draw a parent, or art therapist and young child interaction." This is an ATR-N adaptation of the kinetic family drawing: "Draw your family doing something together" (Burns & Kaufman, 1970). Instead of action, the focus is on intimacy and coregulation. Unlike the kinetic family drawing, which is a projective assessment measure aiming to elicit a family's dynamics, this request seeks to promote the client's insight into, and empathic understanding of, the experience of attuned nonverbal communication.

In order to get a felt experience of what such communication entails, and to support the clinical skill development of those who might be working at early childhood centers, we may ask our group members to manifest such proto-conversation experiences. Using the art to mirror actions or games, such as peekaboo and the hand pile game, the focus is on being mindfully present, in the moment, and responsive to the other. To the older child, turn-

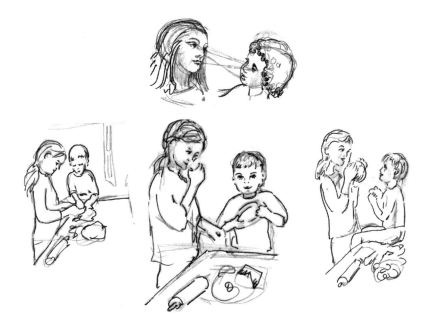

Figure 5.3 *Caregiver-Child Gaze.* Gestures used in the art-making reflect therapist-child co-regulation. Joanna Clyde Findlay

ing to the art material or art object offers a means to take a break and regulate his or her feelings. The child client approaches the art therapist and the art making, withdraws to recompose, and then approaches the therapy process again (Figure 5.3).

In the drawings, the markings may include clues to the parent's or therapist's perceived relationship with the child. This visual trace representation of the therapeutic experience is a metacommunication. It is symbolic of the kind of expression, communication, and reappraisal of emotions that affect regulation entails. The metacommunication assists the therapist in sensing the nonverbal message sent by the client's RH. Such communication has been named a "special realm" (Schore, 2009, p. 178). It occurs via nonverbal micro communication, such as bodily movements, postures, gestures, facial expressions, and intonations. It is likely that this kind of communication is also infused with OXY release (Diamond, 2001). Nonverbal communication and its accompanying biophysical effects vitally inform the interchange between therapist, client, and artwork. This micro communication informs the syntax, semantics, and grammar of the therapist-to-client-to-artwork communication. Furthermore, it has been suggested that adults who maintain long-term secure attachments gain from repeated exposure to OXY, facilitating more rapid stress regulation (Diamond, 2001).

We suggest that art therapists look with their right brains at the art for positive therapeutic gains, as well as for signs of disrupted therapeutic alliances, relational security, and attachment (Chapman, 2014). These may take the form of refusal to make any art, or disconnectedness from the therapist. In these ways, the client's approach to the art, as well as the art itself, can provide insights into the dynamics of attachment and affect regulation. The art making processes provide unique opportunities for developing or sustaining affect regulation.

Experience III: Tree of Life

Drawing on our own experience, we ask each group participant to: "Create a tree of your development." Working side by side on a shared table, each pair of participants creates in a shared space. The co-creation between two close group members will hopefully lead to an experience of co-regulation. Each individual has his or her own paper and collage materials. Our ATR-N collage materials typically include brain-based images, such as neurons, the nervous system and bodily organs. Images of neuronal interlocking dendrites may help participants recall that optimal interpersonal exchanges can shape the social brain throughout the life span. Often, the artists will begin at the base of their Tree of Life and work upward through cutting, pasting, gluing, and drawing. The image of a tree lends structure to the directive, positively suggesting growth and mirroring the individual structure of a neuron branching out. As the participants work next to a trusted other, without talking, they often let the other use a glue stick, pause and look at their neighbor's work, and accommodate each other's movements. This response-based physical isomorphism mimics response art making. Response art making is a general term for using the art to respond to each other in dyadic interaction (Fish, 2012).

> *I figured out that the base of the tree referred to my childhood, and that each branch was expressing a part of my development. It became clear that relationships are the core parts that organize my life. This realization was echoed by my current relationship with Lisa, who was working right alongside me. I liked working next to Lisa as she seemed so focused and calm, and although I often looked at what she made and thought it was better than my work, her calm soothed me. I could then see that my work was progressing also. When we discussed our collages at the end, I really liked that she saw my tree as a strong tree, and I decided to call my collage,* I Can Bend but Not Break. *Jona-than Chris*

The Tree of Life directive is also applicable to older children and parent-child dyads co-creations. For example, therapeutically encouraging a parent and child to create side by side can offer a supportive environment for processing stressful memories, increasing empathic interactions, and shared meaning making. This directive brings forward reflections on personal memories within a relational context. It may evoke positive or negative childhood experiences and provide reparation. In childhood, a secure state of mind is experienced when children receive consistent attuned comfort and encouragement from a caregiver, especially when confronted with a stressor (Siegel & Hartzell, 2003). They experience pleasure and excitation in relationships and learn to find comfort in being with others and relating as they are in the process of learning novel information (Kravits, 2008a). When a child or adult creates an art directive, such as the Tree of Life, in the presence of a significant attachment relationship, they are better able to mobilize strengths (Proulx, 2002a). An emergent property of an attachment relationship, co-regulation can take on diverse forms such as eye contact, touch, smell, or cognition (Hughes et al., 2012). In the ATR-N context, the parent lends actual support in the form of helping with the media and emotional encouragement as the child builds representations of his or her world. Thus, current attachment intimacies and security are reinforced through an attuned connection (Siegel & Hartzell, 2003). Talking about the image further assists in the processing of memories, attitudes, and beliefs. In fact, telling the stories of our experiences is a lifelong process that supports integration of affect and cognitions (Siegel & Payne Bryson, 2012). Not only the child but also the parent can experience side-by-side support (Figure 5.4).

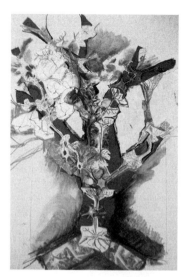

Figure 5.4 *The Tree of My Development.* Brown paper strips form the background for a collage of cutout photocopies of neurons with added accents in red and orange. Shading in blues and greens surrounds the trunk and highlights the spreading network of connecting neurons. Joanna Clyde Findlay

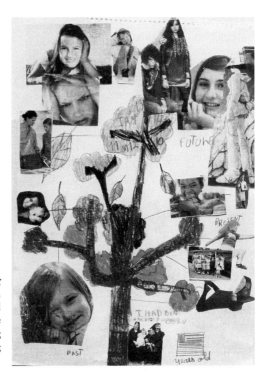

Figure 5.5 *The Tree of My Growing Up.* A green tree trunk extends upwards, becoming brown and gray. Autumnal colored leaves are clustered around the branches. At the branch ends the young artist also glued collage images of young girls at varying ages. Jean Clyde

As Joanna's nine-year-old daughter collaged, she seemed to be attracted to images of people from the collage box. She confidently drew her outlined tree and then decided to have the different branches refer to her significant memories. She placed her birth, and where she was born, at the base, and then identified starting school, getting a dog, and relocating at different ages. At each place, she selected, cut, and glued an image of an appropriately aged child. When she reached the upper parts, she grouped together ages 10 through 14 to express her concerns with the upcoming changes she foresaw. After completing the coloring of the tree with the autumnal colors of the day outside, she added the words past, present, and future, moving from the base to the treetop. The process of talking through her important memories and future concerns in the secure presence of her mother helped Joanna's daughter to manage her mixed feelings about moving to a new city and changing schools (Figure 5.5).

> *My brain felt fizzy going back in time. It felt unusual to do this. It came back to me. I am glad I went back and can remember sad and happy memories. I can see that my memories and feelings can be mixed.* Jean Clyde

The titling of the collage and the verbal processing are co-regulatory processes that can hold and integrate memories and emotions. A gentle discussion of the side-by-side experience and sharing of the work's title or story evokes co-consciousness and promotes shared meaning making. Co-creation within an affirming relationship can support co-regulation. In adults, this takes the form of shared consciousness. We suggest that intentional and attuned, side-by-side creation offers opportunities to practice the kind of micro regulatory social-emotional processes described in the literature (Gavron, 2013; Gillespie, 1994; Proulx, 2002b; Regev, 2014; Snir & Hazut, 2012; Tronik et al, 1998; Tronik, 2001; Tronik & Beeghly, 2011). Although this literature is for the most part focused on children, it applies to adults as well as it is likely that internal working models of attachment are involved. The sharing of the pairs' mutual experience and response art making contributes to increased feelings of social ease within the larger group.

Experience IV: Dual Drawing, a Response Art Regulatory Opportunity

Dual drawings provide an interpersonal opportunity to focus on the delicate interplay of nonverbal discourse; the space of the page becomes a shared and explored territory that can be redivided and redrawn. The marks and lines move toward and away from each other, as they may link, search, withdraw, conflict, or combine. The co-creators may seek or avoid eye contact; one person may lead, the other follow; the tempo may charge or wane; the gestures and movement over the page may bristle with emotion or flow in attunement. When the therapist and client make art together, they embody attuned ATR-N microskills. The therapist ensures that there is sufficient space for the client to create art without overusing the space, and symbolically lends emotional resources.

In pairs, seated across from each other with a large sheet of paper between them, we prepare for a role-play of a client-therapist dual drawing (Gillespie, 1994; Oster & Crone, 2004; Regev, 2014). Each pair receives a child age group and situation to role-play where they choose to use either oil pastels or markers. The pre-established situation is written up and provided to the pair without discussion, allowing all the group members to focus on their partnership. Each therapist and client pair agrees to choose one color and, either with or without a pre-established theme, draw together (Riley, 2001). Following the therapist's guidelines to: "Use marks in order to talk together or to imagine an ideal world together," they first draw without speaking or writing words (Figure 5.6).

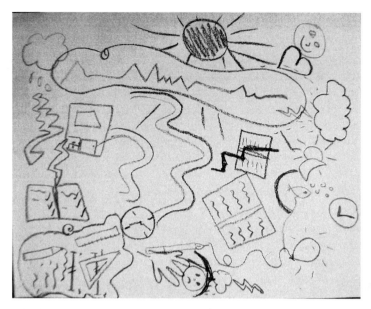

Figure 5.6 *There is Always Someone who Loves You.* Jean's worries about schoolwork are in blue lines while Joanna's comforting lines are in red. Joanna Clyde Findlay and Jean Clyde

I found this relaxing to do. I find that with homework, I have some good times and some bad times, but I know someone is there for me. Whenever I drew sad things, my Mum would draw happy things, which would comfort me. We understood each other without talking. Jean Clyde

At first I struggled with how to let my daughter know that the way I put my lines next to hers was to show that I was there for her. As she drew images of things associated with homework, I realized all I could do was show I had noticed, that I was there. I made an umbrella to shelter her from the storm, but she still drew clouds. It was a visual reminder that I cannot remove her experience of her problems, but I can be available to her. When we came up with our individual titles, she at first called the drawing The Good and Bad Bits of Homework, *and I named it* Being There for You, *but then I asked what we could call it together and I found her title a beautiful summary of our process:* There is Always Someone who Loves You. Joanna Clyde Findlay

Once the drawing is completed, the therapist and the child-client title the drawing separately, and then together, discuss and agree on a shared name and narrative. This titling represents a shift in acknowledging the shared process; it builds in reflective mentalizing and develops a co-created nonverbal experience. Titling is one way in which the therapist seeks to support the client. The role-play partners then discuss their specific exchanges.

The larger group then gathers in a semicircle to look at the images, which are laid out on the floor. The pair shares the dyadic nonverbal exchanges expressed in the visual traces on the sheets of paper with the group, making it a social experience. The lines and marks represent the pair's interactions, moving backward, forward, and across. While the experience may be felt with varying degrees of satisfaction, the pair is provided with the opportunity to describe their process and feelings as well as gain compassionate insight into each other's view. The felt experience is an interpersonal gestalt of regulatory relationships, and the image provides a safe depository for the process. This mutual experience models how the therapist and client use himself or herself, and the art making, to co-create attuned emotional states for the benefit of the therapy. Discussion of the shared creation of the art provides valuable feedback to each dyad and to the group (Figure 5.7).

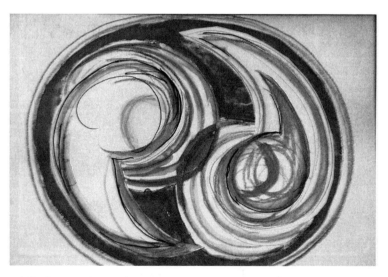

Figure 5.7 *Therapist-Client, and Partner-to-Partner Dance.* In my mind, this image is symbolic of how each person's capacity for co-regulation informs the whole. Embedded on a red background, a dark blue-yellow and a light red-turquoise teardrop balance each other. Joanna Clyde Findlay

My partner was role-playing her feelings for me. I found paying attention to her, being there for her, and listening, just with my blue marker, very powerful. Sometimes she moved her red lines away when I tried to come near. If I made a squiggle echoing hers, sometimes she seemed to like it; sometimes I sensed I was too close. I really felt we were "talking." It was amazing how accurately we both experienced these lines and marks when we talked about it after. Louise Smith

Within the therapeutic setting, mutual regulation of affect needs to be established. A complex, co-constructed procedure evolves between client and therapist (Tronick, 1998). This implicit process of matching, mismatching, reparation of communication, and regulation of physiological homeostatic states is co-created. Within the group, members are asked to take their dyadic drawings and respond with art making to the dyadic shared imagery and symbolism. Response art sharing within a group can be modified for individual work (Chilton, 2014; Franklin, 2010) and for mother child therapy (Gavron, 2014). Gavron's work is interesting as she has developed a variety of art directives to assess dyadic interactions and work with parent-child dyads.

Similar to verbal microskills, the skillful art therapist uses response art in order to query, clarify, interpret, solidify, consolidate, and express connectivity. This is a visual paraphrase and dialogue that embodies attunement. Response art done after session can also be brought to supervision (Fish, 2012) and back to session (Chilton, 2014).

As implicit dyadic states become explicit and co-conscious, shared meaning emerges. This embedded experience of coherent relating is then mentalized and generalized (Tronick, 1998). Thus what began as RH-to-RH intersubjective infant-mother communication evolves into adult-to-adult co-regulation. This co-regulation is both a concrete and mental property of the relationship itself and co-creates itself throughout the life span.

RELATIONAL NEUROSCIENCE: REGULATION

Co-regulation is associated with three interpersonal neurobiology topics and domains. The first is cortical specialization and hemispheric lateralization, specifically, connectivity between the RH and the LH. The second topic relates to how cognitive emotional interactions are expressed via bidirectional, cortical-to-subcortical connections. This frontolimbic connectivity involves the AMY, PFC, and orbitofrontal cortex (OFC). Last, the neurochemistry of good-feeling neurohoromones, namely OXY, DA, and 5-HT, are involved in affect regulation.

Hemispheric Lateralization

Integrated functioning requires coordination of the RH and LH. While the RH and LH share more functions than is commonly believed, dominant lateralized trends are associated with each hemisphere (Carter, 2010). Each hemisphere processes inputs differently, provides specialized outputs, and sometimes competes with the other, and depending on the circumstance, we may call upon one hemisphere more than the other.

Developmentally, the RH dominates in infancy (Siegel & Payne Bryson, 2012). Visual-spatial RH skills are heavily involved in learning how to reach, crawl, or toddle. During middle childhood, the corpus callosum (CC), the wide band of nerves that connects the two hemispheres, enhances change and learning as it thickens, acting as an important neuropathway. The impact of such learning alters and changes neuronal growth and even survival. The LH progresses further during the second year of life, explaining the burst in language skills. By 18 months, the RH has enough sensory and motor maturation that children can focus their energies on the LH and hone their mental capacities. As the LH matures, first in the parietal and then in the frontal lobe, the language centers in the toddler's brain are connected, enabling them to engage in symbolic thought. Until children can use language for self-expression, they borrow the cognitive capacities of an adult to regulate affect and label their experience. Memories and thoughts that are separate from immediate sensory input are generated as the LH matures, allowing children to reflect, intuit, and connect ideas.

Lateralized Brain Functions

RH and LH functions may vary in different individuals, especially in those with histories of neurodevelopmental challenges or in those who have sustained an injury to one side of the brain, in which case the other side may compensate (Stiles, Reilly, Paul, & Moses, 2005). Yet, as a whole, each side of the brain is predisposed to handling certain types of task.

The four principal lobes, the frontal, temporal, parietal, and occipital lobes, are mirrored in each hemisphere. The lobes have shared functions and specialized-lateralized functions listed in the diagram. For example, both the frontal lobes control planning, sequencing, and abstract thought. The left is specialized for the production of speech and the right for the interpretation of facial expressions. In general, the RH favors visual and nonverbal perception and processing. The LH favors verbal analytical processes (Table 5.1).

The linear reasoning functions of language, such as grammar and word production, are often lateralized to the LH of the brain. The LH processes

Table 5.1 Left and Right Hemisphere Functions

LEFT Hemisphere	RIGHT Hemisphere
• organized, objective, cognitive	• implicit, felt social/interpersonal self
• explicit, linguistic self	• holistic, intuitive, synthesizing
• verbalizing, naming, and labeling	• divergent, random thinking
• verbal analytical	• language intonation and emotional emphasis
• logical reasoning	• gestalt processing
• detailed, linear, sequential processing	• kinesthetic
• abstract	• art and music processing in non-artists
• language	• nonverbal perception and processing
• speech/grammar production / syntax	• prosodic auditory and gestural signals
• language comprehension	• visual-spatial processing
• fact retrieval–computation, calculation	• hand-eye coordination
• decision-making processes	• mental rotation of physical shapes
• positive pleasurable experiences biased	• self-regulate social circuitry
• cause and effect	• recognition of facial expression
• avoidance	• negative experiences biased
• mid-range affect	• withdrawal
• neutral of affect	• high affect

verbal memory, language comprehension, and speech output. Fact retrieval and exact arithmetic calculation are left parietal region specializations. Art therapy directives calling for verbal processing of art activities call upon the LH's analytic verbal processing functions. Within the therapeutic relationship, talking about the art product and process may contribute to bilateral integration (Chapman, 2014).

The LH role in affect regulation involves labeling and verbalizing what has been experienced (Lieberman, 2007). Verbal processing seems to engage in a cortical shift from RH to LH, further modulating affect. The LH houses the individual's conscious, linguistic self, and processes information in a detailed, linear, sequential, language-based manner. The LH is implicated in decision-making processes and is more commonly responsible for processing pleasurable experiences (MacNeilage et al., 2009).

Holistic reasoning functions of language, such as intonation and emotional emphasis, are often lateralized to the RH (MacNeilage et al., 2009). The RH, which specializes in understanding the gestalt of things, processes visual, prosodic auditory, and gestural signals that can induce instant emotional effects. Sound and music as well as nonverbal color and sensory stimuli, such as paint, can provide a gateway to RH function as they stir up nonverbal feelings and memories. Through the right parietal lobe, the RH processes visual-spatial perception, involving hand-eye coordination and the mental rotation of physical shapes in the environment. Thus the RH comprises the physical-emotional self of how we relate to and interact with our surroundings. The RH also coordinates an organized sense of the body in space, a function needed to effectively engage in art making.

The RH houses the social-emotional self and holds the frontal structures integral to the interpersonal sense of self, particularly in the right OFC (Schore, 2008). It is biased toward emotional stimuli and communication in a relational context. The OFC is essential in our capacity to self-regulate. This structure is imprinted by stressful misattunement in addition to stress-regulating repair and reattunement in the early developing RH. The right OFC fronto-limbic circuitry is structured by one's emotional and social history. It is central to the ability to empathically understand the states of others and to be able to interpret their intentions. This is the social circuitry that contributes to co-regulation and which is activated by left-to-left eye gaze. In adults, the RH ultimately becomes dominant for the processing of social information.

The RH allows us to recognize facial expressions and changes of voice intonation in the context of emotions (Brück, Kreifelts, & Wildgruber, 2011; Schore, 2008). Attuned RH-to-RH communication allows access to unspoken emotions and supports the active development of affect regulation (Schore, 2003). Dominant in intuition, fantasy, and associational and holistic processing, the RH responds to cues from both internal and external stimuli immediately translated via limbic subcortical structures into emotions. In times of distress, strong affect is processed and communicated via the RH, which dampens LH language functions and logic. For example, speechless states and automatic reactions are characteristic of strong emotional responses. Depression has also been linked to a hyperactive RH. Research suggests that the RH is likely involved in withdrawing from life experience, whereas the LH is more involved in approaching the world (Wager, Phan, Liberzon, & Taylor, 2003). It is important that the therapist be able to communicate in RH language, especially because the RH dominates in avoidant fear-based reactions (Hass-Cohen, 2008a). The RH's extensive connections to midbrain circuitry, is associated with fear and joy. Therefore the RH is more immediately responsive to survival-based danger cues than the LH. RH-based interpretation of the world also forms the basis of our social experience throughout the life span (Schore, 2001b).

The LH functions in the middle range of affect and is biased toward prosocial emotions (Schore, 2001a). In order to achieve cognitive and emotional flexibility, the therapist may therefore encourage the fearful, RH-activated client to engage with art making. At the same time, the therapist may work with the LH-activated client to modulate his or her emotional avoidance

(Hass-Cohen, 2008a,). Image making may directly access the social-emotional self, providing the opportunity to process, self-regulate, and connect.

The art therapist can benefit from knowledge of the role of these brain regions and structures as they contribute to Relational Resonating and co-regulation. RH processes can be intentionally accessed via use of sensory-stimulating media, such as paint, using the left hand (for right handers, for smudging and erasing) and playing music. Sharing the art making space, creating alongside clients, and paying attention to nonverbal exchanges with clients can permit RH-to-RH attunement and reparative experiences of co-regulation. Calling on both RH and LH functions in the making and then the verbal processing of art making supports the development and stabilization of integrated responses.

Bidirectional Cortical Limbic Connections

Early life co-regulatory, face-to-face experiences develop the capacity for trust and self-soothing (Tronick, 2007). Multilateral brain processing supports the interactional co-regulatory experience associated with dyadic and individual meaning making. This integrated emotional and cognitive mentalization capacity uses mental representations for understanding and responding emotionally to others (Vrticka & Vuilleumer, 2012). Central to affect regulation capacities are the connections between the PFC regions and the AMY. Top-down, cortical regulation of limbic emotions contributes to affect regulation, and limbic emotions influence cognitions. The fundamental fronto-limbic brain regions include the OFC, dorsal regions of the PFC, the nucleus accumbens, the AMY, the hippocampus, and the insula (Hughes et al., 2012). The OFC is also implicated in fronto-temporal areas associated with cognitive mentalization, specifically the medial prefrontal cortex, the superior temporal sulcus (STS), and the temporoparietal junction (TPJ). Thus an understanding of a complex feedback loop of fronto-limbic and temporal regions has emerged as a cognitive-emotional amalgam (Vrticka & Vuilleumer, 2012).

Prefrontal Cortex and Amygdala Connections

Connections between the PFC and the AMY serve to modulate response to such fear-based emotions (LeDoux, 2003). Located in the limbic system, the AMY is implicated in affect regulation, as it is responsible for the rapid nervous system fear response. There are direct neural connections between the AMY and the visual cortex, where the AMY prioritizes social-emotional cues received from the visual cortex. The AMY then automatically coordinates affective interpersonal learning experiences, processing facial expressions, and gazing (Schupp et al., 2007). Connected to the hippocampus, the AMY alerts hippocampal-based memories of fear. In general, the PFC acts to evaluate potential threats that may be aroused by emotional triggers such as color, texture, and shape (Hass-Cohen & Loya, 2008, pp. 99–101). The PFC shapes the AMY's stress responses. Infants and young children with limited PFC capacity rely on their parents to evaluate threat. They therefore must use more PFC resources when they have to regulate on their own than they do with parental support. Thus, co-regulation conserves cortical resources. Across the life span, adults and children with low expectations of co-regulation within a secure relationship need to rely on independent self-regulation, which contributes to a depletion of PFC resources (Hughes et al., 2012). This depletion may constrain development as resources and decision making are geared toward survival.

Orbitofrontal Cortex Neural Connections

Specific regions of the PFC have consistently been implicated in emotion regulation and decision-making (Phillips, Ladouceur, & Drevets, 2008). The implicated regions include the OFC and the dorsolateral prefrontal cortex (dlPFC), specifically the dorsomedial prefrontal cortex (dmPFC), the ventrolateral prefrontal cortex (vlPFC), and the anterior cingulate cortex (ACC, Figure 5.8).

Anatomical data support the hypothesis that the OFC may mediate the regulation of important emotional information (Kringelbach & Rolls, 2004). It connects higher-order dlPFC regions, dmPFC, and subcortical limbic

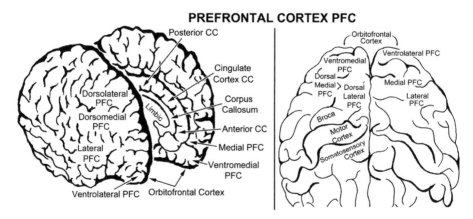

Figure 5.8 *The Prefrontal Cortex.* The dlPFC, the dmPFC, the vlPFC, the OFC, the ventromedial prefrontal cortex (vmPFC), the ACC, and the mPFC.

regions. The OFC is situated where the cortex and subcortex meet. Sitting at the top of the limbic system, just behind the eyes, it is part of a layered network of interconnected limbic regions, which include the AMY and the insula. The insula is considered the fifth lobe. Tucked behind the intersection of the frontal, parietal, and temporal lobes, it connects to physical bodily functions.

Research suggests that attachment experiences, including the nonverbal face-to-face transactions of affect co-regulation between caregiver and infant, directly impact the imprinting of the OFC (Schore, 2000). This fronto-limbic region, which is especially expanded in the RH, has a critical period of growth from around 10 months until the middle to the end of the second year of life. The OFC has a role as a mediator in the control of behavior. It is the bottom-down action of the circuitry in the right OFC that helps to dampen the AMY's reactivity (Phelps, Delgado, Nearing, & LeDoux, 2004).

A complex interplay between genetic, environmental, and epigenetic factors can form neural pathways that can result in dysfunctional stress regulation and fear appraisal strategies. The OFC systems in the RH can be structurally impacted by chaotic experiences of co-regulation in infancy (Schore, 2009). Such psychobiological changes alter the cortical top-down functions of affect regulation. Under stress, the altered OFC inefficiently regulates the limbic physiological processes that underlie emotion. Vulnerability to later psychiatric disorders can be based in impairments to the cortical-subcortical circuitries of this prefrontal system.

Similar to the fronto-limbic circuitry, fronto-temporal circuitry also involves the AMY, striatum, insula, the cingulate cortex, and the hippocampus, which have been identified as active in emotional evaluation and regulation. In addition, within the fronto-temporal areas, the mPFC, STS, the TPJ, and the OFC are dynamically involved in cognitive mentalization (Vrticka & Vuilleumier, 2012). The TPJ is at the juncture of the temporal and parietal lobes. Located within the temporal lobe, the STS activates in response to the human voice and is involved in the perception of gaze, emotion, and motion (Kalat, 2012). Frontotemporal processes regulate and bias emotion-cognition interactions (Ray & Zald, 2012). Neural projections to and from the OFC, the dmPFC, and limbic regions contribute to the regulation of fear-based responses (Phillips et al., 2008). Thus, the OFC system monitors feedback about the current internal state and external changes in order to make assessments of coping capacity. In other words, the OFC has direct links to the autonomic nervous system, where it is central to the homeostatic regulation of bodily and motivational states, as well as to attachment-based affect regulation (Schore, 2009). Based on this review, the interconnection of cortical and limbic brain regions does not support the idea that cognition and emotion form separate processes in different regions of the brain. Shifting cognitions and emotions combine, contributing to novel mental states (Salzman & Fusi, 2010). Moreover, emotional and cognitive linkages support adaptive social behavior.

Neurochemistry

Neurotransmitters, neuropeptides, and hormones (particularly OXY; dopamine, DA; and serotonin, 5-HT) are involved in attachment formation, mood regulation, and behavioral control (Stanley & Siever, 2010). Biologically, the fronto-limbic affect regulation system interfaces with reward-based neurochemistry. Part of the limbic-basal ganglia, the nucleus accumbens, receives major inputs from dopaminergic neurons, connecting experiences of affect regulation, pleasure, addiction, fear, and aggression (Carlson, 2013).

Oxytocin

Produced in the hypothalamus and stored in the pituitary gland, OXY is a neuropeptide found exclusively in mammals (Kalat, 2012). OXY has been implicated in a wide range of mammalian behaviors, including birth, breastfeeding, sexual behavior, maternal behavior, social bonding, and pair bonding (Sbarra & Hazan, 2008). In infants and adults, OXY and the endogenous opioids are implicated in the brain reward systems. Oxytocinergic activity in the hypothalamus, nucleus accumbens, ventral tegmentum, and AMY appear to influence attachment security (Hughes et al., 2012). The physiological reward systems link the neuropeptide OXY and the endogenous opioids in caregiving and pair bond behaviors, which help to regulate the autonomic nervous system and alleviate stress (Diamond, 2001; Machin & Dunbar, 2011). The influence of OXY in adult attachment has been conceptualized in several ways. It increases bonding of sexual partners, reinforces social behavior, acts as a conditioned stimulus in attachment, and attenuates separation distress. In adults, sexual and other intimate behaviors such as cuddling activate OXY and increase mesolimbic and prefrontal DA activity. These systems facilitate pair bond formation. The pleasurable aspects of the release of OXY and opioid system activity via social and sexual contact act as conditioned stimuli when paired with an attachment figure (Sbarra & Hazan, 2008). These associations strengthen and become internal working models through dopaminergically mediated experiences of security (Coan, 2010).

The epigenetic mechanisms, or gene-environment interactions, which can be induced by early life experiences, continue across the life span. In adults, the conditioned association between the rewards of OXY release and the presence of a specific person bears a strong resemblance to the opioid theory of social attachment (Machin & Dunbar, 2011; Sbarra & Hazan, 2008). This model suggests that the rewarding effects of social contact facilitate learning and guide in attachment, making attachment bonds inherently pleasurable, reducing distress, and attenuating responses to social separation. In this way, the neurochemistry reinforces attachment behaviors and promotes resilience to the impact of stress. Impairments in the quality of early experiences seem to have different effects on the oxytocinergic system (Nolte, Guiney, Fonagy, Mayes, & Luyten, 2011). There appear to be gender differences in the effects of OXY; OXY output in the face of stress may be greater in females than in males (Taylor et al., 2000). The estrogen-enhanced antianxiolytic effects of OXY are especially evident in females and may operate to selectively influence women's tending and befriending behaviors. Yet the female need for repair behaviors, some of which may fail, can possibly lead to maintained stress responses over time (Sbarra & Hazan, 2008).

Dopamine

The ventral tegmental area, a group of neurons at the very center of the brain, plays an important role in reward circuitry using the neurotransmitter DA (Carr, 2008a; Kalat, 2012). The release of endorphins in the ACC also embeds attachment experiences in the frontolimbic circuitry (Eisenberger, Taylor, Gable, Hilmert, & Lieberman, 2007; Hughes et al., 2012). Endorphins function as neurotransmitters and are the body's natural opioids and painkillers. Most commonly associated with physical exercise, they are produced in the pituitary gland and stimulated by the hypothalamus, inducing analgesia and a feeling of well-being (Carlson, 2013).

Implicated in all reward-driven learning, DA is a neurotransmitter and a hormone. Movement-related actions, basic emotions, visceral functions, reward-based learning, and decision making emerge from three DA pathways: the mesolimbic, the mesocortical, and the nigrostriatal (Carlson, 2013). Subcortical, mesolimbic DA pathway activation helps motivate feelings and desires and is associated with gaining knowledge and positive relationships. The mesocortical DA pathway modulates higher-order cognitive processes, assigning positive and negative values to emotions, ideas, and experiences. Subcortical, nigrostriatal pathway neurons note errors while a person is predicting rewards. Error detection promotes assessing how to alter goal-oriented behavior (Carr, 2008a). DA pathways have been implicated in attachment research via repeated experiences of pleasure as a positive reinforcer in caregiver-infant bonding. Research on genetic influences on transgenerational patterns of attachment implies that anxious attachment is correlated with a polymorphism of the DRD2 dopamine receptor gene (Vrticka & Vuilleumier, 2012).

Serotonin

The serotonin (5-HT) neurotransmitter is believed to contribute to maintaining homeostasis and restoring internal functioning to baseline (Heisler et al., 2003). It broadly contributes to all aspects of behavior and cognition as well as stabilizing perceptual and cognitive information. 5-HT neurons are clustered in the brain stem, the basal ganglia, the limbic system, and the neocortex (Carlson, 2013). Serotonin receptors are especially concentrated in the AMY and OFC. Well known for its involvement in mood and anxiety disorders, 5-HT has an inhibitory function that suppresses behavior. Food intake, play, and sexual behavior are reduced when 5-HT levels increase. Levels of 5-HT are associated with trust and social relatedness, caring, and grief. The AMY is balanced by 5-HT, helping to reduce the intensity of the startle response. However, it is the balance between 5-HT and another neurotransmitter, norepinephrine (NE), that is important in emotional regulation. While 5-HT modulates impulsive behavior on a cortical level, NE makes the person respond to danger. It appears that raised NE levels and reduced 5-HT levels caused by early life stresses may lead to impulsive adult behavior (Hart, 2008). Variations in the 5-HT transporter gene are implicated in attentional biases. An individual's stress response pattern, including 5-HT action, can be a risk factor for the development of anxiety disorders, which affect attachment patterns (Nolte et al., 2011). Epigenetic processes, or the expression of genes as influenced by experiences and the environment without altering DNA sequence, are increasingly understood to affect the manifestation of early attachment experiences. Avoidant attachment has been associated with a variability of the $5HT_{2A}$ which is a serotonin receptor gene (Vrticka & Vuilleumier, 2012).

CREATE PRINCIPLES AND CLINICAL APPLICATIONS

The primary focus of the ATR-N activities in this co-regulation chapter is the CREATE principle of Relational Resonating. The work focuses on social-emotional co-regulation and co-creation. Image making may directly access the social and emotional self, providing clients with opportunities to process emotions, co-regulate, and self-regulate. We highlight RH function in My Right Hemisphere as central to affect regulation. Affect regulation is mediated by social connectivity.

Relational Resonating ATR-N nonverbal microskills engage the RH and encourage nonverbal RH-to-RH communication, which is central to the development of attuned contingent communication. We have operationalized Relational Resonating to mean co-creation, co-consciousness, and meaning making. We describe a sequence of ATR-N directives, media, and processes that promote Relational Resonating. First, working with color can shift attention to the RH's propensities and sensitivity to a gestalt of sensory information. Listening to quiet scribbling and some background music, and considering art making sounds during the Dual Drawing responsive art making or co-creating of images privileges RH auditory processing. The second directive to draw the dynamic flow between mother and child, Right-to-Right Hemisphere Communication, expands the focus of the experiential to social-emotional processes. During this time, smudging and erasing with the left hand actively promote RH function and track and mirror Relational Resonating. During nonverbal Dual Drawing, marks, gestures, pace, space, rhythm, and eye contact support the development of co-communication skills. Working with clay, extenuates this reflective mentalization (Bat Or, 2010). Third, working side by side to make a personal Tree of Life collage of autobiographical memories further enhances Relational Resonating. Art responses in the shared space give rise to synchronized, coconscious states and enhanced meaning making. Sharing art materials and a creative workspace reinforces attuned nonverbal RH-RH support as well as shared consciousness and meaning. Finally, taking turns to draw in silence during the Dual Drawing encourages reciprocity and RH attunement. Reaching out across the page and sensing whether or not to touch the other's forms during Dual Drawing embodies attuned RH-to-RH communication. Once implicit attunement and understanding are established, titling and discussing the art provides explicit support for the LH cognitive and verbal functions.

Being seen, heard, listened to, and felt by others reinforces clients' affect regulation skills. Sharing art making space, creating alongside clients, tracking nonverbal exchanges with clients, and explicating the processes provide reparative relational experiences. In addition to the responsive art, verbal responses can augment hemispheric connectivity. Knowledge of hemispheric bias allows art therapists to encourage the RH-activated client to express percolating emotions, while engaging in verbal communication, and to work with the LH-activated client to modulate emotional avoidance. This integrative work is supported by client-therapist in-session response art; the therapist responds both verbally and nonverbally in the art to the client's emotive or cognitive expressions. The therapist can also take notes to accurately reflect on the verbalization that was taking place at the same time that the art making was happening. Post session, the therapist's self-art making and the review of transcripts can support the therapist's hemispheric integration.

Embodied Creativity art activities help recall co-regulated moments and life experiences. Prompting a mother to recall holding her infant can bring on strong memories; it activates an IWM of holding, being held, or wishing to be held. Creative embodiment is associated with movement. Fine motor movements, such as leaning forward, moving away, looking up, or meeting the other's eyes, encourage this mentalizing. Representing symbolic and actual movement, art that is made by smudging with the non-dominant hand or with both hands, can arouse these memories. Experiencing and representing positive bodily communication can start a reparative process for clients recalling negative experiences as it sculpts the brain memory centers to reconsolidate the memory differently.

Expressive Communicating of emotions is critical to self and co-regulation (Greenberg, 2011). Implicit and explicit interactions are supported through the use of color, tactile smudging, tangible collage images, and content-rich directives. Opportunities to practice affect regulation of emotions are provided throughout a sequential process. For example, silent expectations and tension that are built up during the Dual Drawing directive which intensify emoting stimulate the need for emotional expressivity. Released during the discussion of the drawing, verbalizing this expression contributes to a sense of emotional togetherness. Similarly, using the non-dominant left hand can contribute to both the expression of the anxiety, confusion, and positive joy that this experience provides. It is during this process that negative emotions can spontaneously be transformed into positive ones. We also use listening to music as a way to stimulate emotional responses.

These ideas also serve to promote Adaptive Responding. As described, the directives can be stressful for some individuals. When these challenges can be resolved, resiliency is supported. The invitation to add color to a drawing can be demanding for some clients as it exposes personal or emotionally vulnerable meaning. The opportunity to discuss this experience and label the aroused feelings can increase a sense of control. Additionally, as previously discussed, sketching the mother-child relationship in Right-to-Right Hemisphere Communication can create tension. Clients, whether mothers or children, can find themselves personally implicated as they may question and reference their own experiences as mothers or of being mothered. Smudging and tracking allow for active changing of the art, which can support a sense of current mastery and internal control. Co-creation also models how communication can be altered.

The challenge of holding an entirely nonverbal exchange based on marks and gestures during the Tree-of-Life and the Dual Drawing activity can be stressful. Participants can doubt their ability to nonverbally read their partner's drawing or be present during these dyadic experiences. Making, and then processing, autobiographical memories in one's Tree of Life within a secure relationship provides opportunities for tolerating difficult memories and leaning on a trusted other's support. Working alongside, or with, a trusted other can ease anxiety as it offers an opportunity to reduce the need to rely on self-resources. Subsequently the discussion of experienced secure attuned interpersonal interactions within a like-minded group of people can facilitate beginning changes in social relating. For example, while visually telling one's personal story with trusted others can aid in self-acceptance. Thus, safe exposure of personally meaningful material within small groups permits participants to progressively build trust within the community. Similarly, the dyadic joining with a family member can be greatly supportive and reinforces reflection, flexibility, and coping. Dyadic work activities such as collaborating to choose a title and post-drawing discussion allow for restitution of troubled connections. In summary, the relational-based ATR-N directives can interrupt the automaticity of anxiety and/or fear-based responses. This may allow higher cortical structures to inhibit and help recondition such reactivity and contribute to the capacity for self-regulation. Repeating such experiences may over time inhibit and help recondition fear-based reactivity and contribute to earned self-regulation.

The CREATE principle of Transformative Integrating is demonstrated by the sequence between the experientials and structured processes within each directive. There are two sequences that promote an integrated autobiographical sense of the social-emotional self. The first moves from representing the intrapersonal social-emotional self (drawing the RH) to IWM representations (mother-infant drawing). The second sequence gives opportunities for co-created implicit and shared meaning-making experiences (mother-child drawing and dual drawings). Several processes within each directive promote lateral and vertical brain integration. Adding color, which is associated with the expression of emotion, to the pencil drawings of the brain helps integrate cognitive and emotive brain centers while consolidating a more expressive understanding of the self. During the mother-child and dyadic drawings, engaging in nonverbal art making, and then in the verbal titling and discussion of the art, contribute to integration of lower ventral brain regions with higher dorsal ones; ventral areas are associated with implicit emotional, cognitive, and interpersonal functions and dorsal ones with explicit function. Likewise, shifting from the nonverbal gestalt of understanding a partner's drawing in the Dual Drawing directive to processing it verbally with the person promotes RH-LH integration.

The CREATE principle of Empathizing and Compassion is central to the experientials of this chapter. Right hemispheric emotional recognition as well as nonverbal communication and expression of emotions pertains to our capacity to understand and empathize with another's emotional experience. Moreover, the group context for art making supports developing a more vibrant empathic appreciation of the differences and similarities of relational experience and creativity. The ATR-N dyadic pairing interventions and processes described can support such sensitivity and attunement. For example, participating in nonverbal Dual Drawing directs attention to how body language, hand gestures, and marking work in sync with one's facial expression, allowing the whole body to convey meaning. Next, gently negotiating the subtleties of creating alongside another in an intimate space, sharing materials, and accommodating another's movement invites mutual consideration and compassion.

Witnessing and discussing the caregiver-child and dyadic drawings facilitates an appreciation of different ways in which implicit attachment can manifest. Perhaps it is the novel experience of nonverbal engagement that can provide a shift toward empathy, especially for clients who are more familiar with engaging in verbal confrontation. Experiences of co-creation can further promote empathic awareness at the level of meaning making and co-consciousness as shared representations are mutually understood.

CHAPTER 6

Relational Resonating: Autobiographical Memory

The year that our youngest, third daughter was born marks the number of years that we have lived in the United States of America, so a quarter of a century and growing. . . . It never ceases to astonish me how long it has been. Some time ago, my cousin asked me if I recall the time she came to visit us in Jerusalem. Our eldest, our son, had just been born. I did not remember. It was the first time that I realized that much of my autobiographical memory of events, whether here or in my country of origin, has been washed away by the impact of our migration. Rather than events, I remember people. Events are veiled by a swishy mixture of grays; a landscape of fluffy clouds. Overall, I have an excellent memory. For example, I can easily recall the art of my clients, and I love and can easily recall information. I tell myself that what is important is that I remember people and can easily recall and bring up the comforting memory of relationships. Noah Hass-Cohen

AUTOBIOGRAPHICAL MEMORY PROVIDES a comprehensive context for further exploration of the CREATE principle of Relational Resonance. Ideally, autobiographical memory is a contained and coherent organized sense of one's history and sense of self. Comprising sensory felt and contextualized memories, and individual emotion-based events, autobiographical recurring memories tend to be abstract, familiar, and integrated (Bluck & Alea, 2005). Autobiographical memories are generally organized as a series of personal episodes that are tied together with temporal, visual, and spatial associations. Across the life span, these self-defining memories are mental signposts of our experiences within a specific time and context. Thus, autobiographical memory holds our unique sense of self in the past, present, and future.

Autobiographical memory is theorized to serve three functions: self, social, and directive (Bluck, 2003; Rasmussen & Habermas, 2011). The self-function consists of internal processes of conceptualizing and managing the self. Also known as theory of mind, these internal processes are used socially and influence the quality of relational connections and communications (Baron-Cohen, Leslie, & Frith, 1985). The directive function, or prospection, guides present actions and plans for the future (Bluck & Alea, 2011). Each function makes a separate contribution to well-being, also known as additive effects (Waters, 2013). Neurobiological research supports the finding that specific autobiographical memories, the use of memories to direct future actions, and interpersonal understanding of others' intentions have an 82% shared neural network (Spreng & Grady, 2010). It seems likely that the three autobiographical memory functions represent multiple, interacting psychological and neurobiological subsystems.

Overall, autobiographical memories inhibit sensory past memories from being experienced as happening right now, by contextually and cognitively anchoring them in time and place. Self-autobiographical memories are broadly categorized into memories about specific life span periods, general events, and specific episodic events (Conway & Pleydell-Pearce, 2000). Sometimes intense episodic or lifetime memories are less well integrated and are either recalled out of context or forgotten. It is as if they are devoid of time and place. It is the balance between contextualized representations and non-contextualized sensory-based representations that contributes to the integrity of memory recall (Brewin, Gregory, Lipton, & Burgess, 2010). In addition, it is our working-memory ability to recall positive and negative emotions and experiences, while maintaining equanimity, which further contributes to effective learning, coping, and adjusting (Blagov & Singer, 2004). Most importantly, the coherent sense of self is bound together by the individual's ability to clearly and consistently hold, narrate, and share self-referential verbal narratives (Singer, Blagov, Berry, & Oost, 2013).

An individual's capacity to access and share autobiographical memories has been directly linked to his or her attachment style. Those with a secure style can take comfort in past positive memories, while those with an insecure style may have difficulty recalling coherent past narratives (Siegel, 2012). Individual life experiences, such as a history of disruptive attachment, post-traumatic stress, and depression, can fragment or distort autobiographical memory. However, different types of distress can have a different impact on autobiographical memory recall. For example, disrupted attachment may fragment the individual's self-narratives, creating inconsistent and incoherent narratives. In contrast, traumatic experiences have a dominant negative narrative that overshadows all other possibilities. Although the narrative is integrated and coherent, it contributes to extreme confusion and dysfunction, as it is not connected to the person's current situation (Follmer, Sun, Bunnell, & Lindboe, 2013). The individual's logic and current functions are held hostage by the memory of the past trauma, and she or he is compelled to reenact it. For example, Holocaust survivors' sense of time and connections between events may be impaired (Langer, 1993). Overall, temporal, causal, and thematic coherence are negatively impacted for people who have experienced trauma (Habermas & de Silveira, 2011). This kind of disrupted coherence, which is linked to relational insecurity and deep mistrust, is most frequently expressed as incorrect causal assumptions (Demiray & Bluck, 2011).

Regardless of how traumatic the experience is, how the experience is interpreted and self-narrated strongly influences the impacts it has on the person's life, his or her sense of self. Hence, although the quality of the memory can be constructive or destructive, the way that the person recalls and narrates the traumatic events are the most significant factor, and the meaning that is drawn from the experience (Hesse, 1999; Rasmussen & Berntsen, 2009). A supportive other, such as a therapist or trusted partner, can provide the secure framework that is needed for making sense of past negative attachment experiences (Siegel, 2006). Clinically, reducing the dominance of negative self-defining memories requires that the therapist employ integration strategies that scaffold the development of clear narration and self-storying.

While the interference of amnesia and new information with active learning has been long established in mobile-accident trauma studies and in memory assessment, it is only recently that the relevance of this phenomenon was explored in animals (Nader, Schafe, & LeDoux, 2000) and human studies (Kindt, Soeter, & Vervliet, 2009). Originally it was thought that memory consolidation does not change over time. We now know that as autobiographical memories are revisited they become labile and can be changed as they reconsolidate (Nader et al., 2000).

The ATR-N experientials included in this chapter are intended to stimulate coherent autobiographical narration, increase a sense of relational security and resiliency and support positive memory reconsolidation or the fading away of negative-based aspects of the original memory. A single self-memory recall directive, the Childhood Cutout, provides the opportunity to revisit a single episodic meaningful event and involves practicing self-regulation. The next experiential, the Autobiographical Timeline, helps the individual to string together memories across a supportive visual line. It is based on a developmentally-based timeline. In fact, from early childhood, drawing a baseline is intuitively embraced as a way to ground expression and provide a perspective of time, place, and space (Lowenfeld, 1987). Two types of Autobiographical Timeline directives are suggested: (a) the Timeline of Episodic Memories, and (b) the Timeline of Relationships. The construction of one episodic memory and the two autobiographical-based timelines can be used for initial therapist-client introductions, as well as for mid points and the end point of therapeutic work. The next experiential directive, the Compassionate Past, Present, and Future Timeline, is drawn from the perspective of being cared for by another. The directive asks to: "Draw your future as it would be seen by someone who loved or cared for you in the past." This directive puts together the self, the other, and the prospective function of memory. It may be useful for working with people who are experiencing a foreshortened sense of the future, which is common for individuals with disruptive attachment styles or trauma histories. Depending on the client's situation, some of the wording might need to be modified. Sometimes, for very isolated individuals, the caring person referred to in this directive may need to be the therapist. Furthermore, because it is often easier to start with caring for another, a necessary first step might be: "Imagine and draw a future for someone you love or care for."

The directives are designed to utilize both nonverbal means of expression and personal storytelling. Our customary sequencing and making of the experientials involves sharing and narrating the art with a trusted group and reflecting on the process by writing updated personal memories within a social context. Hence, they promote the capacity for relational resonance. Our specific directions provide the artist-client with the opportunity to examine, align, and reconsolidate current, past, and future self-defining memories.

AUTOBIOGRAPHICAL MEMORY FUNCTIONS

The three autobiographical memory functions are (1) self-referential, (2) social interactions and relational understanding of others, and (3) prospective and directive, which include thoughts about the future and inform future actions (Bluck, 2003; Spreng & Grady, 2010).

For all three functions, an increased use of personally significant single-event memories has for the most part, been associated with improved well-being, such as perceived positive relationships, feeling that one has a purpose in life, and playing a valuable role in the community (Waters, 2013). Frequent recall of single events is most likely to have a strong emotional impact as these one-time occurrences tend for the most part to be novel and unique. Therefore, remembrance of such events excites and attracts attention to its significance. This can also have a negative effect, as voluntarily or involuntarily recalling recurring traumatizing and non-integrated memories of a single event can be very disturbing (Lanius, Frewen, Vermetten, & Yehuda, 2010). In addition, when a person is seeking to reestablish safety after a traumatic event, vivid memories can drive him or her to avoid the episodic memory or attempt to address the sources of danger (Pillemer, 2003). This behavior may not always be safe or adaptive and requires the self-regulation of emotions.

Episodic memories are explicitly recalled memories of specific single or recurring personal experiences. They comprise sensory and factual details along with an emotional component. However, memories of repeating events play a different role than one-time memories. Repetitious, they tend to be held cognitively and contribute to a sense of stability. One way that autobiographical memory can help with self-regulation and reconsolidation is by using episodic memories to fulfill emotional needs (Touryan et al., 2007). For example, when a person's sense of self or security is threatened, supportive memories can function to offset the effects of disturbing memories (Philippe, Koestner, Beaulieu-Pelletier, Lecours, & Lekes, 2012). From an autobiographical perspective, recalling a time in which needs were met can help offset the impact of times when the person's goals or sense of autonomy, relatedness, and competence are thwarted.

Without experiences of unresolved trauma, autobiographical self-memory functions to increase self-continuity and emotional regulation, which can potentially create a clearer and more coherent sense of self (Bluck & Alea, 2011; Siegel, 2012). Aspects of autobiographical self-continuity include self-concept preservation, enhancement, and change (Bluck, 2003). The sense of consistency provided by autobiographical memory also enhances the self-image, providing the impression "I am the same person as I was before—but better" (Bluck, 2003, p. 116). Temporal proximity, perspective, and adjusted relevance mediate reconsolidation processes. For example, recalling recent positive events is more likely to lead to an enhanced mood. However, the memory of positive events in the distant past can contribute to either a decrease or increase of the impact of present negative experiences. Grief over a loved one is an example of recalling past positive experiences that can increase negative states. In other words, remembering the times spent together and missing the person in the present evokes negativity. Thus, people may also hold on to or distance themselves from past events in order to self-regulate.

Connections between autobiographical memory recall and the sense of self are bidirectional. For example, a desire for an ideal or consistent self-image may alter self-memories. In this case negative memories may be dismissed as old history and irrelevant to the current self, while positive memories remain highly pertinent (Sutin & Robins, 2008; Wilson & Ross, 2003). Such self-enhancing choices may or may not be effective. They may create a conflict with the development and maintenance of a coherent self, depending on the degree of dissonance with individuals' lived experience (Hesse &

Main, 2000). Overall, any change or even the perception of self-change or loss could lead to feelings of sadness, which are associated with a less coherent sense of self (Sutin & Gillath, 2009). These processes depend on individual personalities and family history of attachment dynamics, as well as current circumstances. Thus change, sometimes even positive change, may be difficult as it can be perceived as challenging a person's self-sense of autobiographical consistency, continuity, and coherency.

Coherent autobiographical telling supports the individual's ability to accurately attribute thoughts, desires, and intentions to others, and to predict or explain their actions. This ability, conceptualized as ToM, is built upon layers of previous similar instances, and develops from early childhood (Frith & Frith, 1999). Socially, the sharing of recalled autobiographical memories provides material for interpersonal discourse, makes the conversation more convincing, and is an opportunity for teaching others (Bluck, 2003). The telling of detailed narratives can elicit a supportive reaction from listeners in the form of increased engagement and credulousness, and stronger emotional or attuned and empathic responses (Pillemer, 2003). Thus, problems with autobiographical memory recall, social function, and emotion-based disorders can be interrelated (Fivush, 2011; Williams et al., 2007).

How people share and the effectiveness of their sharing is influenced by a variety of variables such as gender, familiarity, intimacy, and trust. Overall, people tend to share differently with familiar, as opposed to unfamiliar, people. This is a function of attachment, interpersonal security and sometimes gender. In general, women tend to share more intimate details than men. Also, some people have a variety of rich, detailed memories available to share while others tend to recall only in overgeneralized terms (Pillemer, 2001; Warren & Haslam, 2007). This habitual overgeneralization may be due to premature disruption of the recall process, which helps avoid remembering painful or traumatic details (Williams et al., 2007); In other words, generalized recall of a memory precedes detailed recall. Over time, overgeneralized recall can become a habit, and the details of some memories may be completely forgotten. Overgeneralized habitual recall has been associated with psychological problems and depression and may be associated with dismissive attachment strategies (Pillemer, 2001; Warren & Haslam, 2007). Selective overgeneralized recall for painful memories such as a surgery, birth, and so on has protective functional attributes for positive reconsolidation. The lived experiences of bonding can then become stronger and dominate those of the birthing pain.

From an evolutionary perspective, the acquisition of autobiographical memory processes has been helpful to the development of the human species. Societal and individual recorded past memories help us understand and explain the world as well as make direct inferences about what the future will hold, that is, prospection. Stored autobiographical memories direct individuals' attitudes and serve to inform future actions. Some of these self-directive functions include using such stored information in new contexts in order to solve problems, to create and test predictions about the world, and possibly to predict the thought processes and behaviors of others (Bluck, 2003). Again, problems with autobiographical recall have been associated with difficulties in imagining future events (Schacter et al., 2012) as well as with higher levels of depression and rumination (Raes et al., 2006). Neurologically, autobiographical memory functions have been found to be closely linked to one's ability to mentally simulate future and imagined events (Schachter et al., 2012). People appear to use both episodic memory (the memory of personal events) and semantic memory (memories that are anchored in language) to simulate the future. An integrative-reconsolidation memory model has three essential ingredients consisting of autobiographical memories, semantic structures, and aroused emotional responses (Lane, Ryan, Nadel, & Greenberg, 2014). It is likely that facts from semantic memory may help identify the emotive details needed from episodic memory. Being able to create these simulations helps with both emotional regulation, integrated functionality, and solving life problems. Compared to past memories, these imagined future events could be even more important to the sense of self (D'Argembeau, Lardi, & Van der Linden, 2012). This is because, psychologically, future decisions are under the individual's control, whereas the past is not.

Frequently, the directive function of episodic memory can be undervalued, as day-to-day decisions and future planning require the integration of semantic and episodic memory (Pillemer, 2003). Sematic memory, which is associated with facts, maybe be culturally more valued than emotions associated with episodic memories. However, it is the emotional salience and vividness of episodic memories that motivate individuals to approach or avoid future events. Emotional salience can also run a variety of personal interferences to planning. Episodic memories are especially important when one is faced with new situations, or when relevant fact-based knowledge is unavailable. For example, memories of failure can encourage people to maximize their efforts in the future or to avoid these experiences (Pillemer, 2003). In contrast, memories of a supportive parent or trustworthy mentor can influence our ability to approach obstacles. To support a sense of well-being, people also use less momentous vivid memories to provide guidance about their perceived goals and obstacles. Most importantly, originating events, such as remembering when one chose a career, and turning points, such as moving away from home, represent memorable changes in one's life path and impact future decisions (Jansari & Parkin, 1996). Effective use of autobiographical memory to direct behavior is also associated with seeing the future as more open-ended (Bluck & Alea, 2011). Perhaps visualizing future events may be helpful to materializing them (Spreng & Levine, 2012). Most certainly some art therapists have suggested that such imaginary activities are critical to the formation of resiliency (Lahad, 1993; 2000)

SELF-DEFINING MEMORIES AND DEVELOPMENT OVER THE LIFE SPAN

Adults can typically recall autobiographical memories from no earlier than two years of age (Frith & Frith, 2003). However, the processing of past events begins earlier as most parents automatically model ways of reflecting on the past. They tend to ask simple questions about past events, allowing very young children with minimal verbal skills to participate through simple confirmation. In doing so, parents teach their children about the importance of sharing the past and how to reflect on important emotional aspects of it (Fivush, Habermas, Waters, & Zaman, 2011).

Early childhood parental modeling plays a strong role in the developing child's tendency for positive or negative memory processing (Fivush, 2007). Mothers model how to process experiences for their children by reminiscing about them. In terms of immediate recall, young children are better able to describe novel situations when prompted by specific questions and are able to describe repetitive occurrences when asked routine questions (Nelson, 1993). The two styles of mother-to-child memory talk are elaborative versus pragmatic. Elaborative mothers tend to talk about when, what, where, and with whom. On the other hand, pragmatic mothers use memory instrumentally, for example, asking a child where he or she placed a belonging (Fivush, Haden, & Reese, 2006; Nelson, 1993). An elaborative memory style provides the foundation for storytelling, and for constructing narratives about what the parent and child did together. It is also likely that the mother-child conversation provides a platform for memory consolidation, which can be emulated for memory reconsolidation throughout the lifetime. For example, children only remembered objects viewed in a museum if they and their mother had talked about them together. Children of elaborative mothers tend to contribute more recollecting information to conversations about memories than do children of pragmatic mothers (Tessler & Nelson, 1994).

Culturally, mothers from Westernized cultures tend to use more detail and emotions in creating narratives with their children than do mothers from Eastern cultures (Fivush et al., 2011). Their children will then practice their own narratives the same way. These narrative models influence the way children understand their experiences and emotions, teach social norms, and contribute to the growing child's sense of security. Children do not automatically understand how to structure their life stories, as they will tend to relay their narratives in the form of scattered anecdotes. While they may recognize the ongoing effects of certain incidents, they will usually not organize them sequentially or meaningfully. Parents not only help children to make sense of these memories but provide additional information about aspects, such as infancy, that children can integrate into their own narratives (Fivush et al., 2011). An organized sense of self is found more often among children whose mothers discuss negative emotions with them in an elaborate fashion (Bird & Reese, 2006). Recollection of early memories is associated with aspects of well-being, such as self-esteem and self-control. It is also associated with less internal conflict on several dimensions (Alyusheva & Nourkova, 2012). While it is often a mother's role to teach her children how to process emotional incidents by recounting memories of them, helping clients explore their past is an aspect of the therapist's role as a surrogate attachment figure.

During adolescence, children's life narrative starts to reflect on and inform self-identity. They begin to view themselves as the main character in their self-defining memories and narratives, rather than their parents or family. Whereas young children's narrative development is scaffolded by their parents, the coherence of adolescents' narratives is further developed by solitary habits such as keeping a journal or reading others' biographies (Habermas, Ehlert-Lerche, & de Silveira, 2009). Like those of adults, an adolescent's life story incorporates relational, familial, and communal values as well as self-generated external interests, such as formal learning and media (Singer et al., 2013). This identity development influences the construction of autobiographical memories, allowing for more sophisticated meaning making and direction (Fivush et al., 2011).

Adolescents first develop identity by focusing on both continuity and superficial change. Only later, do they begin to introduce the idea of personal transformations of these life experiences (Chandler, Lalonde, Sokol, & Hallett, 2003). When faced with self-behavior that they see as inconsistent with their personalized identity, they tend to explain it in terms of external circumstances or otherwise distance themselves (Pasupathi, Mansour, & Brubaker, 2007). Psychologically, the adolescent capacity for recall of self-defining memories is associated with more insight (Fivush et al., 2011).

Identity is also tied to culturally-based life scripts, which suggest how life is expected to progress. Such life scripts include typical events in their usual sequence, and the time of life that each is expected to occur (Rubin & Berntsen, 2003). Individuals use these directive scripts to help determine how they will structure and present their memories (Alyusheva & Nourkova,

2012). When such life scripts are unavailable for guidance, it can make it difficult for the child or adolescent to develop a coherent personal narrative. Lack of life scripts may impact the coherent formation of an adaptive narrative identity and relational security throughout adulthood (Bohn & Berntsen, 2008).

For adults, self-defining episodic memories also tend to cluster around a reminiscence bump of adolescence and the early 20s (Jansari & Parkin, 1996); When mature adults are cued to recall personal memories, they tend to recall memories of events that happened to them between the ages of 10 and 30 years. Possible explanations of this phenomenon suggest that the novelty and importance of experiences that are encountered during this transitional development are critical aspects of adult identity. The reminiscence bump is specifically connected to the directive function of memory. Over the lifetime adolescent memories and long-existing scripts guide behavior. Thus memories of individual incidents are used to process novel situations (Pillemer, 2001). The development of a narrative identity is an ongoing process that is shaped by the maturation of emotive, cognitive, and social skills (Fivush et al., 2011). Constructed throughout the life cycle, the narrative identity is socially and culturally bound (Habermas & Bluck, 2000; Singer, 2004).

AUTOBIOGRAPHICAL LIFE SCRIPTS AND ATTACHMENT

An individual's capacity to access and share autobiographical memories has been directly linked to his or her attachment style (Hesse, 1999). Thus, a secure attachment style has been linked to coherent self-memory narrations, which serve to continuously self-soothe and support relational intimacy (Bluck, Alea, Habermas, & Rubin, 2005; Josephson, 1996). In contrast, an insecure attachment style has been linked to indistinct, blurry, or unclear autobiographical narrations (see Chapters 4 and 5). This disjointed autobiographical sense of self furthers contradictory self-representations, or random or tangential attention to details; contributing to avoidance, and resulting in a cycle of autobiographical incoherence (Fivush et al., 2011). Then the capacity for self-understanding, creating intimacy with others, and developing sound social relationships can be jeopardized (Robinson & Swanson, 1990).

Individuals with a secure attachment style can compare positive events from the distant past with current negative experiences, take comfort in the former, and transform the current difficulty. It is likely that their internal working models reassure them that their needs will be met again in the future. These assurances can then mitigate the gap between their positive life experiences and a painful present time.

Unlike securely attached individuals, adults with an insecure attachment style may dismiss difficult experiences, most likely because they do not want to experience the emotional pain associated with these memories (Pillemer, 2001). Overall anxiety feels intolerable to them and threatens their sense of self, so they end up distancing themselves from others. Subsequently, this distancing mediates the emotional impact of recalling significant memories or connecting with significant others (Sutin & Gillath, 2009). For example, the person with a dismissive attachment style will tend to generate a self-image that includes cognitive distancing from negative childhood and current adult relationships. Thus the person's need to keep their self-concept intact at all times can overgeneralize, and will continue to undermine their ability to have close relationships. They may also be dismissive of the importance of other events, such as national or international disasters. This dismissive distancing stance also constrains the ability to process new memories. As a result, restricted autobiographical processing ability can cut a person off from cognitive and emotional self-resources. Thus, cognitively, the person may lack the ability to recall an experience in order to estimate the probability of a desired outcome (Pillemer, 2001). Consequently, retrospectively conceptualizing and emotionally evaluating the impact of positive and negative guiding events becomes skewed. This kind of processing provides motivation to work toward that outcome and aids in exploring the nature of anticipated emotions (Singer et al., 2013). Therefore, while protective in the short term, insecure attachment strategies limit the pool of information needed for individuals to envision their future and connect with others.

Alternatively, individuals who grew up in disruptive environments may also have abundant information that is not necessarily adaptive for drawing conclusions. They may have learned that people cannot be trusted and it is impossible to get their needs met. Accordingly, people with an insecure attachment style will gravitate toward recalling familiar negative memories. Many of these memories are related to problematic, disappointing, or non-supportive relationships (Sutin & Gillath, 2009). Repeated activation of a negative memory is likely to have an enduring, undesirable impact on one's well-being (Philippe, Koestner, Beaulieu-Pelletier, & Lecours, 2011). A bias toward recalling adverse experiences further reinforces negative self-perceptions and problems accessing a coherent narrative of unfamiliar positive experiences (Hesse & Main, 2000). This maladaptive reconsolidating cycle contributes to additional relational ruptures, distress, anxiety, loss of self-soothing capacities, and dysfunctional mental health. Incoherent memories contribute to problems with contextualizing current memories, which has been associated with rumination, worry, and clinical anxiety (Siegel, 2012). For people with an anxious attachment style, negative emotional content has been associated with depression. For those with avoidant attachment, the degree of memory coherence and its emotional intensity were associated with a vulnerability to depression and ineffective social coping (Sutin & Gillath, 2009; Raes et al., 2005). Overall, subjective memories and self-constructed autobiographical memories continue to impact individuals' well-being over the life span (Keyes & Ryff, 2000).

AUTOBIOGRAPHICAL NARRATIVES AND MEANING MAKING

Who, what, when, and how, which are the hallmarks of autobiographical memories, organize the recall of attachment history and impact an individual's mental health status. Equally important, beyond just recalling the facts of the memory, is an account of how this event occurred as it did, what it meant, and why it was significant (Fivush et al., 2011). Significant incidents are often recalled as such vivid individual episodes. Strung together, they serve as the foundation for making abstract conclusions and lead to an organized sense of knowing about the self (Knez, 2012). Linking meaningful events to each other and to more remote life events supports the capacity for autobiographical reasoning. Connecting autobiographical origins, events, and outcomes increases and defines personality development (Habermas, 2011) and supports reconsolidation.

Associated with strong feelings, either positive or negative, self-defining autobiographical memories are vivid mental representations, have been thought about many times, and are generally encoded in long-term memory (D'Argembeau et al., 2012). They can start as specific episodic memories, and consolidate in the form of visual images associated with a conceptual context (Conway, 2009). Such salient or recent, sensory and perceptual affective memories become part of long-term memories. They link up to other memories that are similar in theme or content and when one memory is triggered, associated memories activate (Philippe et al., 2012).

Typically, these long-term memories form the conceptual self. They include semantic-factual knowledge, personal values, and a knowledge of self-history. Memories that are at odds with the conceptual self can be maintained either as an anomaly, illustrating a person's character by means of contrast, or function to demonstrate a turning point in the person's life (Pasupathi et al., 2007). Thus, self-defining memories organize into specific and meaningful categories, such as "times I've been to another country" or "the college years." Conceptual self-memories can also illustrate a particular point in time, but they do not have to be dependent on specific memories (Singer et al., 2013). Often, they will be accessible by a repetitive narrative script. Barriers to the development and maintenance of coherent self-conceptualizing memories include experiencing a lack of childhood parental modeling and support, depression, or traumatic events. Making sense of and creating meaning from these experiences, helps change their autobiographical role and negative influences and rebuild the conceptual self.

AUTOBIOGRAPHICAL MEMORY AND PTSD

People who have experienced a traumatic incident often hold it as a vivid landmark in their autobiographical memory. This is particularly pronounced in individuals who develop post-traumatic stress disorder (PTSD) as they are more likely to incorporate the traumatic experience into their self-memory and identity. Unfortunately, other experiences, which may not be directly related to the trauma, may also be tied to the traumatic memory, leading to severe negative cognitive and emotional outcomes (Berntsen, Willert, & Rubin, 2003; Neshat-Doost et al., 2013).

Individuals with PTSD also often experience depression, leading to an overgeneralized recall of events, with fewer specific details being remembered (Williams et al., 2007). In addition, whereas people in general recall positive memories more easily than negative ones, those with depressive symptomology do not exhibit this tendency (Jørgensen et al., 2012). However, under therapeutic conditions, the negative emotional experience of retelling a difficult episodic event can become diffused, and the recall for positive experience enhanced (Segal, Williams, & Teasdale, 2012). As negativity and depression are treated, clients can become more attuned to the meaning and impact of the traumatic events in their life (Allen, 2001). Overall, the ability to find meaning in painful past experiences is associated with positive adjustment (Park, 2010) and optimism (McLean & Pratt, 2006).

TREATMENT IMPLICATIONS: MEMORY RECONSOLIDATION

From an autobiographical perspective, treatment approaches focus on assisting the individual in developing conceptual and emotional coherence (Cozolino, 2010). Coherence has temporal, causal, thematic, and cultural dimensions that can exist together or separately. Temporal coherence emerges from the chronological organization of the story, whereas causal coherence represents a logical explanation of how events led to each other. Causal coherence contributes to the development of a sense of self-cohesiveness and helps clarify seemingly irrational discontinuities. Thematic coherence is a pattern of repeating themes that illustrate something meaningful. Cultural and social status-based coherence represents consistency with expectations of how one's life should progress (Habermas & Bluck, 2000). Collaboratively, the client and therapist can decide which of the dimensions of coherence provides a more effective pathway for building autobiographical continuity or is an obstacle to integrated self-identifying narratives and should be approached with caution. For some, temporal coherency, which entails telling the story in order, might be a better starting point than causal coherence, as the cause of some interpersonal traumas may often be very complex and extremely painful to bear.

The development of autobiographical coherence reflects a person's ability to organize episodic memories and long-term memories into a meaningful new story about the self. The construction of a narrative identity includes two important general processes: (1) memory specificity, or recall of specific sensory memories; and (2) meaning making, or linking memories to the way that the self is currently understood. Memories can be used constructively to explain, illustrate, or stimulate change, thus reforming them. Adaptive meanings are coherent, responsive to new information, and practical rather than unreasonably positive or negative. While people cannot change their past, they can change how they relate to their history, thereby experiencing self-agency and earning coherence. As a result, it can be expected that repeating an account of an incident under positive conditions will help to process and change the memory in a constructive way. The memory of sharing with a familiar or trustworthy person mediates the past memory, and as discussed in Chapter 5, sharing with others has a self-regulatory function. As the interpretation of the memory appears to be more important than the context, supportive others can help reframe painful memories so that the interpretation supports a sense of security and optimism about the future (Hesse, 1999). For example, people who report more personal agency as they tell the story of their therapy tend to experience better therapeutic outcomes (Adler, 2013).

Therapeutic change and an individual's well-being can be expressed as contamination or redemption stories; In the latter, something of value is gained, whereas in contamination stories something of value is lost (McAdams, Diamond, De St. Aubin, & Mansfield, 1997). For example, a person who develops a severe illness may emphasize the loss of functioning or the support he or she received from the community. Contamination stories are associated with depression (McAdams, Reynolds, Lewis, Patten, & Bowman, 2001), while redemption stories and positive interpretations are associated with a variety of aspects of well-being (Singer et al., 2013).

As participants talk about their relational history, the therapist can note the level of contingency and coherence in the autobiographical narrative according to (1) temporal, causal, thematic, or culture dimensions, or (2) bias toward negative or traumatic self-defining memories or contamination stories. Clues as to how people might interact with others include whether or not they can talk with the interviewer without long silences, and without averting their eyes in avoidance, and with the ability to be truthful about past experiences

Table 6.1 Grice's Maxims

Maxim	How it is expressed
Quality	be truthful and have evidence for what you say
Quantity	be succinct, yet complete
Relation	be relevant or perspicacious
Manner	be clear and orderly

Adapted from Grice (1975, 1991).

without dismissing them in order to avoid the pain associated with them (Table 6.1). Assessing for areas of intervention by the therapist can be achieved by paying attention to any lapses in discourse, contingency, and coherence in the autobiographical narrative. The Gricean maxims, which represent qualities that people are assumed to display when communicating comprehensibly, are additional coherence features (Grice, 1975, 1991). They require paying attention to the quality, quantity, and relevance of the narrative identity.

A narrative with causal coherence follows the maxims of quantity and quality, presenting sufficient logical evidence for statements. A narrative with temporal coherence reflects the maxim of manner, relating the incidents in an orderly fashion. A narrative with thematic coherence follows the maxim of relation, only providing information that is relative to the overarching concept.

Until a therapeutic relationship is established, it is important that the therapist not confront what may seem to be untruthful, dismissive reports or dysregulating accounts by the client. These may be expressed in the form of illogical summaries of childhood that are not supported by facts. A client may describe being beaten with a belt by his mother and then conclude that his childhood was pretty normal, violating the maxim of quality, or having evidence for what is said. Processing difficulties may also be identified via nonverbal cues, as in the case of a client who initially relates comfortably to the therapist, but then begins to avert his or her eyes when describing traumatic experiences.

Within the therapeutic relationship, treatment provides an opportunity to both update and revisit the memory differently. This is because each time that we revisit a memory, we are revisiting it, as we told it the last time we thought or talked about it (LeDoux, 1996). The re-telling and re-narrating of the upsetting memory in the therapist's office now includes the therapist's reaction as well as any other reparative information. As mentioned, traditionally it was thought that when we recall a memory, we go back to the original event. However, it has been established that we remember the last time that it was recalled (LeDoux, 1996; Figure 6.1).

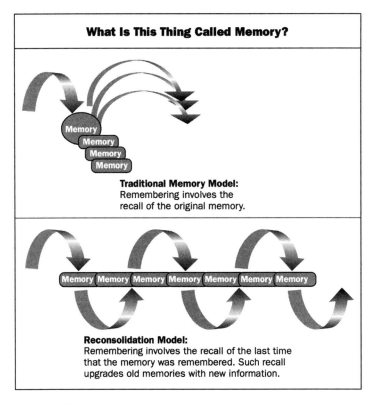

Figure 6.1 Originally it was thought that when a memory is retrieved the original memory of the event is recalled. In fact, it is the last recalled memory of the event that is retrieved.

From an art therapy perspective, several characteristics of self-defining memories can be incorporated into treatment. As is described in the art therapy experientials, sensory vividness, expressive emotionality, and visual linkages to previous memories can be used to update and reconsolidate autobiographical memories. Both clients and therapists can clearly see that the art representations contribute to accessing and making events vivid, coherent, and enduring. As the work progresses, the media properties, combined with creating and making meaning, decrease affective numbing and soothe aroused responses in the here and now. These adaptive states, which are supported by client labeling and narration of the art, further empower clients; as they explore, decide, and reinvent what the image means. The pleasure in this process helps balance reward system functioning by consolidating the beauty and meaning perceived in the art. Fostering contextualization and updating autobiographical memory thus increases clients' sense of self-agency and resiliency. Engaging therapeutic and pleasurable art making while confronting internal fear responses exercises novelty and reward-based processing.

Meanwhile, imagining an optimistic image of the future creates a sense of parasympathetic calm and a view of a future self (Hass-Cohen et al., 2014).

One way to help mitigate the possibility of retraumatization is to encourage clients to represent the trauma from a third-person perspective, which contributes to psychological distancing. A third-person perspective is that of a bystander, for example, the adult who says, "I can see myself as a child cowering before my mother," rather than "I can see my mother looming overhead now." In the art experience, an aerial or bird's-eye view of the event can represent a third-person perspective, which is associated with reduction in anxiety (Brewin et al., 2010). Not to be confused with dissociation or depersonalization, this view mimics the third-person narrative perspective. A bystander or observer position can compartmentalize and contain past and present feelings about a specific memory. For example, a 9/11 survivor drew her memories of waiting to be let into her apartment after the event. From a bird's-eye view, she drew lines around herself to contain that experience (Hass-Cohen, Clyde Findlay, Carr, & Vanderlan, 2014).

Memories viewed from the third-person perspective may be less vivid and emotionally intense. They are more likely to be experienced as more distanced from the self (Sutin & Robins, 2010). Particularly for traumatic memories, this strategy can have a double edge as it can also interfere with the processing of relevant emotions (McIsaac & Eich, 2004). In this case, retrieving memories from the third-person perspective is associated with psychiatric problems and prolonged symptoms, and may be a way of unconscious restricting the painful emotions associated with them (Lau, Moulds, & Richardson, 2009). The difference between the two functions of the third-person perspective is most likely associated with deliberate protective intent as well as the timing in which this occurs. The restriction of dysregulating emotions is often shielding during the initial phases of psychotherapy but can be maladaptive in the long run. In other words, temporary use of this strategy may help make painful memories more accessible to a client who is easily overwhelmed. The third-person perspective may also promote a more abstract consideration of the memory, therefore supporting feelings of continuity with positive past selves rather than negative past selves (Libby, Eibach, & Gilovich, 2005). Overall, it is important to use caution when helping a client to recount a memory. If the client becomes overwhelmed by the recollection and is unable to connect with the positive aspects of the therapeutic relationship, the experience can be retraumatizing rather than helpful (Courtois & Ford, 2013).

Future research may ascertain the type of interventions and conditions that might prevent the traumatic enhanced reconsolidation of a reactivated memory. Alternatively, interventions are needed in order to support the reconsolidation of any balanced and/or faded emotive traumatic memory recall. Because of protein synthesis, these windows of opportunities close within 4–6 hours (Ledoux, 2000). Therefore, there is a need to observe a narrow time for memory reconsolidation-based interventions. Furthermore, it is likely that that successful treatment outcomes usually benefit from a combination of pharmacological and psychological treatments (Schwabe, Nader & Preussner, 2014).

From this perspective, therapeutic change in various theoretical approaches, including art therapy can be conceptualized as contributing to reconsolidating and updating of new memories. As stated earlier, essential components of creating therapeutic change include reactivating old memories, engaging in new emotional experiences that are incorporated in these reactivated memories, and reinforcing the change by practicing a new way of behaving in and experiencing the world in a variety of settings and situations. These therapeutic experiences pave the way to integrate new emotional experience into old memory through the continued process of reactivation, re-encoding, and reconsolidation (Lane, Ryan, Nadel, & Greenberg, 2014). By doing so, new rules or schemas (internal working models) will be updated allowing for more flexible ways of engaging and having emotional response. There is also evidence of an interplay between event memory and semantic structures. The degree to which change will be lasting will vary based on how generalized the reconsolidation of memory is. As the new memory is applied to broader contexts, it strengthens. It is important to note that the changes to memory that are made in psychotherapy are a complete renovation of all past elements of the memory, not just newly created memories or established semantic structures. Therefore, this renovation must include past cognitive schemas and linguistic rules resulting in a new way of experiencing the world. Practice and repetition, in and out of psychotherapy, help achieve and establish this new change. Again, the more contexts and ways in which the person practices these new memories, the stronger the therapeutic change.

EXPERIENTIAL PRACTICES AND DIRECTIVES

Experience I: Episodic Memory Cutouts

The Cutout activity provides an opportunity to demonstrate how internal working models are shaped by our personal attachment histories. Influenced by the Adult Attachment Interview questions (Hesse, 1999), we have structured it in such a way as to elicit an individual's reactions to significant autobiographical events. As stated earlier, adults with an insecure attachment style have difficulty accessing a coherent narrative of the past, especially of positive experiences (Hesse, 1999). Therefore, we ask the artist to create a single-

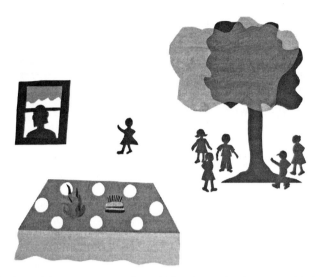

Figure 6.2 *The Birthday Party*, a memory from childhood created with cutouts in black construction paper and colored tissue paper. In the lower right on a pink table, there are white plates and the small orange and yellow tissue paper fire. Behind, a black silhouette of a woman stands at a window with an orange blind. On the upper right, silhouettes of children can be seen at the foot of a tree with green tissue paper. Lisa Cerrina

memory cutout about their experiences of love from their primary caregivers. We suggest that the images focus on episodic memories of caring that relate to childhood worries, illness, loss, anniversaries, and other similar events. The goal is to evoke perceptions of how the participants were cared for at these times (Figure 6.2).

> *The memory of my birthday party is an example of an episodic memory. It is a memory of "being there" that is set in space and time and that re-creates the state of mind that I was in when it happened (Carter, 1998). It is also autobiographical in that it was a specific personal event that happened in my past. . . . My birthday always landed on Labor Day weekend when our family was typically on our annual trip to Oregon to visit our relatives. The result being that I never was able to have a birthday party with friends at home. And, as a general rule, birthdays were usually just a family celebration. One year, I guess I must have talked my mom into letting me have a party, and I invited a few friends. I remembered that the table was set up in the driveway and while my friends and I were playing, the tablecloth caught on fire somehow. Having never had my own party, I remembered having had some anxiety that day over how my party would be*

received. Would my friends think that it was fun or boring? The little fire added some excitement, and I think it relieved some of the pressure I was feeling about whether my party was good enough for everyone. I chose to only represent the most significant images, which were the children, the table in the driveway, the fire, and the presence of my mom in the house. I have always been visually drawn to works of high contrast, so I chose to represent the images on black construction paper. However, I specifically remembered that there was a pink paper tablecloth and so I wanted to express the significance of that memory. And yet, I still wanted to maintain the power and drama of the black and white, so I used tissue paper to add a transparent layer of color, adding accents to the black silhouettes. Lisa Cerrina*

As the participants share the cutouts, we ask them to be aware of any lapses in their discourse. Concurrently, the listeners note the level of contingency and coherence in the autobiographical narrative according to Grice's maxims (1975, 1991; Table 6.1). The artwork above, *The Birthday Party*, called for the inclusion of a reflection on the artist's selfhood. Clearly depicted in the middle of the beautiful cutout is the birthday child, who was curiously absent in the first written reflection. These types of questions can be further explored in follow-up reflections:

I believe that my recollection of this memory was triggered by recent thoughts about my own children and how we have celebrated their birthdays. I have been thinking about how my own personal experience of birthdays may have affected the way that I have recognized my children's birthdays. As I created my artwork, I was performing a rehearsal in my mind of the experience. Although I really couldn't formulate the entire sequence of events, I specifically remember my anxiousness about the party and the excitement of the little fire on the table on the driveway. . . . I had forgotten a lot of the details of the party because the information had not been rehearsed over time. However, because of the art experience and the sharing of it, what I did remember became even further encoded in my brain as an updated memory. Revisiting the experience through both the visual and verbal processes expanded my perception of the memory by inviting me to think about it in new ways and update my memories. Lisa Cerrina

The idea is that while people cannot change the content of their autobiographical memory, healing opportunities are still available. They can change how they relate to their history as well as create a new context for the memory-related event; a safe sharing context. This process supports the acquisition of earned relational security. In accordance with Grice's maxims, the manner in which the art is shared with others is considered in terms of its quality, quantity, and how it relates to the content and the images in the artwork. The goal is to be mindful of any gaps within and between visual, verbal, or written narratives.

Experience II: Autobiographical and Relational Timelines

The autobiographical timeline, a chronologically drawn representation of important events in an individual's life, offers a means of intentionally accessing and exploring episodic memories and reenvisioning autobiographical memory. Drawing a middle line along a roll of unfurled paper, the participant marks important personal events with words, symbols, figures, and colors. Markers or colored pencils allow a flexible yet safe structure for this exploration.

Using the timeline at the beginning of treatment clarifies information related to the person's chronological history and symptomatology. This autobiographical timeline would typically access explicit semantic fact-based memories, such as entering and leaving school, employment, marriage, birth of children, and life cycle marker events, as well as the time when problems started. This plotting process may also reveal inexplicable gaps in temporal or thematic coherence, which provide clues to times of insecurity or disorganization. As the therapeutic relationship progresses during the middle stage of therapy, the autobiographical timeline events can be sorted, reordered, and rewoven by the art maker. Engaging with the timeline can become reparative through gap exploration and significant emotional investment. Updating a self-narrative helps clients and therapists weave together meaningful memories that visually reveal the self and cultural story or "life story schema" (Bluck & Habermas, 2000, p. 122). In addition, this exploration may promote the successful retrieval of forgotten details. Suck retrieval facilitate the development of causal coherence and cohesive life story telling as well as provides a positive sense of control over one's life and memory reconsolidation (Figure 6.3).

In Figure 6.3, Lauryn tells the story of a four-year-long romantic relationship. It spans from the time the two met on a snowy day, to moving in together, to relocating to California together, and to how they presently share professional and interpersonal spaces. There are no significant timeline gaps. The timeline succinctly depicts critical events and therefore has both relevance and meaning. When the person talked about her timeline, nothing was missing or incongruous with her art. Moreover, her discourse was a good fit with the quality, relevance, and manner of her art.

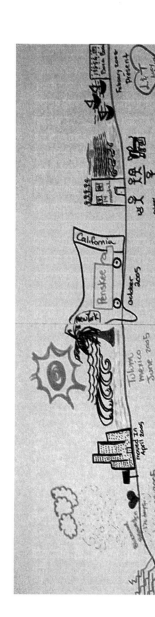

Figure 6.3 *Autobiographical Timeline.* From left to right, drawings of places and buildings are interspersed with colorful symbols: a blue snowy blizzard, a burning orange sun and beach, a seascape, boats, and simple figures. Moving to California. Lauryn Hunter

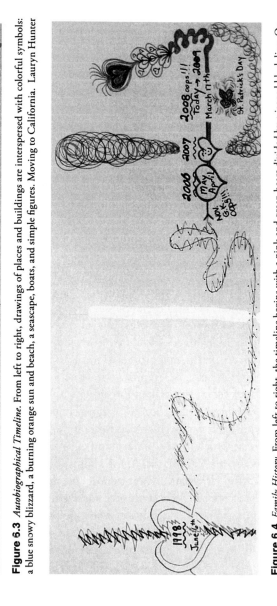

Figure 6.4 *Family History.* From left to right, the timeline begins with a pink and green heart divided by a jagged black line. On the right side, using the same pink, green, and red colors, is a series of smaller hearts and spiraling lines. Anonymous.

Looking at one's timeline requires emotion and affect regulation. This is a second-order experience, in that the participants explore their past while retaining an affective and cognitive hold on who they are now. One way to open a door to visit difficult feelings is to chart relation-based episodic memories. When discussing the autobiographical timeline, we touch upon the interface of attachment, autobiographical memory, and art therapy. The instruction to create an attachment-based timeline and illustrate episodic memories can be used for initial therapist-client introductions as well as for the midpoint and end of therapy work. To assist us in understanding the complexities of the interface of autobiographical memory and attachment history, we suggest viewing the film *Shanghai Ghetto* (Janklowicz-Mann & Mann, 2002).

In an area of approximately one square mile in the Hongkou District of Japanese-occupied Shanghai, about 20,000 Jewish refugees were relocated after fleeing from Nazi oppression in Europe before and during World War II. The refugees were settled in the poorest and most crowded area of Shanghai. Local Jewish families and American Jewish charities aided them with shelter, food, and clothing. The Japanese authorities consistently increased restrictions, but the ghetto was not walled, and the local Chinese residents, whose living conditions were often as bad, did not leave. The filmmakers focus on the stories of four survivors: Heppner and his Illo wife, Fred Fields, and Siegmar Simon. Present-day interviews with these four are intertwined with extraordinary images of Shanghai in the 1930s and 1940s. Survivors vividly describe suffering through the bitter Shanghai winter in rags and homemade sandals. Watching these adults recount their hardships and resilience opens viewers to hearing autobiographical narratives, identifying gaps, assessing attachment challenges, and ultimately working toward transcendent security.

The affective grounding provided by the creative activities allows many participants to state, process, and update a segment of their autobiographical narrative. The second timeline shows an example of difficulty and challenges, where a jagged line represents a history of familial substance abuse, recovery, and loss (Figure 6.4).

The artist deliberately depicted eight years of visual silence, represented by a large gap period. Her verbal timeline discourse met Grice's (1975, 1991) criteria for purposefulness, truthfulness, and coherence (Figure 6.4; Table 6.1). She stated that she did not think it was a good idea at that time to share all of her life history. Instead, she focused on more recent years. This intentional visual editing of the timeline shows her adaptation and resiliency.

During the elaboration of a timeline, the creator is called upon to sensitively notice patterns or gaps and add or rework relational constructs. Processing these kinds of episodic memories increases tolerance for difficult autobiographical information and subsequently consolidates new integrated, coherent narratives. The witnessing of this narrative by a supportive group or an attuned therapist allows the building of a stable self-narrative.

Sometimes we may want to consider questions related to the quality of the communication. As an example, the artists may ask themselves or a trusted other whether the timeline is a truthful depiction of what happened and if there is evidence for what is depicted. In this context, truthfulness means the opposite of dismissal and denial. Other questions pertain to the duration of the narration and quality of the content: "Is it succinct and precise or does the timeline have unexplained jumps and gaps? What is the relationship of the person to what happened? Is it relevant, meaningful or insightful? And does the story include significant others?" Finally, in terms of the manner of the depiction and the narration, "Is it clear and orderly (i.e., are the marks clear or confused)?" These questions promote a temporal, thematic, causal, and cultural understanding of the timeline artist's relational sense of security.

In one particularly illustrative example, Kirsten recounted a need to revisit her worker's compensation claim. Her new lawyer was asking her to resubmit her documented history, and she found herself resisting the task and experiencing some memory gaps. Noah suggested using the timeline to assist her in her process: "Draw a timeline that extends from the time the problem began to now. You can make a line and make symbols on it for each event, but I suggest also adding dates." Kirsten, a graphic designer, used a graph-like format on four 8½ × 11-inch pages fastened to one another with four yellow horizontal lines running at regular intervals. Like the output of an earthquake seismograph, she then plotted her physical and emotional well-being during the preceding year, focusing on the professional and physiological challenges of her arm and back pain and injury. The lines had several dramatic mountains and valleys with visual breaks and gaps. Kirsten provided a distressed narrative revealing a fearful and fragmented autobiographical self. This was the result of her battling physical injury alongside the stress of losing and retaining health coverage and preparing herself for legal action.

Kirsten also shared that the people in her life had always been a source of support. Together, she and Noah looked at the timeline from a relational perspective and saw that there were no people in it. She suggested that she identify what factors and people helped in her story and prompted her to use a positively associated color to fill in her tale. Noah also suggested that Kirsten alternate between fleshing out the timeline and approaching her paperwork task. With the reparative work of intentionally revisiting the memories and timeline to add missing information, helpful people, and resources in a consistent purple color, Kirsten was able to self-comfort and focus.

Hi, Noah. What a great experience. Just looking at the timeline moved me to act. It took me an hour to locate the paperwork I have been avoiding since October. The timeline actually had all the information I needed. I was able to find my case file and open it (sounds so easy!) and look at it to verify dates. I filled out the paperwork for several hours, took a break in the middle, as you suggested, and it all just seemed to happen. I was focused, comfortable, and the drawing itself seemed to support me, like a friend sitting with me. Then, as I filled out the paperwork, I began to add information to the timeline without thinking, then remembered the second directive. I began to draw the positive people/events into the timeline in my purple color. This totally changed the feel of the timeline, and served to weave into it the healing that was always there at every step, even when I felt like I was losing my mind. When I got to the end of the line, I realized the starkness of the red bolt at roughly now, showing my block in doing the paperwork. I thought about the purple, and felt compelled to wash all the red at that end with the purple, as that now felt more accurate. I purpled the bolt, the sweet little house lost to foreclosure, and purpled and spiraled around "new attorney" to change the way I was feeling about "starting over," assuring myself with words around the arrow that it's all okay. This softened my state. The directive allowed me to first complete the victory of moving through the block, and then allowed a place to celebrate it. Most surprising, though, was how just looking at my first timeline gave me whatever it was I was needing to move forward with it. Kristen Anastasia

Experience III: Compassionate Past, Present, and Future Timeline

Different versions of the directives that are related to compassion might be needed for individuals with disruptive attachment or trauma histories as they may have a fear of empathy and a foreshortened sense of the future. Therefore, the third experiential and directive which is to: "Draw your past, present, and future, as it they would be seen by someone who loves or cares for you or from a kind and supportive self-perspective," is sometimes modified.

As it is often easier to start with caring for another, a necessary preliminary step might be needed. For example, "Imagine and draw a future for someone you love or care for." Culturally, and for a traumatized person, it is often more acceptable or easier to care for someone else. These directives help join the self, other, and prospective functions of memory. Depending on the client's situation, the directive wording or sequencing might need to be further adapted, such as, "Draw your future, as it would be foreseen by someone who loved or cared for you in the past." Some very isolated individuals may not be able to identify a current or past caring relationship. Then the caring "person" could be a pet, a beloved person who has passed, or his or her therapist. When created within a safe relationship, this directive helps with revisiting, organizing, and further developing a self-narrative as it provides a source of reliance; the feelings of others who have loved and cared for the person. All variations of the directive include the following guidelines: "Taking three pieces of paper, draw a timeline on each. Each paper is devoted to one period in time: past, present, and future. Starting with any section that you like, make sure to put one event in each time period. See if you can draw each time frame from a compassionate perspective. Particularly for the future, draw something that a person who cares for and loves you might wish for you, or something compassionate that you would wish for yourself" (Figure 6.5).

> *For my first step, an image of my aging mother came to mind. I wished that she would feel tranquil and content with everything that she enjoys—reading, tennis, surfing, the countryside—all there for her within the embrace of the "carousel of time." The carousel is represented by a circle of family and friends. The chain of figures holding hands surrounds her, emitting caring. She embodies acceptance of change and time, realizing that some things will change but many important things remain the same. I felt centered after drawing this.*
> Lisa Smith

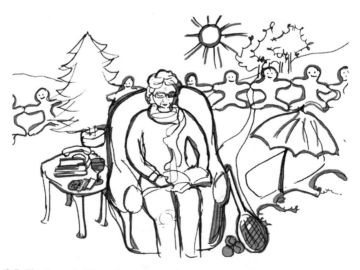

Figure 6.5 *The Carousel of Time*: Draw a future for someone you love or care for. In the center we see an older woman, Lisa's mother, drawn in green, reading. Next to her there are symbols for her pastimes: tennis, bridge, and enjoying the sea. Behind her outlined in orange there is a chain of figures and a bright sun. Lisa Smith

Using markers, each person begins by making their first step, an image of a future for someone they love. They are encouraged to imagine a beloved person or pet and to become aware of how they feel as they make the image. In preparation for drawing the past, present, and future sequences, the studio participants complete a sentence stem written on the back of one of their sheets: "I see my future through the eyes of [blank] because they/I can see my life in a loving manner." This helps them decide who would be wishing a future image for them (Figure 6.6).

When I thought of an image for a past moment on my timeline, I was surprised that I chose a moment 25 years ago when I was single and, unbeknownst to me, was just about to meet my future husband. Located in a park, I have my art materials, a book, and my beloved dog. When working on the past, a very clear image of myself emerged. I first thought that I would represent my family, and then I thought, no, it's clearly me on my own at a transitional moment. I found it harder to represent the present time in one image and was unpleasantly surprised that I was thinking about work. I first made symbols for my work, a laptop and a book, and then tried to find ways to show all the other parts of my life. I added four images for my children, my spouse, and myself, a small Buddha representing meditation practice, our two cats and the dog, a pot for cooking and nourishment, and boots for walking in the country. As I looked at it, I realized that I have accumulated a lot of emotional and physical stuff and drew boxes in the background to represent this cluttered feeling. I notice now how I outlined the symbols that relate to positivity in orange and that these exist across the three time periods such as sunshine and the family members. I also realize that my image for the present is

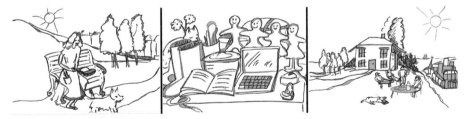

Figure 6.6 *My Sunny Life. Beginnings* (left), *Busy Now* (center), and *Beyond in the Future* (right). On the left, drawn in pale green, there is myself, a woman sitting on a bench in a park with books and a dog under an orange sun. The middle image, drawn in green and orange, is full of objects: a computer, boots, a cooking pot, and symbols of people. On the right, a family group drawn in green sit outside a house on a hill overlooking the sea with an orange sun in the sky. Directive: Draw a timeline for the past present and future. For the future, draw something that a person who cares and loves you might wish for you, or something compassionate that you would wish for yourself. Lisa Smith

crowded with many things, whereas the future has a more global view to it. The experiential reinforces my sense of my priorities and shows me how overwhelming my current life can feel. I began my drawing of the future thinking of what my children would want it to look like. The image is one of sunshine and shared time. The immediate image that came to mind was a welcoming family home with all the things we enjoy. I found this image enjoyable to make, as it could be like a dream with elements that did not relate to my life now. Those include the rural setting, the spacious house, and, more preciously, the time to come together after dinner and look over the mountains to the sea and a boat. It was interesting that I started with this image and then worked my way back. Lisa Smith

The group members then divide into role-play pairs with a familiar partner and share their drawings, switching between playing the therapist and the client. Mindful of the coherence and meaning of the client's narrative, the role-play therapist works with the role-play client to explore the art. One way to explore the art and narrative is to look for hyper-integration around negative meaning, which may be a trauma clue. Additionally, recognizing where there is obvious dissonance and disconnection across the images may provide relational insecurity clues. Conversely, a consistent and meaningful distribution of images across past, present, and future conveys coherence. Repeated positive symbols, which relate a connected story and a meaningful rendition of a future, reflect security and resilience. Being able to contextualize the memories by narrating the story and tolerating difficult emotions, as well as being willing to change the imagery as the story reintegrates, are also security indicators.

As Lisa talked about her autobiographical timeline, it became clear to her that she had avoided looking into her own future, choosing instead to focus on her children as she did for the first step, caring for someone else. The third, future image of a welcoming family home was an image made for others that were loved: the children and family. This allowed the role-play therapist to encourage her to make a new image: "The future that a loving person is imagining for you." Both she and her role-play partner acknowledged that although wonderful, it is easier to think about someone else. However, taking care of the self in the case of motherhood also means being able to take care of another (Figure 6.7).

Having discussed the possibility of making a new image for the future just concerning myself, I felt liberated to visualize myself as the focus. Here I am wearing the walking boots of my image of the present and

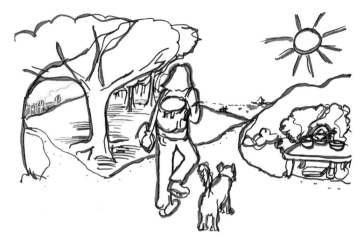

Figure 6.7 *My Future Revisited.* Drawn in blue and green, a woman heads down the right-hand path in a country setting. She is holding a book in her hand and has a dog by her side. To the right there is a small altar with a Buddha, and above her there is a full orange sun. Lisa Smith

am out with my dog in the country. I have my book and art materials and have just left a quiet spot for my meditation. Making this image felt invigorating. I am looking forward to my, and our, future, which is represented by the landscape. Lisa Smith

The therapist and client engage in a series of possible inquiries across different dimensions of autobiographical memory functions. An elaboration-based inquiry asks, "Who else was there, what else happened, and, more precisely, when did this take place and how did it feel?" A meaning-making investigation explores salience: "Why is this so important? What did it mean to you then? What does it mean now? What would this mean in the future?" A related attachment-based inquiry includes: "How does this image relate to your needs being met?" Coherency probes include an investigation of temporal coherence: "Please help me understand more about the order of events across your drawings," as well as an exploration of causal coherence, "Can you tell me a little bit more about how these images relate to each other?" A consideration of thematic coherence asks, "What themes do you think we can see across these drawings? These may be sensory, emotional, or symbolic." Inquiry into cultural and social status-derived coherence can come from questions such as, "In what ways do these images show how you have hoped your life will unfold?" More global, a consistency evaluation calls for further investigation: "How does this show you in the future, as connected to you now, and in the past?" After sharing and in role-play, the therapist asks if the client wants to add any more detail or resources to the images such as using different and supportive colors or redrawing the timeline. Similarly, discarding a page already drawn or adding other connecting pages across time are all options.

> *The exploration of the image from an attachment-based perspective showed me that I repeated the same theme in three of my images. The first step is about my children; the future drawing is about my family; and, in many ways, so is my second present image. The role-play therapist shared that the image of the future created dissonance for her as it seemed about me again caring for others. The image of the past, which clearly depicts myself as independent, is not coherently followed through—raising questions about who I will be when our children eventually grow up and leave home. The issue seems to be not that I do not know who I will be, but rather that I am not seeming to leave space for it. Interestingly, as I experienced this process, I noticed that the sunniness of the sun was carried over from the past to the future. In fact, the sun was in full bloom in the last image I made. Living in a cold climate, this singular sensory feeling carried me through and reminded me of who I was and am.* Lisa Smith

Each participant narrates the experience of how it felt to lay out, engage, and manipulate his or her memories and imagine the future through the eyes of a compassionate, loving other. This experiential seeks to put together the core functions of autobiographical memory, embracing the self, another, the future, and a social context. Self-agency is supported through the creator's active manipulation of the phases of his or her history. The artwork and story are narrated socially with another person, while a loving attachment environment is conjured up to imagine a future. Accordingly, a time can be imagined when the person's needs will be met. The comparisons and connections made across time help to augment change. In this case, it is the representation of the sun and the embodied sense of warmth that seem to carry some of the updated autobiographical narrative.

RELATIONAL NEUROSCIENCE: THE DEFAULT MODE NETWORK

Autobiographical self-memory prospection helps people imagine and direct their actions in the future. It is also involved in mentalizing and ToM, as its functions assist in understanding others. These two functions are neurobiological processes that are distinct from stimulus-dependent thoughts or behaviors. Stimulus-dependent responses are reactions to external events, whereas reminiscent, mentalizing thoughts are related to the self. Thus the self-social-directive prospection that we have discussed requires that the individual generate experiences that are separate from what is being experienced in the present (Spreng & Grady, 2010).

Functional neuroimaging findings further have demonstrated the complexity of autobiographical memory function, as it includes multiple processes: Construction, timing, recollection, and retrieval processes (Mar, 2011). Neuroimaging also provided support for the theory that autobiographical memory prospection and ToM share a common pattern of neural activity (Spreng & Grady, 2010). Self and social references direct the construction of autobiographical memory prospection, which is future oriented. This accounted for 81.42% of the covariance in the data. In another pattern, autobiographical self-memory and prospection were differentiated from ToM, which accounted for 13.75% of the covariance in the data. For example, research participants were first shown a photograph and prompted to remember a similar event from their own past. This resembled the process associated with the recall of autobiographical episodic memory. They were then asked to imagine a future event, engaging in prospection. Finally, they imagined the thoughts and feelings of a person in the photograph, which is a theory-of-mind function. In all three cases, similar patterns of neural activity were identified (Spreng & Grady, 2010).

Autobiographical self-referential processing occurs in the medial prefrontal cortex (mPFC; St. Jacques, 2012). Overall, cortical midline structures such as the mPFC are modulated by a degree of the sense of self in memory retrieval. The set of shared brain structures that are involved in the three functions of autobiographical memory, self-reflection on the past, future thoughts, and social functions, such as understanding the minds of others, are also regions of the default mode network (DMN; Spreng & Grady, 2010). Revealed by neuroimaging, the DMN is active during resting, which are daydream-like states (Catani, Dell'Acqua, & de Schotten, 2013). This neuro-anatomical network includes midline frontal and lateral parietal structures, and medial and lateral temporal-limbic regions (Spreng & Grady, 2010). The dorsal cingulum connects the anterior cingulate-medial prefrontal cortex and the posterior cingulate-precuneus (Catani et al., 2013).

In self-referential, autobiographical, and prospective memory, neuroimaging investigates activity across cortical midline structures. These include the dorsal and ventromedial prefrontal cortex (dmPFC and vmPFC), anterior and posterior cingulate cortex (ACC and PCC), and retrosplenial cortex (RSC), which are regions within the cingulate, the precuneus, which is located between the parietal and occipital lobes; the hippocampus, and the thalamus (St. Jacques, 2012; Summerfield, Hassabis, & Maguire, 2009; Figure 6.8).

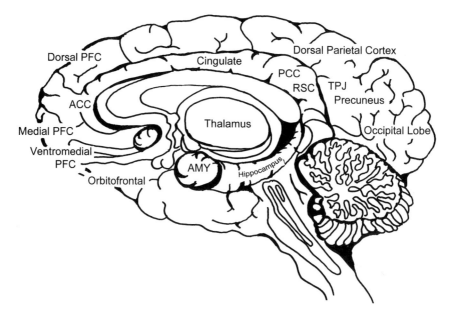

Figure 6.8 *Autobiographical Memory Structures.* The structures are midline frontal and lateral parietal regions, and medial and lateral temporo-limbic regions and occipital lobes. Autobiographical self and prospective memory functions include the dorsal and ventromedial prefrontal cortex (mPFC, dPFC and vmPFC), cingulate (anterior and posterior cingulate cortex, ACC/PCC), retrosplenial cortex (RSC), precuneus, (located in the cuneus, a cortical area between the lateral parietal, and the occipital lobe), hippocampus, and the thalamus. Autobiographical self only functions include the left-lateralized brain regions, lateral prefrontal cortex, dorsal parietal cortex, orbitofrontal cortex and the medial temporal lobe (not shown). Other involved structures are the vmPFC, dmPFC, and the right temporoparietal junction.

The vmPFC is involved in decision making, emotion regulation, and the processing of fear, while the dmPFC is associated with factual reasoning. Autonomic functions, decision-making, and emotion regulation involve the ACC. Linking emotions with autobiographical memory, the PCC is activated in autobiographical memory retrieval. Implicated in various cognitive functions, the RSC is involved in imagination, navigation, planning for the future, and episodic memory functions (Carlson, 2013). Adding to these linkages, is the precuneus that is responsible for integrating self-related information with past experiences and visuospatial processing (Freton et al., 2013). The hippocampus, the memory center, which is part of the limbic system and plays a role in spatial navigation and the consolidation of information from short-term to long-term memory assists in memory reconsolidation. Involved in the regulation of autobiographical sensory information and consciousness, motor control, and relaying information to the cerebral cortex is the thalamus. The linking of thalamic activation and the formation of the autobiographical self and prospective memories may indicate the role of sensory interventions, such as updating memories, connecting them, or decentralizing them through art therapy.

Self-memory retrieval involves left-lateralized brain regions, lateral prefrontal cortex (lPFC), dorsal parietal cortex (dPC), and orbitofrontal cortex (OFC). The lPFC is broadly involved in executive functioning while the dPC is involved in the intake of sensory information, in particular spatial information. Critical to positive autobiographical memory retrieval are the OFC functions (Piefke, Weiss, Zilles, Markowitsch, & Fink, 2003). This is due to its connections with the striatum in the reward system and novel memory formation (Frey & Petrides, 2002). Self-referential processing promotes awareness of the self in time and the construction of memory (St. Jacques, 2012). This ability is associated with understanding another person's perspective (theory of mind), and therefore the neurological components of each process overlap (St. Jacques, 2012). Linking this information suggests that the novel and positive aspects of art making can excite the formation of autobiographical memory updating.

ToM, and other related functions, involve the lateral temporal regions and right temporoparietal junction (Spreng & Grady, 2010). In terms of activity in the temporal lobe, self-referential remembering of the past, or thinking about the future, activates midline and medial temporal lobe structures, whereas other-referential ToM practices activate lateral temporal and parietal structures. There is overlap in brain activity in each experience, as well as some differentiated functions (Spreng & Grady, 2010). In comparison to ToM activation, autobiographical self-memory and prospection activate more frontal and parietal areas. There is also greater hippocampal activation for autobiographical memory and prospection, which may be due to the temporal dimensions of the activities (Spreng & Grady, 2010; St. Jacques, 2012).

The examination of autobiographical self-memory and theory-of-mind function also highlights the role of different parts of the mPFC. The lower region of the vmPFC is related to cognitions about the self, while the top area, the dmPFC is associated with thinking about another, rather than about facts, during theory-of-mind experiences (St. Jacques, 2012). This functional allocation may be due to the distinct difference between re-experiencing autobiographical events or thinking about facts, and shifting perspective to another point of view. In other words, there is a need for interventions that support shifting from retelling the self-story to thinking about others. Such ability to shift is also related to attachment functions. Perhaps for the securely attached individual, this shift happens more quickly.

In people without PTSD, the mPFC, as opposed to the medial temporal lobe network, drives memory construction (St. Jacques, 2012). Therefore, individuals with PTSD whose memory processes are driven by the medial temporal lobe (due to their sensitivity to sensory triggering cues and activation of the amygdala) have, as a result, difficulties with memory construction. This means that emotional regulation such as fears, interfere with memory construction. Therefore if the sensory aspects of art making are not associated with the original traumatic sensory meaning, it is possible that they provide connections with DMN function.

Complex autobiographical memory retrieval involves distinct brain regions that engage in different points in time (St. Jacques, 2012). This is because looking ahead (e.g., prospection or foresight) and here and now executive functions of cognition and memory, overlap (Sestieri, Corbetta, Romani, & Shulman, 2011). Schematically, the frontal regions (right lateral PFC) and midline and limbic regions (RSC, hippocampus), engage first. Then as the posterior regions (precuneus, visual cortex) engage, the frontal regions (left lateral PFC) reengage to process their inputs (St. Jacques, 2012). Shifting from conceptualizing what to draw, then drawing it, re-conceptualizing it, and finally naming the experientials, may activate and be rooted in such neurological processing. Elsewhere, we have also written about the process of shifting from right to left hemisphere as integral to art therapy (Hass-Cohen & Carr, 2008). However, we are not implying that these or other processes are exclusionary.

What is therefore known from these findings is that the allocation of neurological functions is also time dependent. The thalamus, hippocampus, left PFC, and visual cortex are involved in recollection, or re-experiencing and recalling contextual details of events (St. Jacques, 2012). The thalamus plays a strong role in memory recall and recollection, due to the strong connection between the thalamus and midline structures and prefrontal regions, the thalamo-prefrontal cortical network (Carlson, 2013). The hippocampus assists in temporal and spatial context recollection (Ranganath & Ritchey, 2012). It also incorporates sensory information from the thalamus (Pergola & Suchan, 2013). Recollections involve multisensory contexts and the ability to recall details, which depend upon the interaction of the hippocampus and other brain regions. There are additional linkages between the hippocampus and visual cortex for spatial context, and added interaction between the hippocampus and left PFC for temporal context.

Functional memory retrieval imaging which compared activity in regions activated by visual and verbal cuing (St. Jacques, 2012), supports our thinking that visual imagery impacts recollection. Visual autobiographical cues activate the hippocampus and critical regions of the retrieval network, including the lateral PFC, involved in retrieval control; the mPFC, associated with self-referential processing; and the ventral parietal cortex, linked to bottom-up attention processes. Furthermore, visual images amplify autobiographical memory retrieval by increasing connectivity in cognitive retrieval networks. Retrieval networks also activate in response to tasks, such as planning for and making art. These executive function networks are represented by the activation of prefrontal executive function brain areas, typically referred to as the task-positive network (Jung, Mead, Carrasco, & Flores, 2013; Spreng & Grady, 2010). The neural pathway linkages between autobiographical, cognitive, and executive neuronetworks suggest that art therapy may present helpful therapeutic opportunities for processing autobiographical memories.

As stated earlier, emotion also augments autobiographical recollections; there are increased connections between the amygdala, hippocampus, and lateral PFC during autobiographical memory retrieval (St. Jacques, 2012). Thus emotion and memory are connected through frontal, parietal, and limbic connections (Catani et al., 2013). Three functionally different networks are involved: (1) the hippocampus and the entorhinal area above it, which are involved in memory and spatial orientation; (2) the temporal-amygdala-orbitofrontal network, which integrates emotion into behavior and cognition, and is involved in sensory memory; and (3) medial sections of the DMN.

Positive and negative memories activate different areas, resulting in different neurological activity (Piefke et al., 2003). Positive memories result in bilateral activation of the OFC, the temporal pole, and medial temporal areas, along with reward system regions. The entorhinal region has the highest rate of activity, while negative memories increase activity in the right middle temporal gyrus (Piefke et al., 2003). The entorhinal region works in conjunction with the hippocampus and prefrontal connections to code and recall memory. This information may suggest that positive art making influences the updating of memories and self-change.

While autobiographical self-memories and prospection represent personally experienced and relevant information, mentalizing and ToM, are aspects of one's imagination (Summerfield et al., 2009). We have summarized evidence to show that the sense of self in past, foresight, and direction, and mentalizing, the ability to understand others are interrelated neurobiological experiences. It is therefore possible to deduct that there is a correlation between these three functions of autobiographical memory and attachment style. In other words, coherent representations of salient past memories contribute to increased personal ability to successfully put oneself in another's shoes. A secure internal working model of the past allows for feeling secure in one's understanding of another. These findings support the idea that the autobiographical timeline that we designed should indeed put together the three autobiographical functions in each directive. Together with attachment-based interventions, the neuroscience findings also lay the foundation for the theoretical binding of the self and the other in past, present, and future experiences.

CREATE PRINCIPLES AND CLINICAL APPLICATIONS

The primary focus of this chapter revolves around the CREATE principle of Relational Resonating. As stated, we contend that the ordering of the autobiographical art therapy experientials develops the capacity for relational resonance and provides opportunities for memory reconsolidation. We start with making an Episodic Memory Cutout and then linking together several memories to construct the two Autobiographical and Relational Timelines, and finally creating the Compassionate Past, Present, and Future Timeline. These experiences are then processed in a relational context through the sharing and narrating of the art with a trusted group or role-play partner. Throughout treatment, the three functions, self, social, and directive, often present as interrelated and not separate constructs. This means that as clients engage in the exploration of their past, we are, under the right therapeutic conditions, contributing to potential resilience and earned attachment; meaning increasing the clients' ability to see themselves in the future and interact with others.

The Episodic Memory Cutout directive is inherently embedded in the family relationships of the creator, and reveals clients' snapshots of early attachment experiences. The cutout format is particularly suited for this recall activity. This is because memories stemming from childhood through adolescence often present as stand-alone visual images or stories. As explained earlier, the singling out of images may be due to their emotional or developmental significance. Providing quick access to such fleeting personal memories, the immediacy of the cutout only requires an outline and one color. Fittingly, early memories often rely on a single sensory cue, such as a shape or color. What's more, the relationship with the therapist strengthens as the result of the client sharing such an image, helping to integrate into autobiographical memory. Using the cutout techniques is therefore a therapeutic strategy for revisiting positive memories as well as transforming and challenging them.

The Autobiographical Timeline strings together personal events. It provides an opportunity for the client to experiment with coherently narrating the self. In the subsequent reflection process, the client and therapist look at visual gaps and examine narrated incoherencies. This process-oriented, relational work supports reparation by filling in the gaps within a positive therapeutic relationship. In the Relational Timeline, the second type of autobiographical memory timeline, we suggest that the therapist query about positive and supportive relationships. The client then creates a compassionate autobiographical sequence. The directive is, "Imagine and draw your past, present, and future, as it would be seen by someone who loves or cares for you." As explained earlier, the client might be asked, "First imagine and draw a future for someone you love or care for." In creating these images, clients implicitly explore and process their internal working model of attachment. The request to generate and experience loving by others can increase a here-and-now felt sense of relational security. In essence, clients are crowding out negative relational memories and may be able to discard some of them and reconsolidate the memory. As they experience and hold in mind the compassionate witnessing art therapist, this active practice helps develop a secure and supportive working model for relationships. Thus, a client's exploration of autobiographical memories supports a secure relation-based theory-of-mind function. The invitation to experience past, present, and future compassion contributes to these functions; it is a transition from wishful thinking toward reality. The drawing of an autobiographical line, which happens temporally, depicting one event after another, may mimic how the brain processes autobiographical memory, thus effectively updating memory.

A coherent, cognitive, and secure emotional foundation for mentalizing and understanding intentions is needed to accurately attribute thoughts, desires, and objectives to others, and to predict or explain their actions. In that vein, the client has the opportunity to practice mentalizing through the compassionate directive.

Clients' abilities to access and share autobiographical memories will be influenced by their attachment style and history. Those with secure relational histories can use past positive memories for comfort, while those with less secure models or chronic trauma histories may experience difficulty evoking coherent past narratives. In recalling, projecting, and altering the timeline or images of the self in the past, present, and future, the directive function of memory is used to envision future relationships, promoting representations of secure and caring attachment experiences. Sharing with others, being heard, and having one's experience empathically felt reinforce emotional regulation.

Creative Embodiment is solicited in the active, creative processes of the art activities. The memory cutout requires cutting, pasting, and sorting, while the timeline necessitates unfurling, rerolling the paper roll, and revealing and protecting memory, as well as moving between time frames. Just like an old photograph of oneself, time is embodied by the art. In this form of self-generated time travel, clients can viscerally experience different self-perspectives. As autobiographical reminiscing involves visuospatial, parietal processing, the person seems incarnated, having the past join the bodily experience.

Whether or not the client meets this experience with denial or acceptance can be influenced by both timelines. Each one can either assist in transforming past emotional needs with empathy, or taking comfort in the past, which can alter the embodied sense of self. When memories of security are recalled, the emotional component leads to an increase in a sense of well-being. Conversely, when recalling memories of insecurity and of times when needs were unmet, the processing of these recollections with compassion can reduce stress and contribute to self-growth.

Revisiting discrete self-memories evokes Expressive Communicating. Personal, emotional experience is embedded in the representations of the artist's autobiographical memories. For example, the use of color in the Episodic Memory Cutout allows for the expression of basic emotions and supports the exploration of their meaning and impact on one's life. In addition, as one memory is called upon, it can link with others. Clients may be able to explore and understand how a particular childhood memory and others directed their lives. Depending on the impact of such memories, the therapist can assist in making them less, or more, vivid. The Autobiographical and Relational Timelines therefore provide the opportunity for the expression of positive and negative emotions, which also provokes the emergence of conflicts or ambiguity about one's history. After identifying these feelings, reminiscing most likely activates areas of the brain responsible for regulating anxiety. One way that the therapist supports such regulation is by assisting clients in differentiating between a single and a series of memories, identifying supportive affective episodic memories and connecting them together. This type of elaborative remembrance provides a base for secure storytelling and its reconsolidation. Like a parent, the therapist provides the client with additional information about the effects of negative and positive emoting. Using the Relational Timeline and the Compassionate Past, Present, and Future Timeline, in sequence and over time further enhances opportunities to self-regulate. Thus, the cluster of directives in this chapter may be divided into two main categories. The first, the Episodic Memory Cutout and the Autobiographical and Relational Timeline, allow for expression of positive and negative emotions, whereas the second cluster of directives repurposes these memories and assists in self-regulation and memory transformation.

This self-regulation supports Adaptive Responding by using episodic memories to fulfill coping needs. As the Autobiographical and Relational Timelines link significant memories together across a supportive visual line, the client has an opportunity to identify solutions and strengths that helped resolve problems in the past, or to imagine such solutions and apply them in the present. The recognition of whether or not one's security was threatened or one's needs were met reduces the impact of non-explicit fears. More specifically, recording on the timeline when and how self-determined goals, such as autonomy, relatedness, or competence, were met or thwarted at the time, can deactivate short- and long-term stress experiences. This is primarily because the recording of such events may assist in safely locating them in the past. Autobiographical self-memory functions to increase a sense of control, which contributes to create a clearer and more coherent sense of self.

Transformative Integrating of autobiographical memories entails incorporating past memories into the current sense of self while changing the flavor of the experience. This occurs in a therapeutic environment where the negative emotional experience of retelling a difficult episodic event is verbalized and shared, changing its context to a positive one. In other words, the context of the problem is changed. It is temporally connected and accepted through compassion and therapist support. It is also likely that drawing an autobiographical timeline, which happens temporally, depicting one event after the other, may mimic how the brain processes autobiographical memory, thus effectively updating memory. Based on the neurobiology of temporal and limbic connectivity, the hallmark of integrated memories is that they are familiar, abstract, and non-intrusive, meaning that they do not singularly stand out. Thus, as the client's difficult images lose their visual and sensory negative hold through repeated processing and desensitization, they also become integrated. These integrated autobiographical memories can then successfully serve to lead the person into a changed future. Moreover, it increases the capacity to use old information to generate alternatives. It is the clients' ability to clearly and consistently hold, narrate, and share self-referential verbal narratives that will cue the therapist to witness and support their transformation. This integrated change is represented as updated and newly imagined life scripts. For example, as one accepts that some typical developmental sequences may not have occurred, there is a growth in self-identity and control. Salient sensory and perceptual affective memories of art making become part of long-term self-memories and connect to others that are similar in theme or content.

The principle of Empathizing and Compassion is supported through an increased ability to successfully put oneself in one's own shoes as coherent representations of significant past memories are revisited. A secure internal working model of the past allows for feeling secure in one's understanding of another and increasing a sense of life's purposefulness. The compassionate future directive may for many clients, be a novel experience. As such, it has the capacity to call for attention and make a significant impact on the person, contributing to stability. Explicitly including compassion in autobiographical memory processing is particularly important for clients with traumatic memories. Compassion may serve as a protection from difficult memories and may decrease any depression that may arise as a result of the recall.

Thus interpersonal arts-psychology-neuroscience-based platforms that were reviewed and integrated in this chapter provide a practical and theoretical understanding of how the concrete task of autobiographical narrating and exploration support the development of effective mentalizing, and earned secure relationships and compassion for self and others.

CHAPTER 7

Expressive Communicating: Accessing Emotions and the Creative Unconscious

I had seen my daughters paint during various art classes throughout the years, but I hadn't any idea how freeing, seductive, and stimulating paint and brush could be. We became one, as if married. It seemed like a dance to me, I, on the crisp, virgin piece of paper, and the brush, tentatively meeting the paint for the first time. I dipped meekly at first, not quite sure what to expect, then I became bolder with my stroke and colors. I was transported to a more primal form of life.
Marguerite Lathan

EXPRESSIVITY REPRESENTS MOTIVATIONAL AND attention-concentrated states, which may or may not be conscious or explicit. As we focus on the CREATE principle of Expressive Communicating, we emphasize that creativity is an amalgam of fluctuating unconscious and attentive conscious states, which coalesce into novel meaningful expressions. Released from habituated art making, novel creations can have several significant effects. Creativity and expressive communication can help individuals benefit from exploring the complexities of negativity, satisfaction, and joy. Furthermore, engaging in expressive practices charges the brain's reward circuitry and has the potential to increase awareness and insight. Building on the second chapter's introduction of the brain's principle structures, this chapter covers several networks linking the limbic system and cortical regions.

Expressive art making processes can move people to access unconscious and implicit basic emotions. The basic emotions, such as fear, anger, and joy, disgust, and surprise are motivating experiences (Ekman, 1992). Generated by the subcortical brain region's reactions to sensory experiences, and interpreted cognitively in higher cortical regions, emotions are rarely experienced as separate phenomena (Siegel, 2012). In fact, the complexity of human reactions to life experiences interconnects emotions, feelings, and thoughts. Consequently, emotive function is represented by dense connections of subcortical and cortical regions and is experienced as an amalgam of cognitions and felt states. Perhaps this is why emotions can be so confusing and disorienting. Therefore, for the purposes of this chapter, we use the word *emotions* as inclusive of feelings and thoughts. In the same vein, and based on the review of affective and cognitive neuroscience research, we interchange the terms: a) explicit, conscious, and aware cognitions, and b) unconscious, implicit, and imaginative-creative emotions and states.

The intention to access unknown emotions and emergent imagery is innate to ATR-N practices. To demonstrate this innateness, we explore surrealism's techniques. These help capture the unconscious world of daytime dreaming, thus fostering the expression and exploration of emotions while stimulating non-directive and divergent creativity. These CREATE Expressive Communicating activities engage two main processes. One process occurs when random mark making assists people in accessing divergent imagery generated by unconscious or semi-unconscious reflective states. The other process occurs when conscious attention elaborates the same chance-based imagery thus making it explicit. Throughout both implicit and explicit processes, a creative transformation occurs through the transformation of the image.

Image-making techniques that favor chance outcomes provide for an entryway to emotional expressivity. Haphazard creations can free individuals from the constraints of habitual expression or critical art-based judgment or self-perceptions. The results evoke positive or negative basic emotions, as well as feelings of pleasure, surprise, satisfaction, and self-growth. We first focus on three non-representative, process oriented techniques that facilitate accessing and exploring creativity: (a) Scribble Drawing; (b) Dribble Painting, known as Decalomania, the Rorschach Blot, Implement Painting, and Frottage Rubbing; and (c) the Exquisite Corpse Folded Dual Drawing. These directives favor unexpected unconscious outcomes, juxtapositions, and discoveries through image making.

Consciousness expands with the exploration of the results of the unconventional techniques, contrasting images, dribbling paint, smudging, or layering colors. It is during this process that the artist decides what direction is desired for the chance-generated imagery. One example is interpreting what form the scribble suggests and deciding how to consolidate the image into a novel creation. Thus, unconscious-implicit and intentional-explicit expressions of emotions prompt creativity, affect regulation, and personal growth.

PROCESS ART-MAKING

The Surrealist art movement, which emerged in Paris in 1924, paved the way toward an understanding of how to freely express and release the conscious control of reason and art making conventions (Jones, 2012). Rooted in free association, dream analysis, and the unconscious, Freud's work inspired the surrealists to develop methods to liberate imagination and the philosophy and art movement of Dada influenced and espoused anti-rationalist awareness. In accordance, their artistic goals were to expose psychological truth by stripping ordinary objects of their normal meaning, often creating the extraordinary. Often dreamlike, the images formed visual juxtapositions, and had emergent and unexpected content, and nonconventional proportions. Examples include the ethereal imagery of Salvador Dali and René Magritte, and the free-form work of Max Ernst and Joan Miró. In the 1940s and 1950s, Jackson Pollock and Mark Rothko extended the exploration of antirational process art using large canvases and color. Laying his very large canvases on the floor, Pollock dribbled and splashed paint, pushing the limits of fine art boundaries. With no known bottom, top, or side, Pollock's canvases convey a velocity of heightened and changing emotional states. It is as if by using a very large form to hold many drips and dollops, Pollock aspires to release the paint from boundaries and form. The felt sense of his expression, represented by thin, floating blots, crusted small blots, and many other forms, is not cognitively available for interpretation. It is through this process that negative or censored emotions, such as anger or doubt, and exhilarating feelings simultaneously emerge, revealing moment by moment felt experiences.

A similar situation occurs for the observer of Rothko's gigantic, soft maroon-and-black block paintings, surrounded by the spacious canvas, it is as if one is being immersed in unconscious emotions. As Rothko said, "I'm interested only in expressing basic human emotions—tragedy, ecstasy, doom, and so on—and the fact that lots of people break down and cry when confronted with my pictures shows that I communicate these basic human emotions" (Barnes, 1989, p. 22). The focus on color and non-representational large-scale imagery can sidestep both form and the critical, analytical left-brain (Withrow, 2004).

Early in the development of our field, art therapists embraced the idea that deep-seated emotions exist in the unconscious mind in the form of images rather than words. Pioneering art therapist Margaret Naumburg (1973), focused on the use of simple art materials as a way of revealing the implicit. Both Judith Kramer (1971) and Hanna Kwiatkowska (1978) emphasized process art as an entryway into the dynamics of the unconscious. Contemporary Jungian approaches also encourage the stimulation of emergent imagery, as in Steinhardt's (2006) squiggle technique. Such expressive techniques are of great interest for ATR-N practices as they build upon non-rational playfulness to increase emotional expressivity and communication. Free from cognitive control, process art assists in integrating implicit emotions and imagery, embracing both negative and positive emotions, thus facilitating affect regulation.

The neuroscience of emotions seems to support the relevance of the pioneering art therapists' and surrealists' techniques for ATR-N microskills. Unconscious sensory-based and creative experiences closely link with thalamic-cortical activation. Central to mind-body awareness, the right anterior insular cortex filters emotive reactions to sensory inputs. Thalamic, amygdala, and visual cortex information is then propelled forward through the association cortices to frontal brain areas. These areas compute decisions, which influence the interpretation of limbic emergent emotional experiences and give way to expressivity. Cortically, the left hemisphere is biased toward positive emotions. It is highly influenced by functions of the reward system, which are activated by the pleasure of creation (Badenoch, 2008). The right hemisphere is biased toward negativity and avoidance. It is involved in early coordination of nonverbal communication and in determining interpersonal contexts and art-based activities (Chapman, 2014).

Central to understanding the phenomena of creativity is information from clinical neuroscience. Emotions are processed at the intersection of pre-consciousness areas and frontal brain areas responsible for deliberate actions. Then, as the person turns inward, preconscious, default brain areas are activated. This can happen prior to, or just after, engaging with the outside world (Jung, Mead, Carrasco, &. Flores, 2013). After paying attention to new or exciting stimuli, the brain seems to return to a resting state called the default mode network, which holds divergent creative reflections, whereas the frontal brain is responsible for decision making and action. Internal reflection also activates temporoparietal junctions, which are involved in dreamlike states, and divergent and novel thinking. Ethereal states which are processed in temporoparietal regions, and in subcortical and cortical regions contribute to the integration of emergent emotions, and executive decisions. This integrative function characterizes the capacity for creativity. This integrated implicit-explicit amalgam is an ATR-N agent of change, as the processes of approach and effort, reflection, consolidation, and expression generalize into daily life.

EMOTIONS AND THE UNCONSCIOUS

From an evolutionary perspective, emotions govern both behaviors and motivation (Panksepp, 1998). Positive emotions signal behavioral approach and contribute to an increased desire to repeat the experience that generated positive excitation (Harmon-Jones, 2007; Allen, 2012). This is not always a desirable reaction. An example is the craving for more drugs. In contrast, negative affect is associated with behavioral aversion and avoidance, defensiveness, and decreased motivation. Basic emotions have both behavioral and emotional-cognitive motivational functions. For example, while anger or fear can propel people to approach situations aggressively, the underlying motivation is aversive. Norris, Gollan, Berntson, and Cacioppo (2010) describe three models of emotions to explain human experiences: discrete emotions, dimensional emotions, and evaluative constellations.

Discrete emotion theories identify specific emotions, which are associated with specific physiological and behavioral characteristics (Panksepp, 1998). Six discrete emotions accepted by most researchers are happiness, surprise, fear, sadness, anger, and disgust (Ekman, 1992). Other dimensions are (a) designation of a specific emotion as either positive or negative; (b) emotional arousal, indicating high or low intensity (Russell, 2003); (c) emotional-motivational responses, signaling approach or withdrawal (Carver & Harmon-Jones, 2009; Hugdahl & Davidson, 2002); and (d) emotional dominance, indicating the feeling of being in control versus being controlled (Bradley & Lang, 1999).

Categorizing emotions as positive or negative may not fully account for the complex functions of affect expression and emotional experiences (Norris et al., 2010). This is because attractive/positive and aversive/negative emotions can coexist. Therefore, positivity and negativity most likely exist on two separate continua rather than one with two opposite poles. Then as positivity and negativity interface, they affect us independently and mutually affect each other. Quite frequently, oscillating between negative and positive emotions creates a blurred but stable state of ambivalence that can be uncomfortable yet can prepare one for any challenge. Complexity forms as positive or negative reactions are not absolute. For example they are influenced by the preceding emotions. In addition, individuals have a different threshold for negative or positive reactions.

The above framework explains the conflict between approach and avoidant behaviors as coexisting states (Norris et al., 2010). From an evolutionary standpoint, immediate evaluation of a constellation of emotions in any given moment is needed. For example, the bias toward negative emotions is biologically sustained by the evolutionary need to be alert to threat. This aids in recognition and differentiation between threatening or friendly situations. In fact, the human affect system has evolved to be exquisitely attuned to negativity and avoidance (Cozolino, 2010). Such rapid and usually automatic negative reactions happen at a subcortical, unconscious level, which extends across all of the five senses. Applied to varied kinds of nonverbal or verbal stimuli, it affects how a person learns about and responds to the environment. In other words, people are primed to pay greater attention to unpleasant stimuli than to pleasant stimuli (Siegel, 2012). This is the preferred initial information processing response. Surprisingly, in the absence of danger, negativity, or novelty, our default state is to be neutrally curious, which supports positivity and creativity. Enlisting inquisitiveness and a high awareness of resources, this state gives rise to positive emotions and to approach-based rather than avoidance-based behaviors. As stated earlier, individuals have a different threshold for how neutrality, positivity, or negativity coexist and, as a result, may have different meanings attached to emotional situations. As explained in Chapter 4, threshold levels are most likely connected to their attachment history and styles. However, research suggests that for most, there is a slight advantage for the positive default state (Norris et al., 2010). From an art therapy perspective, this understanding explains how the dynamic interplay of negative and positive emotions, and the maintenance of a non-threatening therapeutic environment, can help individuals approach creativity and change.

EMOTIONS, COLOR, AND THE UNCONSCIOUS

Art therapists have acknowledged the important role of color in emotional expression (Hollins, Horrocks, & Sinason, 1998; Kellogg, 2002; Malchiodi, 1998a; Stern, 1955). The attraction to certain colors signifies particular emotional meaning (Burkitt & Newell, 2005; Furth, 1988; Lev-Wiesel & Al-Krenawi, 2000; Wu, Chang, & Chen, 2009). Furthermore, Rorschach (1951) and others (Exner, 1980; Luscher, 1971) have suggested that colors reflect the irrational, unconscious layers of an individual's personality. While color symbolism is closely linked to emotions, there is no universal agreement about the emotional meaning of specific colors (Golomb, 1992; Kersten & van der Vennet, 2010). Biologically, colors are frequently associated with immediate and concrete universal sensory experiences, such as bodily fluids and temperature. The same colors are also imbued with universal and individualized emotional significance, such as red, which may denote not only warmth, but love, passion, and perhaps anger. When combined with other colors, meaning is enhanced or transformed. For instance, red and black often symbolize hurt and pain, whereas red and green signify festivity. Color combinations such as black and white are diametric opposites that are also bound by culture. Black communicates finality, darkness, and weight, while white indicates lightness and expansiveness. In contemporary Western culture, black is thought to conceal, portraying hidden, fearful, or bad experience in addition to symbolizing emptiness, death and mourning. On the contrary, in Chinese traditions, white signifies death and is worn for funerals, and in Native American culture, black is positively associated with fertile soil.

Color can be an indicator of a person's emotional traits or states such as at a particular moment in time (Kellogg, 1992, 2002). Colors and forms bring an individual's patterns of psychological, developmental, and physiological development to light. According to Kellogg's MARI® system, deep red symbolizes mother, while the color blue symbolizes father. When these colors are applied to a target's shape, these colors may be signaling a personal history of conflict during adolescence or any oppositional feelings. The understanding of color as a phenomenon that cannot be separated from form and size prompts the idea that emotions, cognitions, and feelings are also an amalgam. Furthermore, they may change moment by moment and across the life span, contributing to the complex functions of affect expression.

CREATIVITY AND THE UNCONSCIOUS

Unconscious processes play a critical role in creativity (Andreasen, 2011). Creative processes, which are often anecdotally identified, seem to occur when the person is not actively forcing the process. Thus, the creative process is implicit, meaning that it arises from what has been named the unconscious. Historically, an artist or scientist often describes a dreamlike or diffuse state of reverie in which a muse provides inspiration. Furthermore, creative individuals often report that the early stage of art making begins with a gathering of diverse elements or materials. This assembly continues through a type of unfocused and relaxed period of incubation. Shielded from awareness, it is within this gestational period, that connections are made and inspiration arises. From this point forward, awareness becomes conscious insight, a solution or plan of action is found, and such insights are applied (Andreasen, 2011). Art therapist Pat Allen shared how she assembles art materials, setting an intention to be open to the unknown by allowing herself to make marks in a playful way that "lets the painting paint itself" (1995, p. 31). She then sets the art aside to contemplate what was made, the meaning of the colors used, and how her body felt, and then she elaborates on the final image.

An archetypal account of the creative process is illustrated in the story of Archimedes. As he was soaking in the bath, he found a solution to the problem of whether an irregularly shaped golden crown was made of pure gold or an alloy. He had a flash of inspiration, leaping out of the bath shouting, "Eureka!" (Greek for "I have found it!"), running out of his house naked and elated. Did the idea that the amount of water displaced is directly proportionate to the mass of an object come from observation, or was it because he was in a relaxed state in his bath? Like Archimedes, artists may report not knowing where their ideas come from. In addition, clients say that their creativity is uniquely personal and is not linked to other peoples' experiences (Andreasen, 2005). Despite feeling relaxed in this free-floating state, the brain's association cortices are likely working at a neural level. Schematically, association cortices are regions of the brain that run from subcortical sensory processing regions to the higher cognitive areas. They actively connect the soup of verbal and nonverbal visuospatial and tactile associations. Accordingly, it seems that many great insights come when people are relaxing. Newton and Buddha; whose insights reportedly came when one was sitting in water, and the other was sitting under a tree in nature, are historic examples. As explained in the neuroscience section, the oscillation between inward-bound and active outward states generates such visions.

Creativity can initiate and terminate, giving rise to a new cycle. The MARI® Mandala circle of creativity (Kellogg, 2002) exemplifies the cycle of an idea or project running its course, dissipating, and ending through the transformation of symbols. Ideas seed and germinate in the lower half of the circle, which contains the unconscious processes of diffuse cell-like elements. As they spiral and differentiate, the shape of an idea is born. The upper half of the circle contains symmetrical shapes that symbolize the conscious struggle to formulate an idea before it is expressed. These archetypal symbols of the beginning of unconscious processes do not have an identifiable center, and describe a movement from a weblike mesh through a swirl of diffuse elements to a conscious and centered symbol. Fully-fledged forms, such as an intricate petal flower designs, represent the climaxing of creativity. From there, the full bloom slowly fragments, as a center in the symbols disappears, pausing in a divergent, seemingly chaotic state waiting for germination to resume.

Creativity represents the ability to develop new concepts, ideas, and useful inventions, and to make objects or art. Historically, creativity has enabled humankind to discover solutions to environmental challenges. Creating a large number of divergent responses to a novel quest engenders fertile ideas. While initially expressed as multiple possibilities, these responses effectively converge into one solution. These are the moments before putting "pen to paper"; the divergent and creative moments when all possibilities are probable. The process requires a moment of freedom and mentalized reflecting in which the artist turns inward and illuminates in his or her mind all the imaginative options. Creativity continues when the process concretizes to multiple lines, shapes, colors, and then converges to produce one possible solution. The studio experiences described in this chapter illuminate this conceptualization.

EXPERIENTIAL PRACTICES AND DIRECTIVES

Experience I: Accessing Emotions and the Creative Unconscious

Our first surrealism-inspired technique is Automatic Drawing or Scribble Drawing (Steinhardt, 2006). Taking soft lead pencils and a large sheet of paper, our participants are given the invitation to:, "Let your pencil move randomly across the paper without lifting your hand off of the page". Based on variations of traditional art therapy methods (Kramer, 1971; Kwiatkowska, 1978; Naumburg, 1973), we suggest that no deliberate marks are made or forms represented. The artists can turn the page clockwise or counterclockwise with their other hand and draw while looking at a point ahead of them or while closing their eyes in order to turn inward. The idea is that by applying chance and accident to mark-making, the drawing is to some extent freed of rational control. The results can be novel or surprising. It is sometimes necessary to try this technique several times, using large sheets of paper to facilitate the process (Figure 7.1).

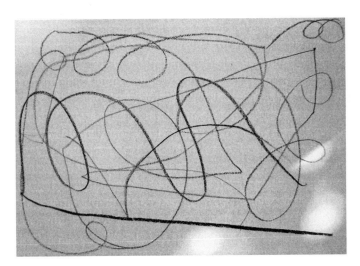

Figure 7.1 *Scribble Drawing.* A tangle of loops and swirls made in charcoal is underlined by a strong horizontal line. Joanna Clyde Findlay

I was deliberate in not looking at the page as I scribbled with my right hand, meanwhile turning the page with my left. When I looked down, I again found the scribble I had made dull and flat looking. It showed me how I had internalized an image of a witty Picasso or Miró scribble, alive with contrast, that I had not achieved. I was left with the reality that random lines may often give uninspiring images. I immediately noticed my attention rushing to find a satisfying symbol or image inside the tangle, as if it was hard to simply be with a frustrating image. So it is maybe that making a scribble and easily accessing the imagination is not so simple. One thought is that I created it alone, without the presence of a therapist. For example, art therapy scribbles are often described by Kramer as a process that the therapist observes or engages with. I am not quite sure. Joanna Clyde Findlay

For the second technique, Decalomania, we pour one dark color of well-mixed liquid paint into a small bottle or paper coffee cup with a pinched rim. We ask the studio participants to: "Dribble or pour paint onto a large sheet of heavyweight white paper. Then cover the first sheet with another sheet and rub them unevenly with your hands in order to spread the paint, and then peel the pages apart to reveal the unplanned blot-like print" (Figure 7.2, left).

Using a series of premixed acrylic paints with different hues moves us into a symbolic exploration of colors and a chance melding of liquid paint, as in Pollock's painting technique (Figure 7.2, right).

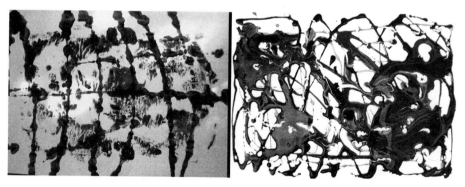

Figure 7.2 *Playing with Paint.* Decalomania, on the left, involves taking a print of the poured paint, resulting in a one-of-a-kind final imprint. Blue and black colors were used. On the right is a gray-and-white dribble painting, where the fluidity of the paint, its thickness and thinness, become the center of attentional focus and manipulation. Joanna Clyde Findlay

I had thought that you just take the paint, pour, blot, or manipulate it. In fact, I found out that I wanted first to play with the suitable consistency of liquid paint, as it greatly affected the results and my feelings about the process and the art. I realized that I enjoyed preparing different pots of paint and became dreamily entranced by the sensory qualities of a thick custardy black, a creamy glossy gray, or a shiny milky white. It was amazing how glossy and wet the black was. I really liked the "wet." It felt like playing with water in a sandbox. When I poured and dribbled, I could not predict or control how the colors would fall, and my attention would be suddenly caught by a lovely dreamlike blend of two liquid tones. I found that the process had different tempos. At times, my attention was deliberate and time seemed to slow down. Then, when my focus was loose, things seemed to happen quickly. When I pulled back the upper page to find the Decalomania print, sometimes I was disappointed that the original dribbles seemed dulled and blotted. It seemed that I was in a hurry to look at it and quickly lost interest in the print-off process, although I was sometimes surprised by the transformed and softened beauty of the skeletal image that emerged. Perhaps because it reminded me of a skeleton of a person, I wanted to distance from it, as I don't really want to see dark spots on an X-ray. In contrast, in the dribble painting I kind of wished it would stay wet and not dry so that the glossiness would not disappear, wanting to hold time in the present. Joanna Clyde Findlay

The consistency of the dribbled paint invites playfulness and the going backward and forward between conscious and unconscious states. This process has been re-envisioned by neuroscience as an oscillation between concentrated attention and default creative resting states. Delving into creativity is supported as diluted paint leaves watery splashes, and creamy paint pours rich and viscous paint splats. Different strands of dribbles can bleed into each other and intermingle, creating unexpected tones, which call our attention to new forms. The process of dribbling paint is an invitation to novel experimentation. Furthermore, the liquid paint provokes strong emotions, capturing attention and concentration. This unpredictable result, often highly contrasted between color tones and the white sheet, calls attention to new associations, while simultaneously creating more associations and increasing creativity. Decalomania dribble art invites a range of small to large movements. Larger sheets allow for expansive arm movements, greater directions in which one can work on the image, and full-body action when placed on the table or floor (Figure 7.3).

Figure 7.3 *Playing with Transparencies.* Made as a mono print with black, blue, and purple diluted blobs and dribbles of paint, different densities of color give the impression of floating forms. Joanna Clyde Findlay

> *I found that the more liquid the paint was, the more the colors would blur and mingle as I poured. When peeling off the upper sheet to form a print, these images would be more diffused and dreamlike. The more transparent the images, the more my associations go to movement and change. My mind seemed to tolerate not finding a "meaning" more easily when the images seemed to float and dance.* Joanna Clyde Findlay

A variation on the Decalomania technique is the third experience, the Rorschach Blot. The directive is: "The page is folded, then opened, and paint is poured onto one side. Then the page is refolded over the paint and smoothed by the hand." When opened, the paper may reveal a Rorschach-like image or partially symmetrical form, like a coronal section of a brain. The image's unexpected graphic nature stimulates positive or negative emotions, compelling some to approach and driving others away, stirring avoidance and a desire to cover it up again. This method differs from the Decalomania technique, as the opening and closing of the page creates symmetry, which is both pleasing and more easily associated with butterflies, faces, and body parts (Figure 7.4).

> *For the Rorschach image, I chose to make multiple prints. This was freeing as each one was fresh and different, and it was exciting to see each one divulge its mystery. The Rorschach-like images were often dramatic and bold, and I found my mind immediately sought to find*

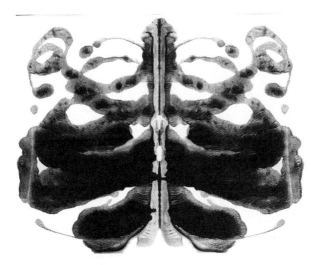

Figure 7.4 *Coronal Brain Rorschach-Like Painting.* Made by pouring thick liquid black paint on one side of a folded page that was then pressed over, then opened, a moth-like image or cross section of a brain with different depths of black and gray can be seen.   Joanna Clyde Findlay

associations: a face, a strange figure, or an animal. This image is to me a magical primitive creature. It reminds me of images in fairy-tale books that I read as child. These books had amazing tangles of black and white silhouettes. So the process took me back to pleasurable childhood experiences, while at the same time edging on the sinister—like children delighting in the possibility of experiencing a thrilling sensation while at the same time knowing that they are safe, as these images are pretend images—in a book, on a page that can be folded over and closed when I do not want to look at them again. As an adult artist, it opens my eyes, or perhaps I should say my inspiration, to images that I would not otherwise access.   Joanna Clyde Findlay

Using another large sheet of paper and liquid color paint, we ask the studio participants to: "Paint with found objects, such as sticks, sponges, knotted string, and buttons, or with the fingers of your non-dominant hand." To avoid being controlled by a pleasing image they turn the page clockwise as they work. In this fourth experience, integrating implements originally designed for other purposes, such as a plastic knife, or using the less skilled hand can also provoke feelings of boredom, frustration, or accomplishment, which may represent a sense of loss or gain of control. Thus the art making illustrates how emotions are associated with the need to define dominance and reflect our evolutionary need to be in control of our environment (Figure 7.5).

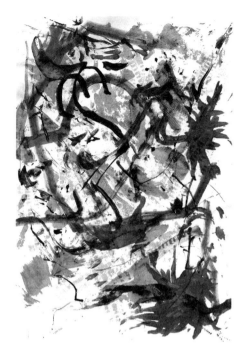

Figure 7.5 *Implement Painting.* In fully saturated primary hues, on a background of light blue patterning, smears of navy blue, dashes of bright yellow, and dashes of black fill the page. In the lower part of the painting, two fiery red explosions dominate. Joanna Clyde Findlay

I found painting with implements surprisingly difficult, as the marks I made often seemed hard to prolong on the page or distinguish. The effect of using sticks or a plastic knife, cut-up sponges, cork, or straws was often disappointing and boring. I did not like feeling bored. . . . I am not sure as to why and what that was about. Perhaps I have these expectations that it should be exciting and that I will always make something satisfying that I can control. I then decided to use my nondominant hand, turn the page simultaneously with the other, and use fully saturated primary colors. When I remembered I could paint with my fingers, I was able to reconnect with the sensory vitality of paint, and I was no longer in my thinking mind, but feeling and playing. It was as if doing so switched my need for intentional control to the surprise of images created by hazard. The image I found at the end had become otherworldly, vibrant, dramatic, and surprising.
Joanna Clyde Findlay

The work of surrealist Max Ernst (1891–1976) inspired the final fifth experience, the Frottage Rubbing technique. He placed objects under a canvas layered in paint, and then scraped back the paint on the corresponding raised areas of the canvas. While paint is an option, we suggested to the artists to: "Take a medium-weight sheet of paper, place it over every day textured

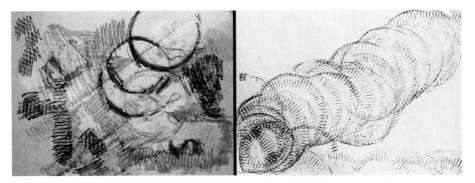

Figure 7.6. *Frottage* (left) *Random Rubbings and Repeated Rubbings* (right). In random rubbings there is a patchwork of aligned shapes made in bright green, yellow orange, and purple. Identifiable objects can be discerned; one can see two pair of scissors, the circular rim of a paper plate, and a box of crayons. In repeated rubbings, lead pencil rubbings from the rim of a paper plate make up the head and body of a plump caterpillar. Joanna Clyde Findlay

surfaces and unusual objects, and then rub the paper with lead pencils or very soft oil pastels." We encourage moving the page, merging rubbings from different surfaces, and overlaying textures, colors, and pressures (Figure 7.6).

> *Making this image brought back memories of childhood trips to old buildings and making rubbings of ancient wooden or stone walls, friezes, and doors with pale waxy crayons. I realize it was more satisfying to rub over an identifiable object like a pair of scissors because I immediately got a recognizable and gratifying image. My exploration of textures provoked my desire to discover rubbings that were pleasing. It was curious how often I found my brain searching for meaning and patterns. Staying with random marks seemed to stir feelings of unease or conflict, as if the pleasure of the act of rubbing was competing with discomfort with images that did not come together. Using the same object as the basis for my second frottage immediately felt restrictive, as I realized I had begun to enjoy the hazard of revelations in my other activities. I felt myself swinging between feeling controlled by only using one object and then becoming drawn into the pleasure of seeing the caterpillar's face emerge out of the layers of rubbings.* Joanna Clyde Findlay

Experience II: Communicating the Unconscious

For the second stage of the activity, each group member gathers together everything that has been created. We ask them to: "Explore each unexpected image by continuing to paint and draw them." We encourage following the emergent images, using emotional processing rather than focusing on the result. Thus, the artists avoid being carried away by finely honed art skills and resist dismissing an image as meaningful because it was made by chance.

Accessed at this level of processing are direct experiences of wanting to approach or deliberately avoid labeling feelings, shapes, colors, and symbols. To remain aware of these shifting perceptions, we suggest that the participants pay attention to which colors they use, what the image looks like upside down, and how their body and breath feel as they add color. Alternatively, defocusing the eyes or closing them retains the connection to the original art process.

Overall, an attitude of gentle discovery retains some of the diffuse, unconscious creative state that was experienced during the original image making. This approach unfolds by way of being aware of both background and foreground, and then working to shift between the gestalt of the form, its details, and the meaning that the art holds. Reworking the art then encourages incorporating a layer of consciousness. Such awareness remains open to possibilities while at the same time actively operating to arrive at a personally significant ending.

Joanna described how adding color and searching for a stable meaning for her Rorschach-like image stirred strong feelings of apprehension. This was because during its creation the dark image kept shifting (Figure 7.7).

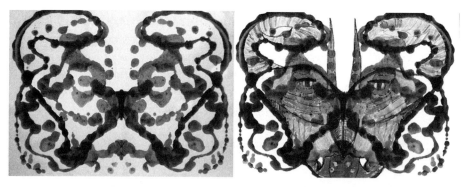

Figure 7.7 *Rorschach Original* (left), and *Rorschach Explored, Her Mask* (right). The Rorschach original is made of liquid black drips of paint in curving lines and blobs. In *Her Mask*, the curving forms have been filled in and textured with gray and brown pencil and pastel. Pointed horns have been added and a face has been elaborated with bright red circling staring eyes and bright red open mouth with fangs. Joanna Clyde Findlay

> *I scanned my Rorschachs with excitement, looking for ones that spoke to me. I found that at the same moment that I would find the image I wanted to make apparent within the dribble, I would lose it and see another form. I simultaneously saw a lion's face, a monster's mask, and rearing scorpions, all aversive and dark. My attention moved back and forward between the indistinct and the clear. Adding deep reds and grays to the black stirred ferocious strong feelings and helped me to access the intensity behind the monster I revealed. This activity was effective in helping me stabilize and relate to my more high-intensity aversive feelings.* Joanna Clyde Findlay

Identifying, recognizing, and responding to symbolism engages the making of visuospatial and cognitive-emotive based connections. For example, Joanna saw her reworked image as a type of mysterious mask. Thus, the second stage embraces the full creative cycle consisting of both the unconscious and the conscious. Once diffuse emotions are recognized, moving to the full spectrum of dimensional and discrete emotions, feelings and thoughts can occur. For example, participants often describe that upon attending and adding to their Rorschach Blot they can identify with one of the six discrete emotions, such as surprise or fear. Tangling lines from the Scribble Drawing are colored with paint, pencils, or pastels, and the images reveal unknown worlds, landscapes, profiles, and creatures of the mind (Figure 7.8).

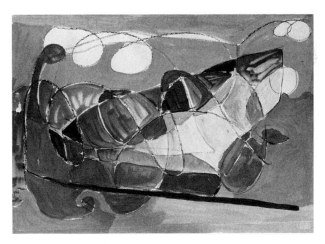

Figure 7.8 *Explored Scribble and Paint.* A blustery seascape can be seen, with a bright blue sea with curving waves in the lower right. A dark brown pier juts out from sandy beaches and grassy green cliffs. Above, a light blue sky holds soft white clouds (see Figure 7.4 for original scribble). Joanna Clyde Findlay

What had been an uninspiring mass of lines became pleasurable to explore with paint. At one point the lines coalesced and I saw a landscape with a cliff, sea, and sky. Filling in blocks of color became a playful, whimsical experience, which was relaxing and enjoyable. Finding an image of a coastal seascape reminded me of recent vacations and agreeable associations with the carefreeness of summertime. It was curious how I had become transported to feelings of spaciousness by adding color and finding meaning. Joanna Clyde Findlay

A textured stimulating surface emerges from patterning, smudging, and crisscrossing implement painting marks. Touching the texture brings direct awareness to the bodily sensations, whether pleasant, unpleasant, or neutral. Now, an internal debate may arise within the artists, perhaps liking the activity and their creation, or not liking it. Various expressions of the pulls and pushes of the positive and negative feelings occur in the process. Reactions can shift between comfortable mastery and an enhanced new vision for an image on the one hand, and a feeling of defeat and even wanting to leave the studio on the other hand (Figure 7.9).

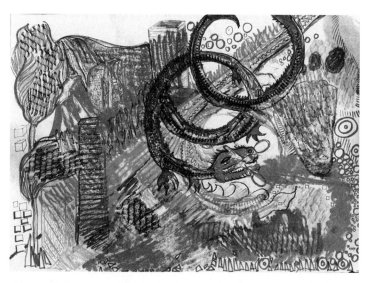

Figure 7.9 *Reworked Implement Drawing Using Colored Pastels and Markers.* A densely worked tapestry of textures in greens, yellow-oranges, and pink reveals a fantastical landscape with buildings and trees to the upper left. In the center, a scaly green dragon with a bright pink head and claws seems ready to pounce. Joanna Clyde Findlay

> *As I allowed my attention to wander from area to area of the frottage drawing, I found I became playful. It was like a puzzle that I could unfold piece by piece, and it did not need to make sense. That sensation was very liberating. It was almost like doodling, letting each area of the image become more detailed and fanciful. I found my attention once more zooming in on details, then pulling back to see the whole. It was relaxing and enjoyable.* Joanna Clyde Findlay

Reflecting in a large group facilitates a discussion about the unique and subtle interplay and creative transformation of emotions. Many group members report being able to distinguish between disliking the product and enjoying the creative process. This dislike and joy are arousal-based reactions. Arousal is provoked by techniques that inspire novelty rather than familiarity. Reflecting on this arousal allows the creators to observe how positive and negative emotions may alternate, and exert or exist in ambiguity.

> *I welcomed the unconstricted flow of paint but was initially ambivalent about the results as they did not seem to be interesting. I immediately loved the process but was critical about the product. As my judgment subsided I playfully manipulated the results. I was able to access a positive emotional state. I found that I can now carry and hold this as my default art making state. My art making was a symbolic climax of these realizations.* Joanna Clyde Findlay

Experience III: Folded Dual Drawings

This folded-paper body-drawing technique is a valuable way to stimulate the connection between feelings and the visual and sensory perception of a body image. For the Exquisite Corpse or Folded Dual Drawing body experiential, the group divides into pairs. "Each group member folds a writing-sized paper into four horizontal strips, like an accordion, and draws a head in the top section" (Figure 7.10).

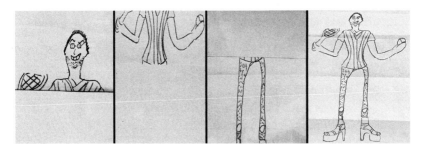

Figure 7.10 *Exquisite Corpse.* Elise Jones and Jennifer Ostin

> *Making the exquisite corpse was familiar to me. This is a game we often play in our family and which always delights our children. I notice that when a bizarre or funny figure is revealed that does not have too peculiar "joins" between the different body parts drawn by each person, we consider it the most successful, as if we are always collectively searching for some coherence in the strange characters that are made. It seems like we enjoy the oddness and unexpected outcomes, but find the images that are too bizarre unsettling. The activity seems to take one to an edge between comfortable and uncomfortable feelings. This one is odd as its gender is ambiguous. The legs are long and skinny, wearing high heels, yet they are very hairy and the genitals are missing.* Jennifer Ostin

Each person then hands the refolded paper to his or her partner in such a way that the head image remains concealed, yet showing some marks that indicate where to continue to draw. The objective is to make as continuous a drawing of a human body as possible, so that each body part connects to the other. This is achieved by folding over the sections to show where the previous drawing ended, without fully disclosing proportions, gender, or color. The partner draws the torso, folds over this section, and exchanges the paper again, continuing partner exchange until the full image has been depicted. Thus, each partner is called upon to imagine and mentalize what the other might have drawn and will draw. The work requires both creativity and the capacity for theory of mind (ToM, Frith & Frith, 2003). Finally, the four sections show the head, torso to hips, hips to knees, and last, knees to feet. The complete drawings will have four linked drawn sections depicting a human form created by the two different artists. When complete, the unfolded image is returned to the person who first drew the head and is opened and named. Then a process of co-reflection augments co-regulation and co-creation.

Upon initially observing the unfolded body, strong reactions may arise and dysregulate. The blindly drawn human bodies can appear grotesque and bizarre. These visceral and unconscious animated affects can contribute to feelings of attraction or, conversely, aversion. The chance creation of distorted or exaggerated body images offers a playful way to access uncomfortable feelings related to body image. The symbolic link to the body is a conduit for experiencing the sensorial discrete emotions of happiness, surprise, fear, sadness, anger, and disgust. It is possible to distance oneself safely from an unsettling image as it was made by chance, as well as to gain support from a trusted other's listening while discussing what reactions arise from the image. Once experienced, words assist in explicitly naming such feelings (Frisch, Franko, & Herzog, 2006; Ki, 2011).

The Exquisite Corpse directive also requires activation of higher social cognitive functions; as each partner is asked to imagine and anticipate what the other person might be creating. The process and its results might be quite different when working with someone that the partner has a relationship with, as opposed to working with a stranger. Inviting an experience of relational curiosity and closeness, the Exquisite Corpse directive requires mirroring, imitating, complementing, and completing the other's work in a playful and non-threatening way. Not attuning to others' images in this case gives rise to laughter and merriment rather than dismay and discomfort. As a result, the discussion fosters a greater closeness, as the object of exploration is, after all, the human body, ourselves.

The artwork inspired by the five experientials is often different from the artist's usual artwork. Consequently, the outcome of divergent imagery is often unexpected and bizarre, evoking basic emotions from the group members. Sometimes their responses are lighthearted in nature, and other times they are somber and dark. Some describe how the use of dark colors for the Dribble Painting led them to make more sinister images than they had before, revealing distorted faces and bizarre forms. Yet, more often, studio participants express surprise or fascination, recounting how pleasurable it was to make images this way and how it can now inform and transform their customary work. The revelation is the ability to create bold and free images despite timidity or lack of fine art skills. The techniques encourage playfulness and liberate intrapersonal creativity as well as interpersonal curiosity and relational connectivity.

RELATIONAL NEUROSCIENCE: CREATIVITY

Exploring the creative unconscious and making it conscious involves neurological processing of integrated sensory-visual and emotive-cognitive experiences. Generally speaking, creative unconscious experiences are implicit neurobiological processes associated with subcortical and midbrain cortical regions, whereas conscious, explicit creative processes are for the most part associated with cortical frontal areas. Creative cognitive processes may or may not be conscious. For example, decision making is a cognitive function that is not always explicitly conscious.

Thus the integrated function of creativity is driven by sensorial felt experiences, implicit and explicit emotions, feelings, cognitions, and thoughts, representing an interconnected function of several specific neural networks (Lusebrink, 2014). Sensory inputs, which are processed by thalamic-amygdala-visual cortex connections, contribute to implicit emotional arousal, as well as to explicit emotional awareness and cognitive insight. For example, implicit bodily reactions are aroused by the processing of sensory-based experiences. This processing activates linkages between the right anterior insula and the sensorimotor strip (Carlson, 2013). Functions of the insula are responsible for the mind-body interface, and the sensorimotor strip holds a representation of all body parts. Activation in the insula also activates the frontal brain areas' cognitive processing. Another example of implicit processing is the neurochemistry of the reward system. It has been associated with the processing of pleasurable implicit information and activation of the left hemisphere in creativity (Jung et al., 2013). As an example of creative explicit processing, the left hemisphere is implicated in the naming and symbolizing of right-hemisphere creative material.

The processing of sensory and body-based experiences arouses negative and positive emotions, which are respectively associated with right- and left-hemisphere function (Carter, 2010). As discussed earlier, neuroimaging findings further suggest that negative and positive emotions can coexist, contributing to the complexity of human experience (Norris et al., 2010). Each category is relegated to dedicated neural pathways that can be activated at the same time. The neurobiology of the reward system supports the finding that these emotions coexist and that discrete catecholamine release is involved for each category. It is as if each category of emotions has its own system.

As demonstrated in this chapter's ATR-N activities, the creative art therapy processes link together creative unconscious processes with conscious explorations and executive decision-making. From a neuroscience perspective, it is likely that oscillation between frontal left-brain areas and the default mode network (DMN) within the temporoparietal lobes form the foundation of creativity. Creativity, imagination, and making the unconscious conscious involves the integrated functions of these regions (Jung et al., 2013).

Making the Unconscious Conscious:
From Sensory Thalamic-Amygdala-Visual Regions to
Sensory Information Processing and Creative Meaning Making

As mentioned above, working with sensory and visual imagery engages thalamic-amygdala-hippocampal and visual cortex linkages. These neural pathways connect subcortical emotional-sensory-based processing, cortical perceptions, and cognitions. All sensory information is received in the thalamus except for olfactory material. Within the thalamus, the lateral geniculate nucleus (LGN) and the pulvinar nuclei engage in complex visual processing (Kaas, 2005; Michael & Buron, 2005). All imagery, especially vague visual cues, are processed for danger, threat, and emotional relevance through the amygdala-thalamic-hippocampal complex (Hass-Cohen & Loya, 2008). The amygdala has direct links to the visual cortex, thus enhancing quick assessment of threat (Adolphs, 2004). This almond-shaped structure, which is nestled in the central brain, fires easily in response to ill-defined shapes, such as a stick mistaken for a snake (Briere & Scott, 2006; LeDoux, 2000). Upon detecting a potentially threatening stimulus, the amygdala can instantly send bodily and emotional alarms. Even in the absence of conscious awareness of the stimulus, the amygdala may activate (Lane & Garfield, 2005). Direct connections between the amygdala and the prefrontal cortex determine emotional and cognitive reactions to sensory information and cognitive processing. Thus the processing of the physical properties of the image, color, texture, shape, and their emotionally safe or unsafe interpretation is integrated (Shaw et al., 2005). From this amalgam, meaning is gathered and can be creatively processed.

Images are processed through two visual pathways, the What and Where streams (Hass-Cohen & Loya, 2008, pp. 95–99; Kalat, 2012). The What stream, which passes through the temporal lobe, determines the content that the image holds, as well as aspects such as texture and color. The temporal association cortex assists in identifying the nature of a visual stimulus. In the Where stream, the parietal lobes are involved in processing the visuospatial environmental aspects. As the associated image is forwarded to higher frontal cognitive structures, meaning emerges. Different brain regions in the frontal association areas are responsible for making decisions about the significance of the image. In addition, it is in frontal regions, specifically in the dorsolateral prefrontal region, that the imagery's connections to the autobiographical self are established, and the planning for appropriate behavioral responses occurs. This description is another way of illuminating the process by which an image or art piece moves from implicit sensorial-visuospatial processing to emotive and cognitive explicit meaning which informs decision making.

Implicit Bodily States: Right Anterior Insular Cortex

The insula lies hidden between the frontal, parietal, and temporal lobes. Considered the fifth lobe, it has a map of visceral, olfactory, gustatory, visual, auditory, and somatosensory areas, which integrates representations of external sensory experience and bodily-somatic states (Craig, 2003). Like a central server, the insula facilitates and regulates communication as it links with the frontal, temporal, and parietal lobes, including the somatosensory cortex. It is also connected with the limbic system's main structures, the nucleus accumbens and the striatum (Nunn, Frampton, Gordon, & Lask, 2008; Shelley & Trimble, 2004).

Surprisingly, the insula has been implicated in emotional processing

(Duerden, Arsalidou, Lee, & Taylor, 2013). This is especially prominent for emotions that are triggered by imagery or the process of memory recall (Shah, Klumpp, Angstadt, Nathan, & Phan, 2009). Insular activation also plays a role in the increased perception of background emotions when emotional stimuli are passively viewed rather than when attention is intentionally inwardly focused (Lane & Garfield, 2005). Subcortically, more activation is also reported for both the cerebellum and insula for negative stimuli as well as in the basal ganglia (including the ventral striatum) for positive stimuli.

It is likely that the insula is involved in associating certain images with visceral bodily feelings such as disgust. The purpose of disgust is to make the implicit knowing a felt experience in order to move it to consciousness. The person is then alerted to taking action. Linked to motivational physical states, these feelings are called vitality affects (Stern, 1985). They are sympathetic or parasympathetic somatosensory feelings that initiate a desire to obtain more or less of an experience or emotion. They represent changes in tensions and cravings and form a dynamic background for our experiences (Lane & Garfield, 2005). Specifically, the right anterior insular cortex appears to be critical in visceral sensory representation, and in the feelings that accompany decision making, such as hunches in the face of uncertainty (Menon & Uddin, 2010). In art therapy, using sensory means to solicit unconscious imagery can therefore access these implicit emotional action-based urges.

Emotions Trigger Implicit and Explicit Motivation: Roles for the Left and Right Hemisphere

On a cognitive level, emotions are perceived as an avoidance of unpleasant, conflicting, or dangerous emotions, and as an approach toward pleasant, motivating emotions (Harmon-Jones, 2007; Allen, 2001). For example, anger that propels one toward action is associated with left lateralization, whereas anger that results in avoidance is associated with a right-hemisphere activation. The right hemisphere mediates the avoidance of unpleasant emotions, whereas the left hemisphere mediates the desire for pleasant emotions (Wager, Phan, Liberzon & Taylor, 2003). Becoming open to diffuse imagery and its associated emotions entails bilateral processes (McNamee, 2003). It is important not to assign a desirable meaning to all positive affect. As stated earlier, wanting more of something can be problematic and can cause approach behaviors to become uncontrollable.

Split-brain research provides a good example of right-left brain lateralization and dominance (Gazzaniga, 2002). After split-brain surgery, patients were observed engaging in discordant avoidant-approach behaviors. The right hand, representing the left hemisphere, desired to pick up an object, while the left hand, which represents the right hemisphere, intervened by pulling the right hand away (Parkin, 1996). When the corpus callosum is severed, the connection between the two hemispheres is lost, resulting in this phenomenon, labeled the alien hand (Carter, 2010). The dominant hemisphere, which for most people is the left hemisphere, loses control over the non-dominant hemisphere, which for most people is the right hemisphere. Then the left hand becomes unresponsive and disobedient. The left hemisphere is responsible for initiating approach-based behaviors. Approach-based emotions are also classified as high dominance, meaning high in control and avoidance, whereas submission-based emotions are classified as low dominance. Additionally, dominance theory quantifies approach and avoidance (Demaree, Everhart, Youngstrom, & Harrison, 2005). Approach behaviors and emotions are associated with positive motivations and expectations as well as positive affect, such as curiosity, interest, and possibly joy.

Neuroimaging studies have recorded individual differences in the propensity for positive or negative affect. Those who have a predisposition for positive affect show increased left frontal activity (Tomarken, Davidson, Wheeler, & Doss, 1992), whereas those with right frontal activity are inclined toward negative affect. This asymmetry has also been documented in individuals diagnosed with major depressive disorder (Allen, Urry, Hitt, & Coan, 2004).

In terms of creativity, asymmetry in right- and left-hemisphere function has been respectively associated with creativity and emotion. Examining lesions in either the left or right hemisphere has been the focus of such research. Lesions will affect the functionality of the region where they are induced. As reviewed by Jung and colleagues (2013), lesions in the right medial prefrontal cortex (MPFC) were found to parallel profound impairment of creativity and originality measures. In addition, originality scores were higher when associated with left inferior frontal and posterior lesions. Therefore, in patients with lesions in the left language areas, the lack of inhibition of the right prefrontal cortex likely facilitates nonverbal expression. As left regions contribute to the production of language and the storage of logical, linear, and automatic knowledge, the activation of language centers may inhibit the formation of novel thought. However, it is important not to simplify these findings and equate creativity with right-hemisphere functions. Left-brain activations were also implicated in creativity (left inferior frontal gyrus, temporoparietal region, and the inferior parietal lobe). The left hemisphere contributes to creativity in a different way than the right, mainly by engaging in verbalization and the interpretation of symbols.

Verbalization helps individuals organize and structure their cognitions and ultimately influences their emotional reactions. Using words to reflect on feelings could help understand one's nonverbal awareness (Jung et al., 2013).

Being able to symbolize and explain emotional trauma in words helps promote the absorption of unconscious bodily memories into conscious self-narratives (van der Kolk & Fisler, 1995). Positive correlations further support the theory that inter-hemispheric connectivity is essential for information integration and the expansion of creative thought (Atchley, Keeney, & Burgess, 1999; Carlsson et al., 1994). Expression joins the hemispheres in building meaning and self-awareness.

Neurocorrelates of Coexisting Negative and Positive Emotions

The suggestion that positive and negative emotions coexist on separate continua is supported by studies on the distinct functions of the reward system, orbitofrontal cortex (OFC), basal ganglia, and cerebellum. The reward system is a neurobiological feedback loop, which continuously updates the strength of the connection between cues and incentivizing outcomes (Vanni-Mercier, Mauguiere, Isnard, & Dreher, 2009). It produces neurotransmitters that contribute to positive and negative emotions. There seems to be a selective involvement of dopamine for positive motivating emotions. Positive emotions primarily activate mesolimbic dopaminergic projections in the brain reward system, ranging from the ventral tegmental to the ventral striatum, including the nucleus accumbens. In contrast, serotonin and acetylcholine are involved in responding to or controlling responses to negative, aversive stimuli (Hoebel, Avena, & Rada, 2007). Negative emotions associated with serotonin release involve the raphe nucleus functions, as it is the primary brain structure responsible for the release of serotonin. As discussed in earlier chapters, there is also a primary activation of the amygdala and hippocampal memory areas of the brain (McNaughton & Gray, 2000).

In the reward system, the raphe nucleus, the locus coeruleus, and the ventral tegmental area connect to the cerebellum, an area responsible for movement. These connections are central to affect processing and positive emotions (Konarski, McIntyre, Grupp, & Kennedy, 2005). The expression of positive emotions such as joy, contentment, and interest broaden the thought-to-action repertoire as well as building cognitive resources for the future (Panksepp & Burgdorf, 2006).

It is also suggested that different subregions of the OFC are involved with emotional processing. The OFC, which is associated with autobiographical processing, activates in the processing of both rewarding and aversive stimuli. Odor pleasantness activates the medial OFC; odor unpleasantness activates the dorsal ACC and mid-OFC (Grabenhorst, Rolls, Margot, da Silva, & Velazco, 2007). Applying the results of this research suggests that both positive and negative memories can coexist at the same time, contributing to an overall autobiographical evaluation by the OFC. Thus, people are capable of simultaneously representing the positive and negative hedonic value of a complex stimulus, thereby contributing to affective decision making. This information is critical for art therapists, as therapeutic art making involves such complexity. There can be both joy and pleasure from the art making and judgment or pain related to the content of issues being brought up. These unique aspects of art therapy deepen clients' meaning-making ability, hones their ability to creatively investigate and act upon emotional responses in a changed way.

Creativity and Prefrontal Function: Conscious Expressivity

Creativity can be measured by, and conceptualized, as divergent conscious thinking. The frontal lobe and associated brain regions are responsible for many such functions that are linked to creativity (Jung et al., 2013). Diverse cognitive abilities regulated by the frontal lobe, such as idea generation and cognitive flexibility, are vital to breaking old conventions and developing new patterns of thinking. Activation in frontal and posterior brain areas, and in the corpus callosum, has shown significant, positive correlation with creativity, as measured by divergent thinking. Such involvement suggests that creativity engages working memory, sustained attention, and cognitive fluency. Increases in white matter suggest that frontal lobe pathways facilitate creative conscious thinking by effective integration of information through several high-level cognitive functions (Takeuchi et al., 2010).

Creativity and the Default Mode Network of the Brain: Unconscious, Reflective States

Within the last 15 years, scientists have discovered the DMN system, associating its functions with creativity (Jung et al., 2013) and with mindfulness (Mars et al., 2012). This chapter introduces the default neural network, which is reviewed in depth as an integral component of mentalizing in Chapter 11.

From an evolutionary perspective, the eyes provide insight into danger, prompting cognitive appraisal. Therefore, different brain regions will engage, depending on the external stimulus source. Surprisingly, Raichle & Snyder (2007) found that once eyes are closed or fixated on a gaze, the brain reverts, as if by default, to the same neural network. By turning inward, people let go of cognitive appraising and default into reflective creative states where divergent thinking and rumination occur. The DMN is the area of the brain that seems to engender wandering thoughts such as those experienced during meditation, and it is most likely also activated when no particular thoughts are happening, as in day dreaming. It is also involved with internal autobiographical self-social-directive functions, described in Chapter 6, and focused self-salient states and reflections (Buckner, Andrews-Hanna, & Schacter, 2008). EEG research also suggests that alpha bands, which are associated with art making, promote lower cortical arousal and relaxed states (Belkofer, Van Hecke, & Konopka, 2014).

Neurologically, default areas were associated with reduced white matter volume (Jung et al., 2013). This seems paradoxical as then decreased cortical thickness in areas corresponding with the DMN pathways are associated with increased human cognitive ability and creativity. More specifically, increased creativity was unexpectedly also associated with decreases in cortical volume in frontal and posterior cortical regions. This is again in contrast with established research showing that more neurons, thicker myelin, and dendritic thickening correspond to higher cognitive capacity (Satz, 1993). As a solution to this enigma, Jung and colleagues (2013) suggested that the flow of information within the prefrontal cortices is gated during time spent in creative divergent thinking. Gating means that neuronal circuitry in this area will not be thickened, that is, increased. It is likely that the anterior insula and the cingulate gyrus block external inputs to allow internal creativity and reflection to occur. The cingulate gyrus is thought to be involved in decision-making (Bush, Luu, & Posner, 2000). More specifically, the dorsal anterior cingulate has been associated with orienting attention to the most relevant environmental stimuli involved with intra- and inter-personal events (Bressler & Menon, 2010). Reduced activity in this area could also account for the lower cortical density associated with dreamlike states of creativity. The DMN region includes areas associated with (a) integration, the posterior cingulate cortex; (b) memory functions, involving the medial temporal lobe; (c) ToM, involving the mPFC; (d) self-referential processing, involving the ventral precuneus; and (e) spatial visual orientation and the association cortices; regions in the parietal cortex (Jones & Bhattacharyaa, 2013; Buckner et al., 2008; Zhang & Li, 2013).

The role of the parietal lobe in the creative arts is also of interest. Neuropsychological studies have contributed to a clear understanding of the roles of the parietal lobe (Goldenberg, 2009; Mitrushina, Boone, Razani, & D'Elia, 2005; Vallar, 2007). These suggest that the right hemisphere of this lobe is involved with processing of visual imagery, visualization of spatial relationships, left-side space, the left side of the body, and drawings on the left side of the page. Additional research suggests that non-artists may not use the parietal lobe exclusively and will instead rely on other right hemispheric functions (Belkofer, Van Hecke & Konopka, 2014). From a creative arts perspective, the left hemisphere of the parietal lobe is associated with understanding symbols and writing.

Returning to the DMN, it is critical that art therapists know that it might be necessary for clients to let go of external visual processing in order to access divergent and creative thinking. Closing the eyes or unfocused gazing can promote this. This is because DMN function is negatively correlated with brain systems that focus on external visual signals. This application is complicated by lack of clear information on how the DMN functions for people with PTSD (Lanius et al., 2010). It is possible that for PTSD clients, DMN activation involves the fear center of the brain, the amygdala. In this case, gazing or contemplating a familiar image might be called for rather than closing the eyes or unfocused gazing. This is because when novelty of stimuli wears off, habituation may also activate the DMN. Keeping in mind that attention to external visual processing can be grounding for such clients is vital (Hass-Cohen, Clyde Findlay, Carr & Vanderlin, 2014).

Creativity: Oscillation Between Conscious and Unconscious Reflective States

Creativity involves exchange between large brain networks, default mode areas, and the highest cognitive and executive regions, including the dorsolateral prefrontal areas of the brain (Jung et al., 2013). As discussed, the DMN is activated when a person is focused internally. A brain that is at wakeful rest shows coherent neuronal oscillations at a rate of less than 0.1 Hz, meaning one oscillation every 10 seconds. Wandering thoughts, which are associated with DMN activation, are also associated with creativity (Baird, 2012). The DMN deactivates during task or external goal-based activity, and the executive decision-making brain regions involving prefrontal areas, in particular the dorsolateral prefrontal area, activate (Fox, Corbetta, Snyder, Vincent, & Raichle, 2006).

Thus, creative art states seem to fluctuate between activation of processes, such as mental flexibility and control, and default modes associated with dreaming, unfocused attention, and the loosening of controls. Such processes associated with the DMN promote insight and divergent reflection. Divergent thinking is associated with the DNM, whereas the ensuing convergent response is associated with higher cognitive functions. Thus, germination of new and useful ideas depends upon alternating between inhibition and excitation of neuronal processes within this core network. The generation of new ideas requires inhibition of singularity in favor of multiplicity, while the execution of such ideas is excitatory and depends upon higher cognitive function. This is consistent with cognitive research showing a role for the dorsolateral prefrontal cortex in implementation of control based-mechanisms, while the anterior cingulate cortex is engaged during the monitoring of performance (MacDonald, Cohen, Stenger, & Carter, 2000). In addition, it is clear that thalamic-visuospatial cortical and parietal networks, described earlier, are critically involved in artistic creation (Drago et al., 2006). Again, in regard to PTSD patients, switching between the DMN and the executive task-oriented brain centers is most likely impaired (Daniels et al., 2010). The five experientials demonstrated in this chapter provide opportunities to explore multiplicity and engender transformative singularity.

CREATE PRINCIPLES AND CLINICAL APPLICATIONS

This chapter has focused on the interplay of unconscious emotions and consciousness as creative ways toward therapeutic change. For each experiential, two phases demonstrate this interaction and explicate the connection with the CREATE principle of Expressive Communicating. In working with clients, the experientials are communicated as directives. The first phase of each experiential includes chance-based image making and unconscious or semiconscious processes. This first phase can help clients let go of judgmental perceptions and thoughts. Directives consist of Scribble Drawing, Dribble Painting (Decalomania), the Rorschach Blot, Implement Painting, and Frottage Rubbing. Moreover, the art processes support the rapid prominence of divergent images, allowing opportunities for positive or negative emotions to arise and subsequently be explored. Accordingly, unexpected results from this kind of art making facilitate the emergence of unfiltered meaning and the emergence of a singular focus. Moving into the second phase further engages conscious image elaboration. Examples include the color reworking of a Scribble Drawing, labeling and naming a Rorschach Blot or Dribble Painting and printing, and the visual organization of a tactile Frottage Rubbing into a coherent symbol. Such exploration requires a shift from a contemplative and gestational state to decisive executive actions. Both phases are needed for creativity and novelty to manifest and inform transformative self-change.

Chance-based image making, which solicits coexisting positive and negative emotions and conflicts, also brings forward ambiguity, a conflicting state. In this case, the art making engages the left-hemisphere positive approach, while at the same time providing an opportunity for the expression of subcortical and right-hemisphere negative emotions. As a reminder, what is meant by left-hemisphere approach is the capacity to make and create rather than avoid. While in verbal therapy negative emotional expression does not require mobility, mobility such as discussed in the Creative Embodiment chapter is an essential feature of the expressive arts. Motion inherently engages the left hemisphere, as there is a positive intention to make something expressive from the media. Dopamine is likely released, providing pleasure and offering a novel way to work with negative emotions. These are some of the unique aspects of art making.

Phases that require assembling materials, playing, and creating imagery, as well as contemplating symbolic meaning, sequentially move the client from unconscious to conscious creative processes. These two, complementary working phases encourage different emotive and expressive experiences. Examples include physiologically felt reactions, an impulse to avoid an image, or a wish to negotiate feelings. Furthermore, a psychological desire to explore the image, as well as the social need to share its meaning with others, may arise. Emotional openness toward exploring this emergent, random imagery supports creativity. It calls for the clients' willingness to change the art or to accept it as meaningful. Using color and sensory-based media enhances our emotional arousal and invites the expression of basic core emotions: happiness, surprise, fear, anger, disgust, and sadness. Clients' responses to chance-based imagery reveal how these positive or negative emotions motivate and signal to either approach or withdraw. Color use mediates high or low arousal in addition to intensity. Thus, the symbolic meaning of color will often depend upon which form it is associated with. Using colorful and sensory-arousing paint may stir ambiguous connotations. In general, painting, which is a less controllable means, can arouse expressivity as well as potential frustration. Elaboration on such outcomes requires developing and maintaining emotional regulation and acceptance, while reworking the associated imagery requires attention, concentration, and decision-making. The contributions of these surrealist and art therapy techniques to creativity are now supported by information from neuroscience. Research shows that a similar vacillation between reflective imaginative states and concentrated states are critical to the emergence of divergent thinking and creativity.

Research on reflective, imaginative neural networks suggests that therapists should also make room to pause and turn inward before consolidating, changing, or exploring the image. Asking art therapists to close their eyes for a moment or fix them on an image can facilitate stimulation of their clients' creativity and potential for change. This is because it allows the client to disengage from visual contact with the therapist and evokes a similar mirrored reaction by the client. The process of calming the brain to a dreamlike state promotes the emergence of divergent options. Then cognitive areas may activate and execute one or more of these options. Encouraging clients and emphasizing the importance of detaching from external stimuli in order to move inward to the default dreamy state for solutions is perhaps the most important ATR-N finding discussed in this chapter. Although some can access this skill naturally, others need to learn it. One means of doing this is to invite an unfocused gaze and deliberately try to slow down thought processes. Practicing how to shift from swift executive functions facilitated by myelinated pathways to the slower processing of unmyelinated default pathways allows self-referential states to emerge. In this way, combining the practice of holding external stimuli at bay and then following up with purposeful exploration increases receptivity to new ideas and creativity. One caveat which we mentioned earlier is working with traumatized clients.

Integrating Expressive Communicating with the CREATE principle of Creative Embodiment demonstrates the utility of working with a large format in the studio, liberating arm gestures through scribbling, dribbling paint from a standing position, and turning the page while drawing or taking a rubbing. As described in the Creative Embodiment chapter, large and fine motor actions bring together the attention, emotive, and imaginative reflective systems. The attention system is linked to the emotional centers of the brain, and to the default imaginative system via the action system. There ensues an integration of actions, emotions, and thoughts, which can contribute to clients' increased motivation and cognition, reducing inactivity and avoidance. On a smaller scale, the paint's fluidity as it swirls and drips from its bottles or cups symbolizes movement and implies potential for change; a dribble becomes an image, and the image continues to evolve.

Scribble making was introduced in Chapter 5 as part of a dyadic relational experience. We described how right-hemisphere (RH) social functions and nonverbal RH-to-RH communication between therapists and clients gives rise to Relational Resonating. In this case, the curious quality of the chance, bizarre, novel, or hard-to-explain scribbles or dribbles calls for therapists and their clients to engage the RH, which responds to novelty and relational cuing. Looking at the stark dark-on-white Rorschach-like imagery stimulates emotional intensity and accesses discrete emotions of surprise, fear, or disgust for both client and therapist. The therapist is asked to remain attuned and flexibly receptive of the client's chance imagery, tolerating whatever is made. Similarly, the Exquisite Corpse or Folded Dual Drawing, which can evoke strong emotional reactions to bodily distortions, requires the therapist's contingent and supportive communication. Clients can talk about what is grotesque or ugly in their mutually made art, safely externalizing it to the image. Made by chance, the art and its associated meanings are therefore a "not me" or "not us" representation. Such moment-to-moment, unplanned experiences infuse the therapeutic relationship with reflection, mentalizing, social intuition, positive emotions, and the integration of lived interactive experience. Tolerating and understanding the emotions provoked by the chance-based-imagery is a function of mentalizing and affect regulation.

While the ability to self-regulate intolerable emotions has its foundations in how our parents modeled and handled such situations, the therapist now intervenes to correct any unsuccessful or maladaptive learned response. The parents' regulated reflection of emotions allowed the child to grasp their own internal states; now the therapist's ability to tolerate the client's response can pave the way to earned, adaptive regulation. Throughout, the elaboration of the imagery promotes a client's ownership of reworked images. As the client moves from the initial automatic art making to a focused and conscious engagement, the relationship between client and therapist shifts. At the forefront of the activities, the art therapist demonstrates the techniques and provides a container for difficult emotions. At the same time, the art evolves into a coherent story, and clients become experts on their own creativity, presumably promoting self-regulation.

Adaptive responding is linked to self-regulation. As described earlier, the experiential can be stressful for clients on multiple levels. For example, the unstructured liquid paint applications may be internally experienced as uncontrollable, contributing to disrupted emotional states. The invitation to dribble paint, use dark colors, and be open to the possibility of surprise imagery provides an opportunity to practice adaptive responses. For some clients, this provokes withdrawal and avoidance but for others, curiosity and approach. The implements or frottage techniques impose restrictions on self-controlled art making, requiring clients to move from comfortable habitual image making in order to adapt to these challenges. As the client moves from the initial imposed techniques to personalized, yet perhaps novel, expressions, a sense of coping ensues and can be made explicit. Structured media (e.g., pencils, markers) can be resources that assist in modulating arousal and in reworking or taming the frottage-inspired image. Adding resources transforms imagery and promotes resiliency (Sarid & Huss, 2011). The lightheartedness of the work can also promote acceptance of these emotions as artists can choose to approach or distance themselves from the results. Even when the ownership of the emotions is denied, they can still be explored. Group or therapist-client discussions about individual experiences of emotional responses further promote coping and self-understanding. Sharing awareness of positive and negative emotions, liking or not liking what one makes, having feelings of mastery or failure, or feelings of boredom, may reveal that competing emotions certainly do exist. For some clients, coexisting polarities are felt as a stable state of ambivalence, while for others the polarity of emotions is experienced as confusing. Labeling and sharing such experiences normalizes, calms, and generates coping strategies.

Recognizing, identifying, and resolving competing positive and negative emotions result in the experience of Transformative Integrating. This happens implicitly through the transformation of the imagery and explicitly through titling and discussion. It is likely that this meaningful change happens by inviting positive experiences and integrating them with older, avoidant responses. The pleasures of art making, even in the face of adverse or uncomfortable emotions, can release good-feeling chemicals that increase prefrontal regulation of limbic responses. Furthermore, the brain's natural reward systems can also generate positive responses. Such a shift from negative to positive responses is a shift from a neuroendocrine-mediated feeling of loss of control to a sympathetic nervous system–based feeling of acceptance or being in control. In the future, neuroimaging research may show that as the fearful, right-hemisphere-activated client is encouraged to approach art making, the left hemisphere is engaged to modulate emotional avoidance. The playfulness and pleasure in the art making support the experience of positive left-hemisphere emotions that broaden perceptions and increase the range of action and social options (Fredrickson, 2004). Positive emotions have also been found to facilitate physical well-being and mental health changes. Therapeutically, these have been further associated with self-mastery, pride, gratitude, and love. The two-phase process promotes hemispheric stimulation and integration as a synthesis of intention, attention, and motivation occurs through sensory experiences and motor control. By moving focus from a diffuse state of awareness to more concentrated outward and body-oriented attention, at the same time as one paints or draws, multiple neural circuits are simultaneously stimulated and integrated.

The ATR-N principle of Empathizing and Compassion is activated during the two-phase implicit to explicit art making. The therapist can first demonstrate the different techniques enlisting human imitative capacities, thus supporting clients' confidence that they can do what they have observed. Attempting a technique and then engaging in the exploration of the emotions stimulated by the chance image making allows them to empathically approach their product. Furthermore, the capacity to experience and direct empathy toward others emerges from self-integration and is enhanced by self-empathy. Requiring tolerance and development, this chapter's suggested techniques are rooted in an unforced attempt to have clients accept somewhat difficult or surprising emotions. Not all the challenges and emotions aroused by the art making can be resolved, which promotes empathy. From this perspective, reworking the imagery permits noteworthy internal processes. It allows for a release of the initial image and process, as well as an understanding and sharing of one's feelings in the release of any attachments to habitual ways of coping and relating to the self.

CHAPTER 8

Expressive Communicating: Interpersonal Touch and Space

When working with the clay, one of the main emotions I felt was fear, and my negative memories associated with it, such as my previous failures with clay. The memory of failure and the idea of fear will present itself as a learned response to the stimuli. From that negative, learned response, the stimuli will continue to produce fear in a person when it is presented, as it is for me when I see, and have to work with, clay. The clay is able to move around and it often does what it wants to do, regardless of what the artist asks it to do. The fear I felt about my piece was that it wouldn't mold into what I had pictured in my mind—that it should look like an ending piece. The only way that I felt safe was because I was in a protected space where I could bare my soul, that place being with my group. Over the past few months, I felt safe and comfortable enough to be able to share a piece of myself with my cohorts. Autumn Cade

TOUCH IS A MAJOR SOURCE of sensory stimulation due to the many nerve-ending receptors in our skin. Therefore, the type and origin of touch, as well as the quality of experience, influences our perceptions of and reactions to stimuli. In Chapter 7, vision was the primary means to learning, whereas for this chapter we invite a focus on the experience of touching and manipulating tangible art materials. This chapter illustrates how art-mediated touch informs the CREATE principle of Expressive Communicating. It also highlights how art-mediated interpersonal touch and space (AMITS) may play out in the room between the therapist and the client (Bat Or, 2010; Hass-Cohen & Kim, 2014). As we describe in the last section, these are "third hand," "third eye," and "second mind" experiences that have the potential to transform internal working models (IWMs) of relationships and contribute to earned attachment. Working with materials like clay serves as a gateway to mental representations of remembered and mentalized touch or emotions, and to the here-and-now experiences of sensory touch. In other words, emotions and memories can be triggered and enhanced by art-mediated touching, and different types of materials evoke different reactions and the associated IWMs. For example, manipulating polymer modeling clay, which can be either smooth or sticky, evokes a different emotion than the experience of earth clay, which clings to hands and fingernails, leaving an earthy odor, which may be reminiscent of playing in the dirt as a child or baking mud-pies with mother. If touching is novel, surprising, or intentional, its processing will involve an amalgam of tactile awareness and emotionality. So the daily experience of touching the fabric of a beloved wool jacket, although comforting, is routine and will therefore not be likely to spark consciousness.

Touch is a fundamental human form of interpersonal communication. The first positive touch sense experienced by an infant, such as maternal stroking and holding, forms early bonding, releases oxytocin, and initiates secure attachment ties. Thus, interpersonal touch provides the most emotional of our sensory experiences, also playing a key role in emotional communication. Even if two people do not know each other, their touching can communicate anger, fear, disgust, love, gratitude, and sympathy as accurately as verbal communication or visual expressions (Hertenstein, Holmes, McCullough, & Keltner, 2009). Interpersonally, touch, or physical contact between people, is a basic psychological need. Touch also releases serotonin, and endorphins, which are good-feeling neurotransmitters (David, 1999). We hypothesize that AMITS may evoke similar bodily sensations and biochemical reactions. In fact, our sense of self and the environment is highly informed by visual and haptic processing of personal and interpersonal information. For example, personal haptic holding of attachment objects, such as a teddy bear or blanket, might include interpersonal memories. Conversely, a mother might keep her son's childhood teddy bear for his own son. Non-directed and directed playful dyadic interactions, which use soft familiar materials, provide opportunities for attachment reparations (Jernberg & Booth, 1999).

Interpersonal haptic touching involves friendly touching as well as the memory and the IWM of touching. Both physical and symbolic interpersonal haptic experiences also inform our sense of interpersonal space. Friendly, romantic, or sexual touching activate regions of the brain responsible for spatial and bodily processing. Mediated by culture, our sense of interpersonal space is survival based (Zur & Nordmarken, 2011). For example, since we cannot see behind us, any unexpected touching from outside our scope of vision may alarm us, causing an impulse to move away or turn around. All touching calls upon brain areas responsible for the spatial and cognitive processing of sensory information, including thalamic-limbic regions that connect with the parietal lobe and right frontal areas (Kalat, 2012). Such haptic processing also necessitates insular lobe–mediated bodily sensations, thereby stimulating memories based on environmental, bodily, and psychological experiences. Thus adjunctive therapies such as soft massage may be important and needed interventions that could be included as recommendations.

For some, a persistent lack of touch can be isolating and painful. For others, touch has traumatic connotations, as it can be a reminder of punitive or abusive touch. Hence, sometimes, without knowing, tactile touch can trigger insight into negative interpersonal memories. For example, the wet residue of clay on fingers and clothes may be a reminder of punishment or even abuse by a parental figure, activating an amygdala fear and avoidance response. Conversely, touching and molding the soft, yielding texture of the clay can be a reminder of a positive childhood experience of playing with mud. Smelling the clay's earthiness or sensing its symbolic colors can bring about joy, another amygdala function. With deliberate therapeutic intervention, the fear of touching that can be aroused by tactile media can be cognitively accessed through the higher sensory cortex rather than simply from the amygdala's unconscious reaction. Thus by activating the prefrontal regions of the brain, the amygdala response will be less able to activate (LeDoux, 2003b). Touching the media and verbalizing its effects assist clients in cortical processing of these implicit basic emotions, and unrecognized dimensional feelings. In this chapter, we review this psychoneurobiological interpersonal hub of processing.

Our group members are asked to work with different kinds of clay. We discuss such clay-based objects as mental self-representations of haptic associations and IWM connotations. For our purposes, three types of clay are used: earth-based clay, nondrying oil-based modeling clay (Plastilina), and delicate polymer clay. Earth-based clay evokes strong intrapersonal reactions and transparent group experiences. Here we ask clients to create a Personal Object. Due to the media, these objects are usually large. As they are easily seen by others, their creation facilitates a social environment. Oil-based, easily manipulated, and colorful, the Clay Doodling experiential recruits interpersonal communication by way of making Human Figurines. Here, the use of Plastilina, which is a type of very malleable oil-based clay, aptly connotes interpersonal neurobiology-based changes and plasticity. Finally, polymer clay, Sculpey, may give rise to reflections on reparative touching of fragile connections associated with the frequent fragmentation and burning of this delicate medium during its baking. We facilitate this intrapersonal reparative work by a request for a representation of An Imagined Loved Landscape or Place.

ART-MEDIATED INTERPERSONAL TOUCH AND SPACE

Symbolic and physical AMITS are some of our art therapy field's advantages (Hass-Cohen & Kim, 2014). This is partially because therapist-client touching of any kind is actively discouraged. Such touching presents a high risk to clients with a history of abuse, an aversion to touch, a cultural difference, or a prohibition regarding touching the opposite sex. Positive and safe AMITS include sharing materials and touching one's own artwork or a client's artwork, as well as expressing a positive interest in the tactile aspects of artwork. Several opportunities exist to express closeness, interest, curiosity, and support in this way. In the early stages of a therapeutic relationship, the art therapist may ask or suggest that the client touch a smudged pastel area on the therapist's own page. Alternatively, he or she might ask to touch a client's page to stabilize it as the client's scribbling moves it, or ask to hold a ball of clay made by a client to sense its weight and power. As art therapists show child clients how to wash a brush properly, manipulate the clay, prepare paper strips to make papier-mâché, smooth hands over mono-prints, or wrap precious objects to take home, we ask ourselves about the accidental touch of therapists' and clients' hands. Alternately, the use of dual play with puppets allows for safe touching experiences, as the cloth is a barrier to direct touching. These examples illuminate types of touching, yet, importantly, they also exemplify how AMITS defines the boundaries of interpersonal space.

Symbolically, fingertips brushing another person's fingertips is an example of how the art therapist's "third hand" (Kramer, 1986) can provide reassurance, comfort, and security. In dual drawings, therapists and clients touch the same page as they gesture to each other to co-create. Images of hand representations and their decorations have important therapeutic contributions. For example, a master of interpersonal touching, the late Shirley Riley, used to ask students in her class to draw around one hand and decorate it as a symbol for themselves. They then cut it out and place it with the drawn hands of the other new students, touching or not, to make a mural of connection. She and we use this activity for purposes of a confidentiality statement; it is not unlike a handshake promising to keep each other's information private. More importantly, it creates intimacy, closeness, and assists in positively updating IWM of attachments. The simulation of touch is not limited to touching materials that arouse symbolic mentalization of holding, touching and being touched in a supportive way. Dyadic games, which are common in play therapy, provide another source of here and now touching. Examples are the passing of cotton balls between mother child, holding a large rubber ball between father and child without letting it fall and so on. These are the kind of touches that we ascribe to in a relational setting and that are congruent with family-based attachment treatment interventions (Hughes, 2004). The process of discussing such group or dyadic art provides opportunities for active mentalizing (Bat-Or, 2010; Gavron, 2013; 2014a; Harel, Kaplan, Avimeir-Patt, & Ben-Aaron, 2006).

Exploring the phenomena of touch led us to create a list of touch types and related art therapy microskills that offer unique reparative opportunities through different types of touching. These include accidental, task-related, and appreciative types of touch. Each conveys a different meaning through haptic experience. Of particular interest to art therapists are active and intentional task-related touches, which are examples of several kinds of interpersonal touches and gestures (Jones, 1994). Positive touches are supportive and appreciative, and are associated with togetherness and affection. On the contrary, negative touches represent control of another, infliction of pain, or anger. Sexual and playful touches can be either positive or negative. Ritualistic touches of acknowledgment, such as welcome or departure greetings and handshakes, are gender and culturally driven. From an ATR-N perspective, the psychobiological foundations for deliberate physical or symbolic touching are interpersonal art therapy haptic skills. Table 8.1 describes each type of touch in general, with modifications specific to art therapy (Jones, 1994).

Our purpose in describing these various types of touch is to heighten our awareness of them as therapeutic tools. It is notable that all touching types can be playful or not and for the most part they can all be neutral, positive, negative, or ambivalent. Together, AMITS form a package of interpersonal microskills. Specifically, we suggest accompanying AMITS with nonverbal gestures and verbal expression, which has the potential to reduce interpersonal misunderstandings. Verbal expression can happen concurrently with AMITS or can follow up. Sensorimotor psychotherapy (Ogden et al., 2006) is a form of therapy that actively focuses on nonverbal gestures, specifically on incomplete sensorimotor actions associated with trauma. The practices of this approach teach clients to self-regulate by mindfully contacting, tracking, and articulating sensorimotor processes. Among other techniques, the art therapist pays attention to gestures that the client has difficulties completing, or ones he or she may avoid because they are associated with the experience of emotional pain (Sholt & Gavron, 2006). Oftentimes art making will evoke those gestures.

As we have discussed, interpersonal touch is a core human need that is mediated by visual, verbal, and emotional memory (Konijn & Van Vugt, 2008). The meaning of touch is wide-ranging. Mediated by our skin, which is our largest bodily organ, tactile touch is a sensory perceptual mechanism that transfers afferent, incoming, external stimuli for the brain to process (Kalat, 2012). The phenomenon of interpersonal touch is an amalgam that

Table 8.1 A Range of Touching Types

Types of Interpersonal-Social Touch	Description/Micro-Skills	
	General	Art therapy
Reference to features and appearance	Touching and talking that point out a body part or artifact that the person might be wearing; the person notices a friend's haircut, sweater, jewelry, and/or other personal effects and says something like: "this is pretty, soft, and silky"	Reference to the art or media qualities by client or therapist that can be accomplished by a combination of pointing, touching, and talking; can also be positive or negative reference to the self of client
Task and instrumental	Touch that accomplishes a task in itself; the meaning is clear from the touch itself, but secondary positive meaning may be implied; assisting a person in putting on a coat; placing a hand on a person's forehead to check for fever (implies support)	Assisting a client in achieving his or her intentions; positive if the therapist does not overpower with his or her intent (e.g., helping support clay objects in process or holding paper while the client engages in art making)
Accidental and incidental	Touching that occurs as an unnecessary part of the accomplishment of a task; mainly hand-to-hand contacts; here, touch can accomplish a secondary message of interest or friendliness; most common is handing an object to someone and allowing hand-to-hand contact (e.g., a clerk returning change)	Most common is handing an object to someone and allowing hand-to-hand contact; most safe when working with children; can be negatively experienced by client; if accidentally happens, needs to be acknowledged; symbolically touching the same paper as the client, helping to stabilize the artwork such as in taping it down, can be experienced as very supportive
Directive or controlling	Attempts to direct behavior, aim for compliance, direct or request mental or perceptual attention; may be experienced as supportive or coercive and controlling even if subtle or well intentioned; often dictated by culture; may or may not require a response	Examples include therapist touching the page and turning it vertically or horizontally, touching a brush or paint, indicating a preference for color through gesture and so on; verbal directives fall into this category as in art therapy all directives invite touch; directive touch differs from instrumental touch as it is broader and may or may not stem from clients' self-goals; however the differences between the two are subtle

Adapted from Jones (1994).

includes actual physical or social touch intertwined with the mental representation of repeated patterns of somatosensory firing. Throughout our growth
and development, body-based touch experiences become laced with emotional and cognitive memories, as touch is social and anchored in the needs
of our species (Gallace & Spence, 2010). Interpersonal touch occurs in a
relational context. Therefore, it is plausible that the memories of interpersonal encounters embedded in here-and-now tactile touch give rise to (a)
unconscious reactions, such as fear, joy, disgust, or anger; and (b) cognitive
awareness of loss, longing, anticipation, pleasure, and specific memories.
These touch-based memories will also determine how we handle interpersonal space. Handling and making objects accesses mental and symbolic
representations in these memory systems. Over a lifetime, this circuitry is
connected to the individual's relational experiences, emotions, feelings, and
cognitions.

AMITS and verbal expression assist individuals in constructing a coherent sense of past and present. Experiencing therapeutic symbolic touch via
art media can strengthen new neural pathways. Furthermore, examining cortical processing of sensory touch seems to provide insight into the meaning
and social construction of interpersonal touch (Murray & Wallace, 2011).
The interface between emotions and cognitions, which involves structures
within the limbic system and the neocortex, is central to understanding how
social touching leads to awareness of fear of touch versus celebration of social
closeness.

EXPERIENTIAL PRACTICES AND DIRECTIVES

Experience I: Earthy Clay

> *The earth is in my hands. It is soft and cold to the touch. Memories of
> childhood reenter my mind as I squeeze and allow it to gush through
> the tiny openings between my fingers. It reminds me of my first discov-
> ery, or taste for that matter, of earth. It reminds me of sandcastles and
> "sandwiches" on Muizenberg beach, of mud pies and dams at the end
> of the driveway, of the quest for gold beneath the soil of my feet. What
> the earth does for me is ground me and remind me of my roots. I am
> free to be with the earth again. It's quite enlivening. I spend my time
> playing with the clay. I have no intended shape or form for it, since I
> know that the clay will ultimately form itself. I close my eyes, still
> "warming" the clay for myself, and allow a form to transpire, for my
> art to unfold.* Janine Stuppel

The size of the objects mediates the kind of interpersonal space and touching that occurs. Larger clay forms are transparent as everyone can view them, whereas the artist can choose whether and when to share the smaller polymer clay objects that can be hidden in the palm of the hand. However, the decision to share small objects can create a heightened state of intimacy. This is because personal space becomes interpersonal. To begin the work with clay we therefore invite our group members to: "Use three different clays to make three personal art pieces in small, medium, and large sizes." The invitation to play with size structures aligns well with the types of media offered. For example, the earthy clay lends itself to larger organic forms, whereas the delicate polymer clay is better suited for smaller, more detailed forms. Variation in size provides an intimacy of scale that defines the interpersonal space. People will peer at the tiny objects held on the palms of their peers or even ask to hold a creator's art piece. As objects are revealed, there are many references to the art features and excited verbal exchanges. Symbolic interpersonal touch enhances the tangible experience of working with the three clays. Notably, studio artists report that working with various clay types on the same day heightens awareness of their personal reactions to its properties and their interpersonal interactions.

To facilitate this process, we also organize the shared creative space into three centers. One center has large lumps of gray and terracotta earthy water-based clay, wooden boards, and newspaper. At the next center, trays hold colorful oil-based modeling clay, paper plates, cardboard flats, and utensils. Some trays contain bright, medium-sized square chunks of new and still-wrapped clay, while others hold lumps of reused clay with bled colors. At the third center, polymer fine-grained clay is found in small squares. Plastic-based, it lends itself to the manipulation of fine details. Found three-dimensional objects can be incorporated into any of the clay selections. Just as in the original setup of the art therapist's media table, the presentation of the clay material on center-based tables elicits subtle but important meanings. Whether the oil-based clay or polymer clay is wrapped or unwrapped, has mixed-up colors, or has pristine candy-like appeal, the material offers a level of symbolic meta-communication that touches our IWMs. For example, wrapped clay may send the message that its use requires permission to touch. If the clay seems virgin and new it can bring about excitement, fear of failure, or feelings of unworthiness. Used media can, in contrast, connate social sharing or disgust at touching media that have been touched by others. Thus the medium offers a vehicle for inquiry, flexible reflection, and self-expression and also opens a gateway to interpersonal tangible and symbolic touch. We appreciate the center arrangement for underscoring the relational underpinning of our studio art therapy approach. As in group art therapy, working with the same media, sharing water and utensils, offering support, and providing encouragement enhance relational interactions, and mentalizing thus shaping the interpersonal space.

Occasionally, we set the stage for this AMITS work by asking our milieu's participants to bring in a personal inspiring and meaningful handheld object or symbol. Some suggested items to make are handheld objects, a hand or other body part, and a personal or universal symbol, such as a power animal, which they can then replicate and modify. Maribel selected the clay in order to make a clay nest for a precious stone egg that she brought from home (Figure 8.1).

I chose to create around my found object, [and] I immediately felt a sense of joy and calmness. . . . Immediately I recalled the many times in the past when it was just me and the clay, at times not knowing what would emerge from the clump of clay, and at times going into it with clear intentions. I enjoy watching the forms evolve in front of me and at times losing control and welcoming a wonderful accident. As I worked, I looked to my hippocampus for my stored knowledge of the techniques useful for working with the medium. I relied on my thalamus and basal ganglia to guide my movement. A few moments of slight anxiety were provided, courtesy of my amygdala, when I thought my piece would collapse, but soon the same structure, after further processing, provided me with a renewed calmness. I successfully completed the new home for my found object, which is a safe nest for my precious egg. Maribel Sandoval

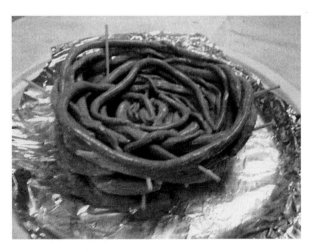

Figure 8.1 *Safety.* Maribel Sandoval

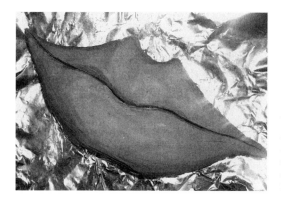

Figure 8.2 *Mysterious Expression.* The smile is somewhat mysterious, like the Mona Lisa smile. The mouth is not open to a full smile and the lips are pursed together. I wonder what emotion is behind this expression? Rachel Tate

In contrast, Rachel opted to present a mouth. It is curious that the experience of touching the clay brought forward an image of a part of us that is so central to sensory experiences. As discussed in the upcoming neuroscience section, the neurobiological representation of the mouth is one of the larger regions in the sensory strip. It is as if touching intuitively mediated this for Rachel. In her writing, she connects her sculpting with pleasurable feelings (Figure 8.2).

> *I first began working at the earth clay table. Grabbing a handful of clay, I sat down at my space and began to knead the clay together with my hands. The cold, textured clay was messy, but fun to play with. My hands were masked in the mud-like clay and as the clay dried on my hands, it turned into crumbles that became flaky. The mud-like smell of the clay brought back pleasant memories of ceramics art class when I was younger. After molding the clay in my hands for a while, I decided to make an anatomical body part—a mouth. I had been reading the beautiful Carter book and remembered an illustration of a mouth as part of a chapter on the correlation of emotion and expression in the brain. I formed the lips into a smile.* Rachel Tate

Clay inherently pulls us into a broad sensory experience that involves movement, muscles, sensation, touch, sight, and smell. Most people will likely prefer to work with the earth clay by standing up, pressing down the rather large lumps with deliberate touch. Wet clay inherently allows contact with greater weight and mass and a cooler temperature. The initial act of helping oneself to a chunk of clay involves peeling back the plastic sleeve around the block of clay and slicing a slab of it with the wire cutter. For some, this tugging bodily movement is dynamic and invigorating, while for others, it can be intimidating. Tactile touch incorporates pressure, temperature, pleasure, pain, joint position, muscle sense, and movement. Sometimes, we ask artists to shut off visual processing by closing their eyes. This facilitates experiencing the primacy of our sense of touch and the challenges in defining what is involved in touching.

At the earthy clay table, group members discuss the experience of touching, kneading, and forming the wet clay. This organic substance provides a very powerful means of eliciting and modulating intrapersonal basic emotions, primarily pleasure or disgust. Some of the artists report that they are very much attracted to the earthy clay, whereas others would rather not touch it. Clay artists share that the medium has two qualities that inherently contribute to this reaction. The first is the grainy, cool, and moist quality of the clay that quite quickly dries on the hands, which can irritate the skin or soothe it. The same is true of its unique smell. Second, the problem that earthy clay poses is that it requires a strong intuition of its qualities in order to create a sturdy form. It can be slippery and unwieldy, and large forms are prone to collapsing. These organic qualities contribute to visual and emotional ambiguity that may trigger a fear response initiated by the amygdala. Indeed, most art therapy perspectives postulate that the unstructured nature of clay may evoke a felt sense of lack of safety and control (Malchiodi, 1998a). The triggering of an alarm response depends on each artist's personal history and familiarity with the media. However, we hypothesize that when experience with the clay is increased, the fear center response is altered into joy; the amygdala fear area is deactivated, and the areas responsible for coping and joy are activated and connected to the trigger.

From an ATR-N perspective, no single or specific medium provokes the same reactions of safety, control, fear, or pleasure for every individual. Rather each person's reaction is triggered by familiarity with the media and by personal and interpersonal memories. Some of our artists report that they find the contact with wet clay pleasurable and novel, as well as stress relieving through the processes of rolling and kneading. Others say that it is not malleable, controllable, or clean—meaning it is messy, dirty, hard to manipulate, and difficult to control. They disclosed that it triggers reminders of times when they felt they lacked control over their environment, sparking a discomfort in touching the clay. Perhaps it was the "yucky" cool, wet clay that dried on their hands, or the "gooey" oil-based clay that stained their fingers. These sensations may have funneled hopeless feelings at the gap between what they perceived as childlike productions and their creative goals. Others might be reminded of times when they were chastised for getting dirty. In contrast, many are delighted at the discovery of the minute fine motor skills required when working in plastic clay and the physical pleasure inherent in rolling, squeezing, and handling large masses of clay. Issues around actual and perceived control are commonly discussed. Many artists comment on the need to surrender to the clay's fluidity, even if it means ending up with a mud pie for a sculpture. This process may resonate with one's IWM and life experiences. Soothing touching of the watery mess can support accepting this process and with therapeutic support, the process can start to feel good and be therapeutic. As this surrendering experience is supported and accepted, it provides stress reduction and relief, updating of IWMs and valuable opportunities for a diversity of ATR-N interactions.

Experience II: Oil-Based Colorful Clay

Playing with colorful clay has the potential to stir childhood memories as well as invite pleasurable feelings and positive bonding with others. We ask the group members to start by doodling with the colorful Plastilina. Soft, malleable, and never hardening, this type of oil-based medium promotes handling. Little preparation is needed to roll, squeeze, or play with it. Spirals, snakes, balls, or stacks of globes that may resemble a pile or a snowman quickly emerge. All the forms are rounded and organic, and the clay's immediacy requires less attention, leaving room for socializing. Thus, the invitation to let their fingers lead and the ability to rapidly produce artwork relaxes the group members and supports group cohesion and bonding. As in a knitting group, people's fingers mimic each other's hand movements, mirroring mutual fine motor movement. Often there is a type of contagion as one person begins to roll the clay with her fingers and others pick up the motion. In addition, rolling the clay often results in squiggly tubes and coils. Perhaps the childlike nature of the gesture supports the emergence of such spirals and snakes, butterflies and abstract doodles. There is very little pressure to perform when doodling with the oil-based clay. For some who may have had disrupted childhoods, or may not like to play, observing the group members may bring forward a sense of loss or longing for playfulness. Moreover, such pleasurable bodily interactions are associated with the release of oxytocin and reward circuitry chemicals.

> *I usually get really irritated if I see someone copy what I am making, but when we were playing with the plastilina, I thought it was inspiring and comforting how we all ended up making similar shapes. It felt uniquely human; it also reminded me of carefree playful times as a child and adult.* Olivia Stern

Oil-based clay tends to get softer as it is handled and does not have much structure. Therefore, working with this type of clay can also bring up issues of control. Negative reactions to the polymer clays are usually more on the neutral side and focus on frustration with the lack of ability to bring sharp definitions to the clay forms. Cut-up plastic stirrers or wooden toothpicks can provide structure, similar to armatures.

As experimentation progresses, some of the doodles will naturally turn into small figures, and everyone is asked to: "Create small figurines." As these figures emerge, the chatter often quiets and groupings of human figurines begin to cluster. We then ask participants to: "Position the figures in relation to each other: sitting, standing, and touching." Role-playing with the figures may ensue, quickly moving into the interpersonal realm. This is in part because one can construct such figures so rapidly out of the oil-based clay. It is also quite easy to change the appearance of the figurines, have them hold hands, and interchange figures with one another. Similar to play therapy, this work provides an opportunity for therapeutic projections, mentalizing and reflections (Bat-Or, 2010; Sholt & Gavron, 2006). Changing the figurine's features and adding decorative personal touches, such as a baseball cap turned backward or buttons, alters and makes the figurines personal. As such an idiosyncratic personal body schema develops, it is possible that the insula, the fifth lobe that connects the mind to the body and is implicated in touch, may be stimulated. Our sculptors report that they try to figure out how a body works in order to make their figure stand up or sit. The process stimulates connecting with one's own body in order to find such solutions (Figure 8.3).

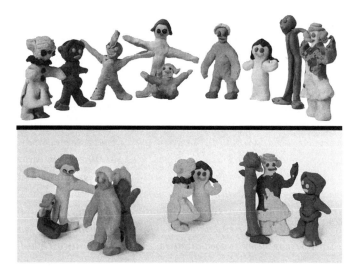

Figure 8.3 *Group configurations. Parade of Figurines* (left) and *Relational Pairings* (right).

As I played with the clay, I thought to myself that I could represent myself in this figurine group. I added a yellow cap to my red figure. For me, it represented my ginger hair, which as an adolescent I had tried to cover up. Now red is my favorite color. I identify with its symbolic qualities. Much to my delight, the group at the table immediately picked this up, asking if the figure was me. It felt supportive. They did not know about my past, but they sure see me in the present. Olivia Stern

It is inevitable that as the figurine groups emerge, made-up families, groups, or couples emerge; touching, holding, or reaching out to each other. In small clusters, each participant first places his or her figurines in families or groups. Accordingly, relationships can be described suggesting closeness or tension. Our late colleague, Shirley, elegantly employed AMITS by using simple clay figures to explore and demonstrate relational dynamics. Her students always experimented with repositioning figurines they had made in order to achieve a felt sense of family dynamics. This directive is also reminiscent of Virginia Satir's (1988) family sculpting. She used the live family sculptures to evoke emotion and connectivity. Ahead of her time, she recognized how emotions and positivity can promote systemic changes. Influenced by Satir's interventions, group members request each other's permission to touch, move, or change the posture of their figurines. For example, Olivia adjusted Mary's figurine arms so that they could embrace each other. Exploring Satir's model in the small groups and how it translated into clay work in the studio promotes a deep understanding of mentalizing systemic art therapy approaches.

We then suggest a final theme to: "Make a real or imagined place that you love with the oil-based clay," which we attribute to Rachel. In Rachel's case, she did not include human figurines (Figure 8.4).

The next table I went to was the Plastilina table. There were many bright colors to choose from, and I first chose a light blue color. As I pulled away a handful of the modeling clay, I could immediately tell the difference between the earth clay and this plastilina. This clay was smooth, but hard, felt a little sticky, and left an oily residue on my hands. I thought about my handheld object—the little tree that I had bought during my trip to Brazil. The memories of being in the rainforest and seeing the amazing Iguazu Falls came back to me and I decided to create a personal object; to re-create a waterfall after the memories invoked by my handheld object. I started with red and brown clay, resembling the earthlike, rocky base of the falls and the

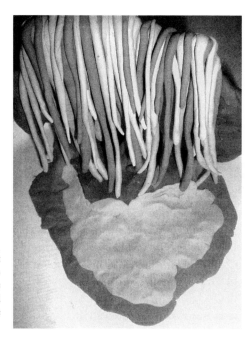

Figure 8.4 *Waterfall.* A personal object reflecting a pleasant memory of a trip to Iguazu Falls, Brazil. The bright blue colors and the malleability of modeling clay enabled me to capture downward movement of the falls. Rachel Tate

back wall of the falls. I used popsicle sticks as a support to prop up the brown clay for the background of the waterfall. Then, taking a handful of bright blue clay and with the light blue clay, I rolled the clay into thin pieces of varying lengths and attached them to the top of the base and wall. The layers of blue clays were molded to represent the downward movement and force of the huge amounts of water gushing from the falls that coalesce into a pool of water below. Rachel Tate

Tactile touch of objects and body can be presented as a chain of associative images or can form one cognitive visual amalgam, as illustrated by Rachel's waterfall. The qualities of this oily clay lend themselves to the representation of memory-based touch, such as Rachel's experience of the gushing waterfall and deep pool. Attempts to accurately represent one's memories will frequently stimulate a squashing, smearing, and blending of colors. Then longing for soothing, comforting touch can be represented via imagined warm beachscapes. In this way, the real-time pleasure of touching the easily moved clay, combined with the imagined well-being in a loved environment, results in an experience of safe, supportive touch. Transitioning from a Personal Object and Clay Doodling, to a Human Figurine, to a representation of an Imagined Loved Place allows the creative artists presents IWM that are mediated by AMITS. The kinds of touches that this work inspires run the gamut of the types of touches possible. Task-related touching as well as accidental or form-controlling touch happens as the group members help each other. Moreover, referencing and discussing the art further expands opportunities for interpersonal touch.

Experience III: Polymer Clays

Similar to talismans, handheld and symbolically felt, Personal Objects have multiple therapeutic uses. They serve in this capacity as reminders of safe experiences, connections to nature, and souvenirs from people and places. Many group members will disclose that they have collections of such objects stored in boxes, or displayed as part of small personal altars. We ask group members to use the delicate polymer clay in order to: "Create a personally meaningful object." Some examples are gritty beach shells, little pieces of soft driftwood from dry riverbeds in summer, or wind-polished granite pebbles from a desert. As described earlier, Maribel's object was a precious egg. She had originally made a safe clay nest for it and then transitioned to describing how she made delicate clay feathers for the nest's lining. The floating green-and-white leaves, and the small heart she named Comfort, convey the tactile pleasure experienced from pressing, squishing, bending, and fine-tuning polymer clay into a representation of the egg, nest, and feathers. They are also mental representations of safety and self-care generated during the artist's manipulation of clay (Figure 8.5).

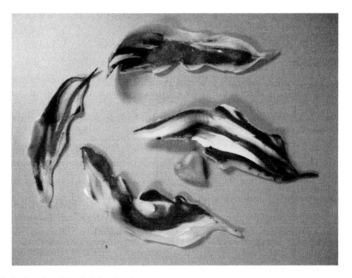

Figure 8.5 *Comfort.* Maribel Sandoval

Using Sculpey I decided to continue with my theme of home and safety for my precious egg. I thought about the colors that would evoke feelings of safety, warmth, and comfort. I chose a light fleshy pink. I rolled it out and then introduced strands of a soothing green into it and meshed them together. Light white clay, which resembled moonlight to me, caught my eye, and with the feelings of serenity that I feel when I recall the moonlight, I immediately reached for it and incorporated it into my work. I associate light as a symbol of safety, guidance, and hope. After some time of rolling the Sculpey into one, I then began to tear it apart to create feathers. I plan to line the nest with them. Maribel Sandoval

The polymer-based clay can hold a form, and it allows finer control in smaller dimensions. However, although polymer clay can easily be baked and hardened to a permanent form, it is fragile and risks burning and loss of fine details. Studio participants can feel the sting of disappointment when a figure cracks or breaks upon baking, or when frustration besets an ambitious goal.

My friend had turned the oven up too high and burned her little clay scorpion, and when it finally came out of the oven, two of the delicate legs had broken off. Our studio facilitator took on the role of the therapist and embodied a third hand in guiding and assisting her through the process of fixing her object without influencing her process. Paint was added to the image and the burned section of the clay became an intentional color black. Then, the legs were carefully attached with tacky glue. Together, they discussed what this experience meant for her. She said that this experience gave her scorpion a quality of being able to sustain and survive [being burned in the oven]. I found this very empowering. Jessica Plotin

Within an interpersonal safe space, the therapist's or peer's "third hand" can offer technical support, comfort, and a mutual experience. As the work progresses, the artists continue to discover the significance of this interpersonal "hand." Therapeutically, the role of the therapist as a third hand (Allen, 1995; Kramer, 1986) is expanded into the realm of the social-interpersonal milieu. As group members respond to the demands of drying or baking their polymer pieces, which require shoring up and support, they also witness and experience the soothing assistance modeled by a friend or the studio facilitator. An example involves the artist or support person wrapping the earth clay so that it dries slowly. Treating the drying processes with loving attention by carefully wrapping the clay with layers of wet cloth and plastic provides opportunities for supportive touching. Making space for the clay sculpture on the drying shelf and taking care that it does not touch neighboring projects is symbolic of a secure interpersonal space. The artist and the studio facilitator revisit this space after one week. As they check the progress of the project by carefully touching and looking at the sculpture, they are reminded of the time when it was made and of its meaning. As a group, we witness how patching, securing, and supporting three-dimensional art making products become interpersonal exchanges.

Sometimes group members will ask for others' help, asking, for example, "Can you please hold this part here while I tuck in some supports underneath it?" Others will offer help and support in the form of aluminum foil or similar props that hold the object while it dries, or that will lighten top-heavy parts. Alternatively, some may prefer that their work remain untouched. Thus, during this process each group member may behold, comment upon, and touch others' art, resulting in interpersonal closeness and a united small-group experience. In other words, we actively advocate for looking at and experiencing technical strategies as interpersonal supports. These interpersonal strategies run the full gamut of generating ideas, working on the project, and finishing it. For example, the process of making Olivia's dragon required flexibly adjusting to the clay's properties. Such challenges allowed for exchanges around making the dragon safe and comfortable, which are also conversations about art-mediated intrapersonal safety, attachment based IWM and tactile touch (Figure 8.6).

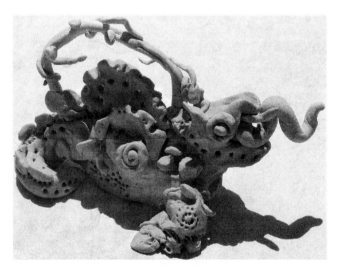

Figure 8.6 *The Fierce and Loving Dragon.*

I decided to make a dragon. I have always considered it my power animal. I love the shape of the fire-breathing hoarding European dragon and imbue it with the Chinese dragon's good luck. Originally, I had thought to make this wonderful fire-fighting dragon with its wings wide spread, about to take off. As pieces of my intricate wings started to break from the main body of the dragon, my friend said, "Why don't you use strands of clay to make your dragon fire?" Slowly, the image transformed to this decorative dragon, which I strongly identify with. Olivia Stern

Maribel's final comments mention the group as she reflects on the process:

In the end it was agreed that during our art experiential our emotions were heightened as we visually enjoyed the colors, took in the scents of the clay, and experienced the feel of the clay on our hands.

Overall, the clay experiences allow the studio participants to foresee therapeutic choices that enable different levels of perceived control and interpersonal touch. They also report on an increased sense of safety and empowerment. One contributing factor is that the art assists in organizing the interpersonal space and reducing unpredicted spatial movements in the room. The artists expect that those working at the earth clay center will move around, handling the large accessories such large lumps of clay, wooden boards, and water pails; this anticipation and acceptance contributes to an internal sense of safety. More importantly, we all anticipate that group members will wander around the room looking, touching, and talking about the media and the art. The emergence and completion of sculptures trigger curiosity, movement, socializing, and thus interpersonal space.

I knew that they were coming to see my dragon so I was not particularly startled by their accidental touching of me or the bits of clay lying around him. I was happy that no one touched him but was not startled by them coming really close by to me. In fact, I was flattered and it made me feel good. It freed me to go and visit other people's sculptures. Some asked me to feel how hard the edges of their baked clay had become. That was surprising. I learned much about myself and others through touch. Olivia Stern

RELATIONAL NEUROSCIENCE: INTERPERSONAL TOUCH

Humans and other mammals seem to have a great need for touch. Harlow's (1958) research demonstrated that baby monkeys sought comfort from a terry cloth mother even when it did not provide food (Harlow & Zimmerman, 1959). Interpersonal touch is a complex psychological phenomenon with beginnings early on in life. Orphans raised in substandard institutions with minimal caregiving and touch may experience difficulties in cognitive, social, and neural development (Kravits, 2008b). Conversely, stable intensive care that includes touch for preterm infants has been associated with increased weight gain, improved developmental outcomes, and reduced duration and number of hospital visits (Field, 2004). In fact, skin-to-skin touching between mother and newborn was found to reduce cortisol measures of stress in babies and improved breast-feeding outcomes (Field, 2004). Based in animal research, touch continues to emerge as an important sensory modality that facilitates growth and development in the young (Ardiel & Rankin, 2010).

In the previously provided neurobiological overview (Chapter 2), as well as in other chapters, we introduced most of the critical structures, brain areas, and functions. Here, we expand and build upon that schematic information and further examine how subcortical and cortical circuitry work together (Christian, 2008). This is particularly relevant to the study of fear and interpersonal touch and space. In the upcoming sections, we discuss some aspects of the neurobiological interface between fear, control, and interpersonal touch. In a nutshell, it is plausible that the meaningful manipulation of clay, which involves emotive expression, is influenced by the brain's fear center, the amygdala. Clay work also involves controlled voluntary movement, a function of the motor system that increases cognitive functions. Cognitive awareness and emotional expression are further heightened by integrated functions of the somatosensory strip, thalamus, parietal lobe, insula, and other prefrontal regions. From an art therapy perspective, the formation of imagery, which involves kinesthetic and sensory manipulation, directly shapes memory over the life span (Lusebrink, 2014).

The Amygdala

Neuroscience research suggests that emotions and cognitions are not isolated from each other. Both Damasio (2005) and LeDoux (2002) have shown that amygdala-based emotions involve neural processes that crisscross limbic, cortical, and lower brain regions. Findings from case studies of people with damage in the prefrontal cortex suggested that emotional and cognitive processing are interlinked (Damasio, 2005). Brain damage in cognitive processing areas is linked to expected cognitive dysfunction, yet emotion and personality are also heavily affected. Conversely, in cases of damage to the amygdala (AMY), cognitive functioning can also become diminished or compromised because of this impaired emotional function (Phelps & LeDoux, 2005). It is also likely that how people react is culturally and language driven. For example, in Pali, which was the language used by the Budhha, there is no separate word for *cognition* and *emotion*, and for *brain* and *heart*. Our Westernized culture and language may account for some of the mind-body dichotomies that we experience. As described above, neuroscience research continues to suggest that these dichotomies may not be valid.

Similarly, the AMY, which receives messages from the senses is sensitive to experiences of both fear and joy (Koelsch et al., 2013). Thus, tactile stimuli associated with particular pleasant or unpleasant memories can trigger AMY responses. Due to the AMY connections to the hippocampus, the memory center, memories triggered by touching can activate the AMY. The touching of media is processed by the thalamus with inputs to both the AMY and reward circuitry. These inputs contribute to an evaluation of the stimuli as either dangerous or safe and pleasurable. Tactile sensations and emotional memories are often bi-directionally associated (Vance & Wahlin, 2008).

While benign signals are first sent to the neocortex, the AMY receives fear-arousing visual signals before they are processed by the neocortex (LeDoux, 2002). The same is true for ambiguous tactile signals and for amalgams of visual, tactile, and verbal stimuli, which are difficult to label as safe or unsafe. In fact, the AMY houses memories of such stimuli. Therefore, at times, a person is likely to feel and then act, before the neocortex has had time to process the information. Generally, circuitry conveying fear responses (LeDoux, 2002) departs from the AMY on two possible pathways. One is a lower path that goes down into the body, and the other is a higher path that engages cortical and reasoning areas. When acting on thalamic sensory-based messages interpreted as threatening, the AMY immediately sends messages along the low road to alert the body. It also sends and receives messages from the sensory cortex that confirm or negate the fear response via the high road (Kravits, 2008a). However, the lower pathways associated with subcortical structures and autonomic functions react quicker than the high-road recipients do. As multiple bodily and neural sensors respond to touch via pressure, temperature, pain, joint position, muscle sense, and movement, they forward information to the thalamic-amygdala projections, resulting in such immediate automatic reactions (Kalat, 2012). For example, a person will most likely dart away from ambiguous stimuli or avoid a vague sensory trauma reminder, such as the sticky feel of clay. It is only when the high-road cortical response conveys that the stickiness is only a texture that the stimuli ceases to cause unease. In fact, sometimes the AMY fear response is so urgent, that the neocortex is not involved until after danger has passed. This is one of the reasons touching clients with a history of sexual abuse is contraindicated. Their cortical higher-pathway responses are weakened (Hass-Cohen et al., 2014).

Four general areas of the AMY are involved in fear response: the top, two areas in the center, and a bottom area. When a fear stimulus activates the top part, the dorsal lateral region (D-LA), it stimulates the central nucleus (CeN) of the AMY and/or the bed nucleus of the stria terminalis (BNST), considered part of the extended AMY. The CeN or the BNST activates the hypothalamus to bring on the fight, flight, or freeze response. This deactivates the bottom area, which is associated with coping (LeDoux, 2003a; Panzer, Viljoen, & Roos, 2007). A fear response often results from a conditioned stimulus response (CSR). A CSR occurs when one associates neutral stimuli, like watery clay, with an evocative stimulus, like a childhood memory of being scolded for getting one's hands dirty. For example, in rat studies in which a sound was paired with an electrical shock, the same sound eventually elicited a freeze response in the rats even when presented without the electrical shock (LeDoux, 1996). This kind of fear-based response triggers the top, D-LA, which is exquisitely sensitive to conditioned fear-based stimuli. Fear-based responses further sensitize connections between the D-LA and the CeN, causing a bias toward passive coping (Figure 8.7). Over time, this D-LA fear-based CSR inhibits active basal-coping responses. However, if, over a period, the trigger for the CSR is repeated without the shock, the conditioned

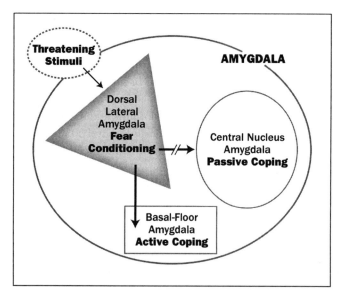

Figure 8.7 *Three Areas of Amygdala Function.* The dorsolateral amygdala (D-LA) and the central nucleus (CeN) or the bed nucleus of the stria terminalis (BNST) can become conditioned to fearful or anxiety-promoting stimuli, causing a conditioned stimulus response, which weakens connections to the basal lateral AMY involved in active coping responses (updated from Ledoux, 2003a; Panzer et al., 2007).

response may be subsequently extinguished and the AMY's ability to produce the fear response decreases (LeDoux, 1996). The AMY connects to the medial prefrontal cortex (mPFC) which can dampen the emotive reaction. Its superficial region has been also associated with activation by social stimuli (Baeken et al., 2014). Future research may continue to shed light on the possible importance of this information for clinical applications.

The AMY is also connected to the anterior cingulate cortex (ACC) and the right hemisphere orbitofrontal cortex (OFC). Both are involved in autobiographical memory and directly inhibit the AMY (LeDoux, 2003). In other words, when an individual draws a representation of a CSR related to a traumatic autobiographical memory, and the OFC or ACC inhibits AMY responses, there are no evocative consequences. With this association weakened, an extinction of the traumatic response can begin to occur. "It's an image of my stepfather shouting at me, but it's only on paper and there will not be an adrenalizing, negative abusive consequence here and now. It's only a red-and-black image of a shout on paper." Unfortunately, even after the extinction of a response, lower storage cells in the basal lateral and central nucleus of the AMY seem to store the trigger and can be re-sensitized to react. Clinically, this may mean that a diversity of interventions is needed to help calm the person (Hass-Cohen, 2015a, 2015b).

Motor Responses

We suggested in Chapter 3 that intentional fine motor activity may activate a sense of control that can mitigate fearful, unsafe feelings and thereby assist in the expression and exploration of basic emotions. Such therapeutic assistance is grounded in the interface of the motor system with the CeN fight, flight, or freeze response (LeDoux, 2003). Motor movements help resolve the fear response, for example, clay pounding and lifting. These movements involve fine and gross motor activity. Activating older reptilian areas, specifically cerebellar-motor-system outputs and involving the basal ganglia engages involuntary and voluntary movements. It also brings online cognitive processes, such as working memory and the planning of future behavior (Strick, 2002). In support of these ideas, research suggests that dysfunction in the basal ganglia or the cerebellum may contribute to behavioral problems associated with depression and autism (Hoshi, Tremblay, Feger, Carras, & Strick, 2005; Timmann & Daum, 2007). Thus it is plausible that large and fine motor movements, such as tapping can calm a fear response (King-West & Hass-Cohen, 2008).

Furthermore, the research of Panzer and colleagues (2007) indicates that there are most likely no direct neural pathways between the lateral prefrontal cortex (lPFC), and the AMY. lPFC activities which are responsible for higher thinking and executive decision making are supported by verbal discourse. Therefore, in order to support change, insight-based verbal therapies must accompany somatic and behavior-based therapies (Ogden et al., 2006; Panzer et al., 2007). Recall of fear-based memories, which can be triggered by touching, are survival oriented. Rooted in the primitive brain, they are more likely to invoke unconscious, nonverbal automatic responses. Therapeutically, verbalizing these experiences helps integrate them with higher cognitive, stabilizing prefrontal functions.

Somatosensory Strip

The processing of sensory information generated by touch has been associated with the function of the sensory cortex, which is composed of the primary somatosensory area (S1) and the secondary somatosensory area (S2). The organization of the somatosensory cortex, includes both S1 and S2. This is similar to the motor cortex found in the frontal lobe, underscoring structural communality in the important relationship between touch and movement. Both S1 and S2 activate in reaction to physical tactile stimulation (Kalat, 2012). The S1 is activated by mental representation of tactile sensations, which explains why amputees report sensations in phantom limbs (Ramachandran & Rogers-Ramachandran, 2000). Activation of the S2 has been associated with the functioning of the AMY, insula, and hippocampus. It is involved in tactile learning and memory, such as recognizing handheld objects. The S1 is located within the post central gyrus of the parietal lobe (Carlson, 2013). S1 is the main receptive area for creating the sense of touch. The S2 is responsible for the integration of sensory information through connections with higher-order functions in the parietal cortex, the insula, and indirectly, the premotor cortex. It is tucked just behind the S1. There is a map of sensory space called a homunculus at the area of the S1. Meaning "little human" in Latin, the homunculus is a scaled representation of the human body (Figure 8.8).

The size of the brain map devoted to certain areas of the body is not proportional to the size of each body region, but instead depends on the amount or importance of somatosensory input from that area. For example, a large area of S1 is devoted to sensation in the hands and lips, while the area devoted to the back is much smaller. Rachel's *Mysterious Expression*, a pair of large lips made out of clay (Figure 8.2), intuits this neurobiological phenomenon. Thus the manipulation of the clay may provide implicit access to nonverbal knowledge. This speaks to the mind-body bridge afforded by art therapy, which can contribute to the profession's effectiveness.

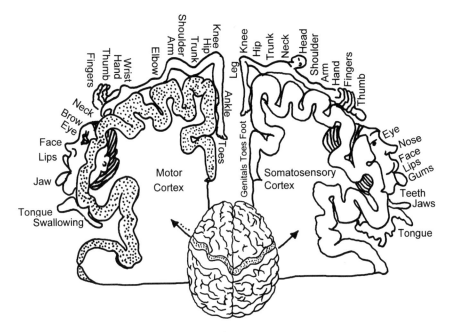

Figure 8.8 *The Brain Represented as a Homunculus.*

Curiously, Rachel's art process reveals how we are primed to access and represent the proportionally larger areas of the somatosensory homunculus. It is as if pressing and touching the clay stimulates ancient dispositions that explain the artist's yearning to draw, paint, and sculpt hands and facial elements as fine art objects. This priming also explains why, as art viewers, we are drawn to portraits and depictions of hands and facial elements. Most evocatively, it offers insight into the fascination that classic images have for viewers, such as Mary holding Jesus and Mona Lisa's smile. Both actual sensory experiences and somatosensory mental representations inform the brain.

Somatosensory cortex activation is foundational for the awareness and processing of sensory information. However, it seems to be an insufficient condition for the mental awareness of touch. It is likely that the reciprocal interactions between the entire somatosensory cortex and other cortical brain areas create awareness, processing, and storage of tactile information (Berry & Hansen, 1996; Gallace & Spence, 2010). Thus, sensations are transmitted from the skin through various afferent neural pathways to the thalamus, which distributes them to the limbic area and specifically the AMY. They are then transmitted onward to areas involving S1 and S2 as well as the parietal and frontal areas of the cerebral cortex.

The Parietal Lobe

Parietal areas interpret touch sensations and forward this information to cognitive areas thus informing us of where we are spatially. Parietal processing integrates touch, vision, and audition (Kalat, 2012). Interestingly, visual information from the occipital lobe of the cerebral cortex has a strong influence on our awareness of the intensity of tactile information. This influence is due to the ongoing repetitive association between visual and tactile stimuli. Thus, the somatosensory neurons respond to visual stimuli associated with tactile stimuli received from the posterior parietal cortex, where both tactile and visual information are processed. The parietal lobe also associates tactile sensations with bodily positions. As we proceed through space, our journey is regulated so that we can choose to touch gently, forcibly, or not at all. This makes personal space around us a felt experience similar to actually touching an object. Positions in space are related to physical touch, which can be environmental, interpersonal, or both. For example, although we cannot see our backs, we can know what is behind us based on tactile information. We know without seeing that when we are seated, there is a chair back behind us. Another example involves negotiating space in a crowded city subway or bus. This requires both maintaining a sense of the space so that one does not fall on another person, and avoiding skin-to-skin contact. The involvement of both subcortical and cortical areas is necessary for tactile consciousness, meaning that managing physical and interpersonal space may become conscious to us only during frontal lobe processes or when necessary. Cognitive, cortical association of tactile information is similar to association of visual stimuli, where the integration of projections from the occipital lobe to the frontal lobes comprises the phenomenon we call seeing (Hass-Cohen & Loya, 2008). This integration of cortical and subcortical functions may explain why we normally experience touch as a unitary sense. Another conclusion from the reviewed neuroscience is that the brain areas involved in the memory for tactile stimuli (anterior and ventrolateral prefrontal cortex, OFC, posterior parietal cortex, putamen, perirhinal cortex, the insula, and the lateral occipital complex) are also most likely involved in the remembered social aspects of touch (Gallace & Spence, 2010). For example, observing professionals as they come into a conference reveals similar nonverbal negotiation. First, they pause, scanning the space and seating options. Then, depending on whether they have come alone or with other colleagues, they will strive to leave an empty seat between them and the next person, or secure seats close to their colleagues. Seeking or avoiding touch is thus part and parcel of interpersonal socialized space.

Finally, tactile processing is strongly influenced by verbal processing

(Tanaka, Fukushina, Okanoya, & Myowa-Uamakoshi, 2014). The conglomerate of touch, vision, and auditory information forms the sensory backbone of verbalized social memories.

> *The sensory memory of my mother sitting on her stairs and stroking my hair, brushing it again and again, in a valiant yet critical effort to keep those curls in check, gives me goose bumps. The close quarters of the cool marble stairs, shielded from the blazing heat, which led out from her kitchen to the back yard, are now long gone. But the daily strokes of my hairbrush going in and out and the memory of marble on the soles of my feet and the stories that I tell myself about her are here with me as I paint long and tangly strips of brown paint.* Noah Hass-Cohen

The Insula

Insula function is another example of the connection to bodily sensations. Considered the fifth lobe of the cerebral cortex, it is responsible for processing stimuli that arise within the body. The insula also notices ongoing bodily conditions in others, contributing to our ability to understand and to empathize with others. Furthermore, its cortex plays a part in regulating extreme emotions, awareness, and expressions of bodily states, such as disgust and pain (Carlson, 2013).

Body image is composed of primarily visual characteristics, whereas the body schema has proprioceptive, tactile, and kinetic aspects. The two are intertwined and usually inseparable, yet each contributes differently to the awareness of bodily and interpersonal touch. Researchers studying the neural correlates of the affective aspects of tactile processing implicated the insular cortex in our emotional and hormonal responses to tactile contact (Wessberg, Olausson, Fernstrom, & Vallbo, 2003).

Neurotransmitters

Breast-feeding, social grooming, and other occurrences of nurturing interpersonal touch can activate a number of neurotransmitters, including norepinephrine and serotonin, as well as oxytocin, known as the bonding hormone (Kravits, 2008b). Lack of touch has been linked to a cycle of reduction in serotonin circulation and maladaptive outcomes, such as feelings of depression. Norepinephrine depletion may mean that high levels of dopamine and the accompanying impulsive behavior will not be checked or inhibited, a result often linked to aggression in children. Field (2004), a primary researcher in the area of touch for children, suggests that massage therapy can increase norepinephrine and serotonin levels, which in turn may inhibit such excessive dopamine release.

CREATE PRINCIPLES AND CLINICAL APPLICATIONS

The primary focus of the studio art therapy activities in this chapter is the CREATE principle of Expressive Communicating of pleasant, unpleasant, or even fear-based experiences. In this context, group members sculpted a series of personal representations, making large, medium, and small objects, with three different clays. We also discussed the different types of touch and hypothesized on the therapeutic advantages and neuroscience of AMITS.

From the very beginning, clients experience different types of art therapy precursors to touch, which engage a variety of relational and emotional dynamics. For example, the rise of unconscious emotional reactions may be elicited by even the simple presentation of materials. Opening a package of Plastilina or Sculpey may be experienced as a gift, something special, either an enticement or something not to be touched. The block of wet clay may appear approachable, or too dirty, or with a definite odor. These internal provocations predispose the clients' emotional senses and, at times, may also raise feelings of safety or danger, depending on the associated memories.

We postulate that engaging limbic structures, such as the AMY, in the sensorial stimulation of working with clays provides access to basic emotions. Deliberately working with clay stimulates the rich interaction of limbic, cortical, and bodily sensorial pathways, permitting access to implicit emotional memories. Handling the different clays can trigger a wealth of emotional expression through physical contact and movements, including tearing, pushing, punching, slapping, and piercing wet clay, as well as rolling, flattening, modeling, and sculpting finer clays. These expressions can also be accompanied by a variety of smells. The vividness of colored clays, such as the oil-based clays, stimulates further emotional reactions and processing.

The sensory stimulation of working with clay models also engages motor system skills, bodily awareness, and motivation, which are Creative Embodiment advantages. The different qualities of the three kinds of clay require clients to use a variety of motor skills, ranging from large gestures needed for picking up and kneading the earth clay to fine motor manipulation for the intricate modeling of polymer clay. Experimenting with the object sizes also requires the practice of a variety of motor skills that contribute to emotional and cognitive familiarity, and a sense of empowerment and accomplishment. The motor movements involved in handling clay promote sensory haptic experiences that access clients' memories associated with interpersonal touch and space. As discussed, beholding the art and the art making initiates movement and organizes how group members move around within the space. In addition, as clients navigate the shared space of the studio, moving among the tables that hold clay, the toaster oven that bakes the polymer clay, and areas such as cabinets where the earth clay dries, they begin to accommodate everyone's personal space and needs. Similarly, at each table, the sharing of materials calls forth gestures and motions supporting real or symbolic touching of each other's productions. Opportunities spontaneously arise through this movement for accidental and instrumental touch, which shape the interpersonal space. Symbolically, the playful manipulation, touching, and placing of the self-made Human Figurines can invite clients to experiment with sharing and controlling interpersonal space. Modulation of interpersonal space via mirrored touching, gesturing, sitting close or far, and turning toward or away from others further complements the attuned therapist's ATR-N microskill set.

The CREATE principle of Relational Resonating is deeply embedded in the experientials' focus on touch. The request to represent Personal Objects and Human Figurines creates a contagious social environment that is infused with personal meaning, mentalizing and reflection. Therapists can aid this therapeutic and creative expression by anticipating and structuring the process by thinking ahead, foreseeing the pitfalls of unfamiliar media, and attuning to technical mishaps. The art therapist's microskills can promote a strong sense of safety and emotional comfort for clients. To illustrate, we advocate advising clients to start by taking hold of portions of clay that feel just the right size in the palm. The manageable size combined with the direct sensory experience can aid in the self-regulation of comfort. We offer soft pieces of cloth to work on, which contain dry fallout from the clay and permit easy handling and removal of the work from a surface. Propping up a delicate piece of clay work with foil gives it support, while painting white carpenter's glue or acrylic paint on wet clay assists the drying process, prevents cracking, and gives color and sheen. Explicitly referencing and verbalizing the type of touch, such as, "May I hold and support your clay sculpture?" brings awareness of the dyadic nature of the client-therapist-client relationships. Thus, awareness of interpersonal touch and space becomes an experience of symbolic and concrete relational connectivity. Salient emotional meaning may then be instilled into activities, such as placing Plastilina in a cool place where it will not fade or melt, wrapping ceramic objects so that they dry as slowly as they need to, and talking through an ambitious construction.

The ATR-N therapist's microskills described in this chapter are much more than the skills of a craftsman. They have critical therapeutic meaning as they embody the maker's "third hand" and "third eye," and perhaps even a "second mind." The third hand represents the task, and the third eye leads to intuiting what kinds of supportive touching are needed, whereas the "second mind," a term that we came up with, is the social mind that knows what the other intends to represent. It is a practical application of theory-of-mind constructs (Frith & Frith, 1999; 2003; 2006).

Working with clay can also readily access attachment IWM and memories. Affect based autobiographical memories are seated in the limbic system and linked to the OFC brain region, an area that has a key role in the regulation of affect and attunement. Such linked areas are also appraisal centers for visual and sensory-haptic inputs. Instrumental and task-oriented touch, as in the handling and exchange of materials, provides a way for the therapist to touch subcortical and cortical-symbolic levels of representation, connect emotionally, and reach implicit affect regulation states with the client while deliberately developing intentional relational attunement. The therapist is intimately present, touching the self of the client via her or his self-objects, and providing a container for emotional and sensory experiences.

Working with the variety of different clays can be a challenge. Each kind of clay requires different handling and skills that are often demanding, eliciting the CREATE principle of Adaptive Responding. The challenge of making complex clay sculptures, or having one's work witnessed by others, stimulates discussions about fear and performance anxiety. Offering a variety of different clay types is an ATR-N clinical skill, providing the opportunity to practice coping skills. A range of structured to less structured safe art therapy media provides contexts where modeling highly controllable plastic-based clay can calm and focus. In contrast, messy water-based clay may excite or stimulate uncertainty and fearfulness (Malchiodi, 1998a). Stimulation from touching as well as exchanging the media may engage sympathetic nervous system responses that are alarming or excitatory, or inhibitory parasympathetic coping responses. The therapist's guidance and task-oriented touching support coping and the building of increased tolerance for affect, whereas incidental or controlling touches may create the opposite effect. The Imagined Loved Landscape environment provides opportunities to revisit sensory-based memories of times and places where support was available or experienced.

The opportunities for supporting the CREATE principle of Transformative Integrating are present within the relational context of working with clay along with others or a therapist. Within a safe therapeutic relationship, the kinesthetic, emotional, and meta-higher-cognitive processing involved in working with clay supports integrated meaning making and elaboration of coherent narratives of self and other.

Experiences of felt and anticipated aid support the emergence of Empathizing and Compassion. The therapist, who is the "third hand," "third eye," and "second mind," overtly and symbolically empathizes with the client's needs. In addition, mirroring, echoing, and imitating clients' hand gestures form a language that conveys understanding and empathy. Different types of touching, such as reference to features and appearance and pointing, as well as talking about the art, convey relational interest and caring. In essence, these microskills model compassion building. Instrumental touch, the intent of which is to help convey prosocial meanings, is augmented by task-supportive touch. Furthermore, mindful attention to types of touch supports mutual empathy, insight, and compassion. The client also has the opportunity to mimic the therapist's hand gestures and work, forming a language that conveys understanding and empathy. Such reciprocal dialogue moves the client toward experiences of felt and anticipated aid and the CREATE principle of Empathizing and Compassion. We expand on these last ideas in Chapter 13.

CHAPTER 9

Adaptive Responding:
Fear and Stress

I remember the first time that I heard about the long-term stress response and its ill consequences. My first reaction was disbelief, guilt, and then fear because I know that I carry and create a great deal of stress; for myself and, at times, for others. In the decade or more since then, I have seen my art therapy students and clients go through the same kind of reaction. In my case, I have been able to figure out that when I feel confident that I can do what I set out to do, the stressors then do not seem to get to me. However, when I am overwhelmed and do not feel in control, or when I experience my significant others as distancing themselves from me, I can literally feel cortisol coursing through my veins, pecking holes in my memory, bruising my muscles, and inflaming my skin. I have learned to physically and emotionally recognize this phenomenon. I am not sure how my students can experience less stress since it seems to be an integral part of the demands of getting a higher education. I try to encourage them to be part-time students, usually without success. I am learning to observe my stress ebb and flow. I still need to learn how to do less, accept it as "my stress," look inward, reach out to others, and learn to live with my stress peacefully. Noah Hass-Cohen

Through the art, the client can gain a sense of control over the stress-arousing subject matter, especially by using structured media. Making art can also help bring the perception of the stressor and one's response to it to a higher road by repeatedly and safely exposing the client to the arousing stimuli and creating newer, calmer associations to it. Tamara Cates

STRESS RESPONSES MAY PRESENT ON multiple levels, ranging from short-lived to long-term and chronic stress. A short-term stress reaction can transform to a long-term stress response and in time take the form of a post-traumatic stress disorder. Types of stressors also vary from an expected day-to-day stressor to a single unexpected, or a reoccurring expected traumatic event. We expand on the CREATE principle of Adaptive Responding in this chapter and the next. Here we discuss short- to long-term stress responses, whereas Chapter 10 focuses on chronic stress and complex trauma reactions.

Adaptation happens as a result of an individual's attempt to control his or her environment via fight, flight, or freeze cycles, or by turning to others. Tending or befriending others by seeking social support is recognized as a preferred female stress response (Taylor et al., 2000). Thus, relational options can provide alternatives or additions to the natural inclination toward fighting others, running away, or freezing. Such viable relational options also include turning to others or turning inward to the self, and finding a literal or internal safe place (Sapolsky, 2004). This is particularly true given increasingly urban, physically restrictive environments. Unlike life in the ancestral jungle environment, in modern life we cannot run away from our jobs, our families, and our cities. While Taylor has found that it is mostly females that turn to others, the role of social interaction in mitigating the stress response has now been established (Davidson & McEwen, 2012).

Governed by the brain and the nervous system's checks and balances, the adaptation to stress involves the stabilization of basic life functions. From survival and psychological perspectives, adaptation contributes to a sense of safety, self-control, acceptance, and resiliency. Furthermore, as adaptation requires a change in our relationship to the stressor long-term changes in how we respond to stressors may occur. For example, an anxious traveler can control panic attacks, a short-term stress response, by regulating breathing, and this knowledge can help establish a sense of safety for future airplane rides. Adaptive responses to long-term stressors, however, require a more complicated relationship. For instance, while a bereaved husband who lost his wife to a chronic disease may slowly reach out to others and start to integrate the loss into his daily life, he may still experience a longing for her. Physiologically, his nervous system echoes this change, and there may still be short bouts of hyper-arousal in which he wants to flee from the empty house or hide in their bed. Yet he can now eat, sleep, and read in their home. He is no longer frequently ill with colds and aches, and finds himself more interested in others, as evidenced by generally being able to enjoy things that he previously liked. He is therefore surprised when, on the second anniversary of his wife's death, he again feels frozen, as if dead himself, for a few days, just going through the motions of daily life.

The magnitude of natural disasters like Hurricane Katrina, human-instigated disasters like the 9/11 terrorist attacks, interpersonal violence such as rape, abuse, and domestic violence, as well as combat-related post-traumatic stress disorder (PTSD) play an important role. However, despite the undeniable and unavoidable effects of such trauma, it is probable that an individual's history of distress and perception and felt sense of a particular stressor, trauma, or problem is the most important indicator of how the response will manifest (Lanius, Bluhm, & Frewen, (2011). Frequently a person's attachment history, as well as the immediate reaction to the stressor, will influence the nature of such a reaction (Siegel, 2012). This information is often tricky to convey to ourselves and to others as it may be interpreted as finding fault with our own or others' reactions. Developing compassion toward self and others may hold the key to the transfer and use of this knowledge.

To engage with the cycles of stress, safety, and resilience, our creative milieu members first engage in a quick drawing of a stressful moment or a problem. As stress-based memories are nonverbal, these are critical learning experiences; working with the sensory arts may easily reactivate a vivid memory from a difficult time and facilitate this work. In the second experiential, members transition to considering the relational aspects of the stress response by making an Adaptation Container. The expressive container represents internal, or implicit, and external, or explicit, responses, many of which are encoded in attachment based internal working models (IWMs). Accordingly, the creation of a container may lead participants to consider the differences between what they present to others and what they may experience internally. As they describe and detail their containers, infuse them with meaning, reflect and change what needs to be altered, they are acquiring coping skills. Comparing between inner and outer representations of the container can also lead to a mixed sense of perceived control and resiliency and hopelessness as well as sadness, which can be a stepping-stone toward mourning and resolution. In the third and fourth experientials, we reflect on how drawing a Safe Relationship and Turning toward Others image, can further foster a sense of a safe haven and comfort as an antidote to both short-term and long-term stress responses. The next experiential requires the participants to reconsolidate this information by envisioning an ongoing stressor, and to represent turning toward others as a coping response.

EXPERIENTIAL PRACTICES AND DIRECTIVES

Experience I: Stressful Moment

Alerting the stress response, we start the group with a request for: "Draw an image of a vivid stressful moment that you have experienced." The chosen moment should be a short-term stressful experience that feels safe to visually or verbally disclose. Mimicking the quick, millisecond-long flight-or-fight response, the drawings will be executed rapidly (Figure 9.1).

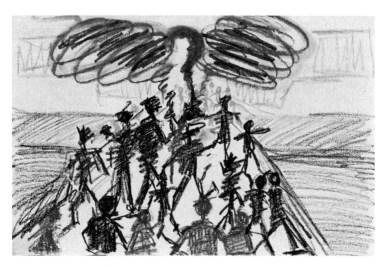

Figure 9.1 *Short-Term Stress Reaction.* A crowd of gray and black figures move across a bridge. In the distance, a bright pink-and-orange tornado lands on a small lost figure in the distance. Joanna Clyde Findlay

I vividly remember being out with my family in a crowded public place crossing a bridge when my husband and I realized we had lost sight of our son. I recall the rapid panic, the crowd becoming a gray blur, and my attention flashing everywhere, desperately searching for him. Suddenly, I saw his shape and found him and I knew that he was safe. It was as if all of the people fell away and I could breathe again. Joanna Clyde Findlay

Suddenly, a palpable tension fills the air as the theme and time limit inject the studio with edginess. Some group members will fumble in their media art boxes for materials, while others rise to stand in front of their tables. There is sudden quiet and an intensity of gestures. As the work time ends, members look up as if suddenly pulled away from a private world. The reminder to title their art and put materials away facilitates the shift to sharing their work as a group.

We then form a semicircle and reflect upon the drawings that are laid out on the floor. Black, gray, and urgent reds and oranges frequently dominate the art. Lines are often jagged and the pressure of the crayons, pencils, or markers exerted while drawing may be readily visible (Figures 9.1).

Within the group, the levels of self-disclosure may vary. However, most members share relief in not being alone in their art making stress reactions and in finding out that others have also experienced sweaty palms, breathing tension, and/or increased heart rates. Some of the Stressful Moment drawings seem more automatic and abstract, with bursts of intense color and shape, while others are more narrative, with discernible progression in content and form. Automatic drawings use limbic system language, are less form-based, and tend to utilize color, line, and movement. These images transmit a powerful sense of striving for control. Conversely, planned and processed drawings are more thought out and appear to have a story line.

Studio participants also relay how their bodily responses differed when they made images of short-term versus ongoing stressors. One young woman described feeling a sudden twist of instant stress in her gut as she drew her vivid, stressful memory. This is opposed to the heavy tension of constant worry in the neck and upper back associated with long-term distress, which was reported by others. Short-term stress images may be identifiable as episodic, sensory memories clearly situated in space and time. Long-term stress images seem to evoke repetitive, endless road-like symbols and diffuse uneasy imagery (Figure 9.2).

> *The drawing on the left shows my short-term stress response with my tendency to want to hide when faced with a stressful situation. The drawing on the right shows my effort to manage my response to long-term stress by treating it as a journey with many obstacles, but a steady path to follow.* Rachel Tate

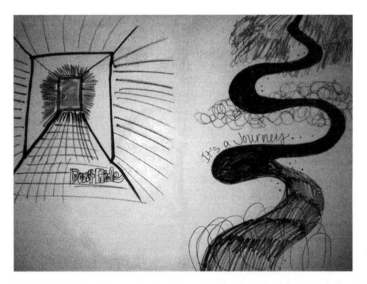

Figure 9.2 *Don't Hide/It's a Journey.* On the right, a bright yellow door is found at the end of a corridor. The door is outlined in red and emanates orange lines. On the right, a twisting path winds its way through first blue, then green and red looping lines. Rachel Tate

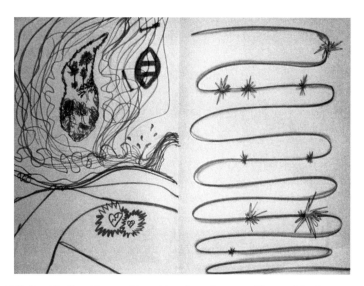

Figure 9.3 *Fear.* The Short-Term and Long-Term Stress-Response. The top of the drawing represents the rushing blue river, a small island, and the orange canoe. On the lower left, two hearts in red depict the artist and her father by the side, watching the river. The image on the right shows a winding green and yellow line intersected irregularly by flashes of orange and red. Tamara Cates.

We also talk about how to phrase a stress-informed directive. For example, the open-ended directive, "Draw what happened," can lead to a fear-based limbic response. On the contrary, the directive, "Draw your specific reaction to your stress or stressor," labels the experience and focuses on the reaction to the incident (Figure 9.3).

> *My art was about a river-rafting trip that I took with my family when we went down the biggest rapid and we all fell out of the raft and landed in the white water. My sympathetic nervous system and fight-or-flight response went immediately into action, and my dad and I swam as hard as we could to the shore. At one point I looked back and saw my mom and brother, who were not swimming; they were just looking stunned and scared, and floating down the river. My dad and I stood on the shore, waiting and waiting. . . . I depicted the two of us in my art by drawing two broken hearts. I was aware of how scared I was, but I did not actually feel scared.* Tamara Cates

Although commonly used as synonyms, stress is the reaction to a stressor. Stress itself also acts as a stressor to which we react. Another orienting directive, "Draw what you came to see me for or why you are here today?" locates the focus in the here and now and points to the resources available in the clinical setting. We also discuss the impact of media choice. Furthermore, when we restrict the media to structured tools such as pencils and crayons, it allows for more control of emotions. This is in contrast to the use of fluid tools, such as paint, which support the spilling over of affect. In the same vein, using paper with small dimensions versus large formats reflects the artists' quest for control.

> *The media (markers and paper) felt safe because it was easy to use and it provided me with a lot of control over what I was creating. However, the subject matter and the actual activity felt less safe. Being asked to remember and portray a specific stressful situation actually brought back some of the feelings I experienced when the real situation took place. Many other participants used the same kind of energy I did to portray their short-term stress responses. The artworks had similarities in color as well. I noticed that many of us used red to depict the stress.* Lisa Kandros

Experience II: Adaptation Container

Our second art experience focuses on the development of stress management and adaptability resources. For the Adaptation Container experiential, we ask the studio participants to: "Choose a box of any size, ranging from one small enough to fit in the palm of your hand to large enough to carry with both hands. Then decorate it inside and out, representing your private intrapersonal self on the inside, and your social interpersonal self on the outside." Often called an inside-outside box, the Adaptation Container directive has been used many times by art therapists. It is psychodynamically oriented, with the outside thought to represent the conscious level and the inside representing the unconscious; the internal versus external self. Our name for the directive reflects the ATR-N approach as we are interested in how the implicit-explicit and internal-external representations function to support interpersonal and social adaptation. The relationship between the inside and outside representations can reveal our ways of responding, as well as our ways of coming up with resilient coping responses. Some may be apparent to other people, others just to ourselves.

We discuss how adaptive responses and internal working models (IWMs) of security are evoked when we take thoughtful ownership of our inner space through artistic expression. This can be accomplished by adding inspiring images, symbols of faith, love, connection to special others, small tokens, and soothing colors or textures. For some, such a connection becomes a touch point for future resources. Sometimes real or symbolic places and people are

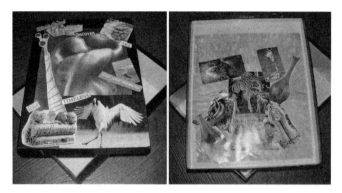

Figure 9.4 *My Inside and Outside Boxes.* My internal and external self are reflected in the symbols I chose for the lid of the box. On the box lid, on the left, there is a central photograph of a brass sculpture, above which there are symbols for the sun and moon, and the natural world. The lower half of the collage shows images of puppies and a bird. The image on the right shows the collage glued inside the pink interior of the box. On a radiant yellow image, various photographs can be seen representing closeness or touch: hands in prayer, two figures embracing, pairs of animals touching. Channie Thal

referenced, which can create a private sanctuary space. We explore the relationship between the inside and outside of the boxes because it provides clues to the person's position on the continuum of striving for control, feeling in control, or a loss of control (Henry & Wang 1999). Accordingly, the box can reveal the successful fit between the inside and outside of the self as the person achieves a balanced, self-compassionate, and adaptive response to his or her environment. The Adaptation Container is a holding environment for these dynamics and can also be used for containing and safekeeping of artwork (Figure 9.4).

When the inside and outside do not fit, such disharmony can indicate a feeling of loss of control, and risks a long-term, enduring stress reaction. The process of making the Adaptation Container not only helps the person recognize this discrepancy, but it also provides an opportunity to address it in a creative, constructive way. A softening process may occur in which self-understanding and compassion may foster resources and allow the person to tend to herself.

The cultural majority tends to value strong individual identity, while minorities have varying ideas of the value of one's inner world (McGoldrick, Giordano, & Garcia-Preto, 2005). For some studio participants, it may be important to develop transparency between the internal and external. Others may experience the inside-outside binary as a culturally driven idea. From a psychological perspective, some are often reluctant to share their inner landscape, leaving their box closed. It may then be important to keep the internal and external separate. This is valuable information about a person and his or her access to stress-coping resources.

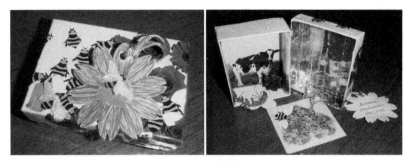

Figure 9.5 *Adaptation Box.* Decorated lid with red flowers and yellow bees on left. On right, the inside of the box is decorated with personal symbols. The bees, on the lid, represent external industriousness, whereas as the black-and-white cow is a symbol for immobile, internal calm. Kazuko Numato

The inherent qualities of a box that can be opened, closed, filled, emptied, or locked lend themselves to a great range of possibilities for experiencing control, loving self-care, and safety (Figure 9.5). Symbolically these are mentalizing processes. Studio participants anticipate and learn from others as they see boxes tied with ribbons, hinged, or sealed. Indeed, the different methods in which boxes are decorated provide important relational insights.

> *Everyone was able to both conceal and reveal any past memories, future hopes and different parts of herself. Initially I was not sure if I felt safe—yet when my box was completed, I felt a sense of ease and acceptance as I had managed not to listen to my inner critic while I was creating. I actually created something that I was proud of. A sense of safety emerged together with relief and pride emerged. It was as if the environment became more secure. This studio feels so much better than art school because we focus on the process and on us as a group.*
> Lisa Kandaros

Experience III: Draw a Safe Relationship

The third studio art experience, Safe Relationship, focuses on the expression of a perceived sense of safety. To promote a sense of security, the media choices are arranged within easy reach and include paper, oil pastels, markers, and drawing materials, as well as unused paper plates. We then invite each participant in our creative community to pay attention to how their body feels. Sometimes we add more specifics, such as grounding interventions that include paying attention to the sitting posture, contact of the back and legs against the chair, and the natural movement of breath in the belly and chest. The directive asks for each person to: "Represent a safe relationship with a living or deceased person, or a beloved pet." Group members are invited to feel the comfort, reassurance, and acceptance this relationship offers. Other senses are also involved, including associated colors seen, sounds heard, the setting in which they are present, and the temperature evoked.

For Draw a Safe Relationship, artists can choose to create within a circular containing frame (Jung, 1963) which can safely contain the image. We reassure them that the image may be an abstract representation, as often people will struggle with whether or not to draw realistic images. Most often, warm or pastel colors with soft curved lines, marks, shapes, and colors can access the relationship more intuitively. Whether realistic or abstract, the vivid elaboration of the setting or environment in which the relationship occurs is encouraged. It's as if we are ingraining the support that the safe relationship offers in our memory. It is this directive that helps develop a gentle and kind attitude to self, to what has happened to the self, to mistakes made, or to things that have happened outside the sphere of the individual's control. Once the drawing has been completed, group members write a title on the back, place their images on the floor in a semicircle, and gather around to share. Sometimes, given the highly personal content of the imagery, it works best to begin sharing more generally about the form and color (Figure 9.6).

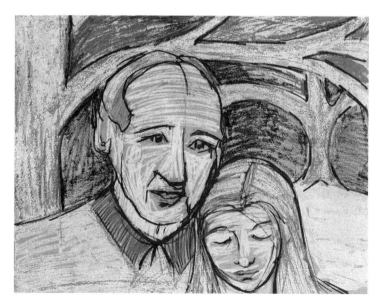

Figure 9.6 *My Safe Relationship.* An image of being held. Set in a nurturing landscape of trees, a father holds a daughter close as she rests her head on his shoulder, peacefully shutting her eyes. Joanna Clyde Findlay

As I focused on my felt sense of safety, it became clear to me that I was reexperiencing the comfort and trust that a child may have in a caregiver. This image evokes the comfort of closeness, being in my father's arms as a young child, closing my eyes and relaxing as he watches over me. The background describes the ease of summer warmth in the rural setting of my childhood. I drew the blue contours first. I then deliberately added color in flat planes to emphasize a childlike image, like pieces of a puzzle that add up to a complete rosy image. Joanna Clyde Findlay

In this way, the three creative experientials progress from a request: Depict a Stressful Moment, involving a sense of loss of control and a fight-or-flight coping response, to the Adaptation Container, in which control or striving for control-based representations is encouraged. Then, there is an invitation to: Draw a Safe Relationship, which is a preservative image based on a remembered sense of security. The fourth experiential, described below, exemplifies the value of actively turning toward and tending to others.

Experience IV: Turning Toward Others

Turning toward others is a little less-recognized component of the stress response. In preparation for learning about the continuum of stress and relational support, we ask each group member to represent a long-term stress response: "Draw your reaction to an ongoing life stressor, such as loss, illness, a relational problem, or a social hardship." Once this first part of the directive is complete, the learners are invited to: "Add an image that represents a turning toward and/or tending to others." In other words, a different response to the stress is requested. The art making associated with this dialogue between the two images usually takes some time. In some cases, the two parts of the art request become one whole image, especially when they are placed or drawn side by side (Figure 9.7).

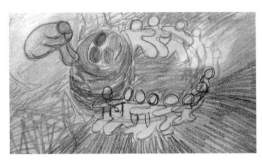

Figure 9.7 *Moving Toward Others: Expanding to Connection.* In the upper left, a gray figure is hunched over, hiding her face. Next to her there is a multicolored cocoon with red, blue, yellow, and green ovals inside. The right side of the image shows a chain of human figures in dark green, red, orange, purple, blue, light green, orange, and yellow. Joanna Clyde Findlay

This image represents withdrawal in the face of loss and distress and the healing effect of reaching out to others. My initial reaction was to hold my wound alone, as seen in the isolated figure on the left, but then the progress toward the right shows my needed connection to others. At first I sought solace within the small huddle of family safety, then I was able to open to the wider embrace of a supportive community of friends and relationships. As I connected and told my story, and was supported by these safe others, I became linked to the warmth of a rainbow of colors and feelings. In the context of the nervous system and the HPA axis, the purple gray perhaps represents damping of energy. This is in contrast to the bright energy radiating from the rainbow, brought by the release from long stress effects. Joanna Clyde Findlay

When processing the feelings that this sequence of directives may have evoked, many participants report fatigue and discomfort, as well as comfort. The damaging sense of loss of control, which is associated with long-term stress responses, can be balanced by the affiliated attachment behavior of turning toward others. Other reactions range from those who divulge life-long coping challenges and remarkable resilience, to those who feel fragile and prefer not to share detailed accounts of their burdens. Nonetheless, the second directive generally invites a conversation on how the transformed image represents resources (Sarid & Huss, 2011). Relational exchanges, family, community, and friendships are potent resources for perseverance, faith, and hope. Sometimes the studio itself is experienced as a healing environment for the participants. For example, one of the groups made a request to leave the relational images of connection and movement toward others on display in the studio. They wanted the images to continue to act as powerful interpersonal symbols. The group said that this was an important resource for repairing the ill effects of stressors and stress.

Stressors that we experience as threatening or novel may initiate either new or remembered stress responses (Cozolino, 2010). These stressors may be external circumstances or internal processes, and can activate memories of unpleasant, unknown, or threatening events. Stress responses can be triggered by visual, auditory, tactile, and proprioceptive/nociceptive sensory information. Proprioception is a felt sense of bodily position that comes from within. Nociception, on the other hand, is a response to external stimuli. In other words, painful, gustatory, vestibular, and olfactory stimuli can also be triggers. These triggers may be stimulated via the art and in the presence of caring therapists. With sufficient relational resonance, structure, and support, the potential stress response can be processed. Such a successful outcome can become a source of coping. As a result, art therapists are uniquely poised to access and process stress-based material in a safe and resourceful way.

In our ATR-N view, there is a key difference between talking about a stressor and making a changed, transformed art piece about the stressor (Hass-Cohen & Clyde Findlay, 2009). As stress is triggered, the in vivo experience evokes pleasure, achievement, and, most importantly, the sense of control that accompanies art making, contributing to a person's cache of resources. In addition to the safe presence of the therapist, it is perhaps the recruitment of executive functioning necessary for art making that can recondition the stress response. In this experiential, we therefore lead the work from forming an image of the stressful experience to actively imagining turning toward or tending to others.

RELATIONAL NEUROSCIENCE: THE SHORT- AND LONG-TERM STRESS RESPONSE

Over time, the stress response may have a severe impact on a person's sense of well-being, contributing to immune system dysfunctions and other health issues. Therefore, it is critical that people who suffer from the ill effects of day-to-day stress have access to information on the stress response. While we have described the neurobiology of the stress response in greater detail in elsewhere (Hass-Cohen, 2015a; Hass-Cohen & Carr, 2008; Hass-Cohen & Clyde Findlay, 2009; King-West & Hass-Cohen, 2008; Kravitz, 2008b), here we provide an overview that is geared toward psychoeducation.

In general the stress response can be comprised of (a) a freezing and shaking response, like a deer caught in the headlights of an oncoming car (Levine, 1997); (b) a flight-or-fight response such as running away, like a zebra from a lion, and/or fighting like a male baboon (Sapolsky, 2004); or (c) a turning to safe others and places, like cubs returning to mother's den. The first response is a very primitive immobilizing response associated with hyperactivation of the parasympathetic nervous system. The flight and fight responses are excitatory, sympathetic nervous system reactions, whereas the third response (c) is social and friendly, a turning to others response, which involves a parasympathetic balanced calming response.

In urban environments, solutions to freeze, flight-or-fight responses, which represent immediate efforts to gain relief, may not be available. For example, it is difficult to find a place in which to hide safely from, fight with, or run away from a demanding employer. Therefore, it becomes difficult to reduce and regulate stress. Thus rather than externalizing our responses to stress and resolving them quickly, they are internalized in the body (Scaer,

2001). Although freeze is an automatic response that can be protective, it can also be detrimental, as it represents an out-of-control reaction that can spiral into dissociation, flashbacks, and depersonalization. In contrast, turning to safe and soothing resources can reduce the potentially toxic physiological and psychological effects of chronic, overwhelming, or long-term stress. Examples include a tending or befriending response, such as finding comfort in sharing with a loved one, or the give and take and comforting touch of an embrace (Taylor et al., 2000). Other comforting options include seeking out a pet, a favorite place, or, alternatively, finding comfort within.

In the context of the stress response, we like to share the Buddhist "Two Arrows" parable. The first arrow is the experience of suffering, such as pain, illness, death, or personal or social injustice. The first arrow often catches us by surprise, since we have little control over it. The second arrow is our reaction to the first arrow. While the first arrow can elicit an immediate stress response, it is the second arrow that most often significantly contributes to long-term stress. This secondary reaction is more in our control, and yet we sometimes, understandably, continue to stab ourselves with second arrows. (The Buddha's parable of the two arrows can be found in the Samyutta Nikaya, 36.6, the Sallatha Sutta).

We emphasize the issue of control because it is the perceived lack of control that is the most damaging to our bodies and is a risk factor for stress-related health problems and mental health disorders. Sensory stimuli can unconsciously trigger and quickly activate the relaying of information along a direct stress response path. However, distress responses are activated not only by events that happen to us, but also by our internal perceptions, thoughts, and emotions (Barlow, 2002). Clinical conditions, like generalized anxiety, phobias, and PTSD, can manifest as a result of this mechanism (Shin & Liberzon, 2010; Ströhle & Holsboer, 2003). For example, sensory stimuli associated with past threatening experiences can trigger an automatic stress response before the conscious mind can interfere and decide whether to place the memory in the past or react to it in the present. In other words, the speed of responses that are relayed by the direct path works both to our advantage and disadvantage. This is how sensory impulses connect to an indirect path toward the frontal lobes. This allows for a slower, more cognitive evaluation of the stimuli (LeDoux & Muller, 1997).

Below, we discuss several kinds of stress- and trauma-based responses, which involve one or more bodily systems. They are listed in fairly evolutionary order: the freeze response, the short-term fight-or-flight response, and, last, the long-term stress response. Each response is followed by its function, which is then expanded upon neurobiologically.

The Freeze Response

The freeze response, which is shared by insects, animals, and humans, is a protective, evolved response to threat akin to playing dead. It can present as a feeling of rapid immobilization, and is activated by such events as thinking someone has broken into your home or an earthquake. Some people report that the experience feels as though their heart has stopped, which can quite literally happen. This crisis response of freezing is brought on by the vagal nerve, which is mediated by the reptilian brain system (Porges, 2001). Originally articulated by Walter Cannon (1942), who reported that shamans could induce heart stopping, has also been dubbed the "voodoo deaths."

This kind of heart-stopping freeze response is associated with the vagal nerve function, whose widely distributed presence in the body is signified by its Latin name, as *vagus* means wandering. On a day-to-day basis, the vagal nerve regulates the gut, encourages healthy digestion, and tips people off about their gut feelings. For example, we tend to feel nauseous when we remember traumatic experiences (Allison & Friedman, 2004). Vagal nerve regulation plays a role in both freeze and relaxation responses. It is also implicated in stress-related loss of appetite and in the development of ulcers.

Located in the vagus system, the vagal nerve is comprised of the two longest cranial nerves. The top part of the vagus system is known as the dorsal vagal complex (DVC), and the bottom part is known as the ventral vagal complex (VVC; Kalat, 2012; Porges, 2001). The DVC is the branch that is primarily responsible for the immobilization response. Stimulation of the DVC is essentially automatic and unaffected by cortical control, meaning that it is not under conscious control. Conservation of bodily resources through behavioral strategies such as immobilization and avoidance is the function of the DVC (Porges, 2001). In contrast, the VVC plays a role in social engagement and involves the bonding hormone oxytocin (Porges, 2001).

Thus, the polyvagal theory (Porges, 2001, 2011) also postulates a connection between the vagus nerve and a balanced relaxation response. When the parasympathetic nervous system is activated to relieve the body of a sympathetic stress response, the vagus nerve contributes by carrying information throughout the body, thereby enhancing the relaxation response. This information is communicated effectively due to the wandering length of the vagal nerve. Its stimulation is thought to promote social interaction as a result of its influence on heart rate, facial expression, breathing, listening, and vocalization (Porges, 1998). The polyvagal theory also proposes that the VVC regulates the lifting of the eyelids and tensing of the middle ear muscles when we listen to others. By attuning to someone's voice and linking it to verbal expression, the VVC cues our gut reactions. VVC stimulation also allows for reduction in heart rate. For example, when we are excited to be with someone and enjoy his or her company, our heart beats fast. Giving a friend a hug most often slows the heart rate, supporting perceptions of calm and enhancing the possibility of positive social interaction (Porges, 2001). Those who have personally experienced the freeze response a few times find the dual function of the vagal system quite fascinating and the knowledge comforting.

> *Freezing has happened me when I have had to say good-bye to an intense, short-term social interaction, such as a weeklong family event or even workshop. I have learned that these moments tell me that I just experienced irrevocable, relational loss. For example, when I was just out of undergraduate school I was an art facilitator at an overnight youth camp for two weeks. A fortnight of art, music, and drama with like-minded others had just finished, and I could not get out of the car that was taking me home. My legs were like rubber. Supported by research, I now think of these experiences as vagal system social responses. It helps; I know that turning to others at such times will mediate this rather strange and somewhat uncomfortable bodily response.* Noah Hass-Cohen

The Fight-or-Flight Response

The evolutionary fight-or-flight short-term stress response activates adrenaline and readies the individual for action. Such instinctive responses protect us, such as when we instinctively jump to the side when a car drives too close to us, or when we want to hide in our office for time away from pressures. One of the more common antidotes to stress is exercise, which provides many benefits, including raising adrenaline levels.

The central nervous system, which is composed of the brain and the spinal cord, works in tandem with the peripheral nervous system to orchestrate the short-term stress response. The peripheral nervous system has two main parts: the somatic nervous system and the autonomic nervous system. The somatic nervous system is the voluntary component of the peripheral nervous system, and governs conscious responses to sensory stimuli. Cranial nerves and spinal nerves receive and send sensory information, which may trigger an autonomic nervous system response.

Further dividing the nervous system, the sympathetic nervous system is responsible for the fight-or-flight response, whereas the parasympathetic nervous system allows the same response to subside by returning us to more relaxed, ordinary functioning. As discussed, the fight-or-flight response is mediated by the amygdala and the sympathetic/adrenomedullary axis (SAM). The adrenal medulla is the core of the adrenal gland, which sits on top of the kidneys. This axis involves epinephrine and norepinephrine, which stimulate organs, such as the heart, to pump more blood into larger muscles. This increased blood flow primes muscles for running or fighting. When the perceived danger has passed, the parasympathetic nervous system stimulates the relaxation response.

A quick and immediate SAM response has been conceptualized as functionally signaling a person's attempts to be in control (Henry & Wang, 1999). In this regard, the organism's priority is self-preservation. In fact, more recently, stress response systems that can have negative effects on the immune system and aging have been re-conceptualized as malleable over the life span (McEwen, 2013). The sympathetic and parasympathetic nervous systems work together, allowing our internal bodily states to shift between mild variations of excitation and relaxation as we respond to the environment. Thus, for the most part, the stress response is automatic and influenced by rapid transmission of impulses from sensory inputs to the limbic system. Sensory impulses are forwarded along a quick, direct path (LeDoux & Muller, 1997) from the thalamus directly to the amygdala. The amygdala processes the impulses and relays information through the SAM system, initiating the flight, fight, freeze, and social engagement responses (Porges, 2001).

As discussed in Chapter 8, it is thought that four general areas of the amygdala are involved in the fear response: top, bottom, and the two areas in the center. When a fear stimulus activates the central nucleus of the amygdala and/or the bed nucleus of the stria terminalis, considered part of the extended amygdala, the central nucleus and/or the bed nucleus activate the hypothalamus. This activates the quick short-term stress pathway: the fight, flight, or freeze response (LeDoux, 2003a; Panzer et al., 2007; Figure 8.7). In contrast, the indirect path is significantly longer. Information leaves the thalamus, travels to the primary sensory cortex, the entorhinal cortex, the OFC, the hippocampus, and finally to the lateral amygdala. This indirect path involves many more neurons and therefore unfolds more slowly. The result is the engagement of cortical areas where analysis, judgment, and resulting modification of our responses occur. The reevaluation of relevant implicit and explicit memories is thus routed to appropriate systems for action (LeDoux & Muller, 1997).

The transformation of a negative response into a positive or assertive response can result in a shift from a neuroendocrine-mediated feeling of loss of control to a sympathetic nervous system–based feeling of being in control. This dual function is mirrored in the fight-or-flight response, which initially increases immune function, then diminishes it (Sapolsky, 2004). While these are adaptive responses, over time, repeated and chronic over-arousal transforms into long-term stress and can manifest on the continuum of anxiety, depression, trauma, and health disorders.

The functional description of the short-term stress response provided above allows art therapists to understand the sympathetic nervous system and adrenal medulla axis response as an adaptive response. In art therapy sessions, refusals to draw, or hurried marks on the page, are behaviors that portray visual imprints of an adaptive response. Alternatively, drawings made with large gestures, or drawings that embody the fantasy of fight or flight, are creations that increase the sense of control and calm.

> *I recall working with middle school children before the Columbine High School shooting tragedy happened. That event understandably resulted in a legitimate shift in the level of tolerance of violent expressions in art making. Before then, the children in the school art therapy groups often chose to draw spontaneous images of daggers, blood, arrows, and angry words, suggesting that they were perhaps relieving fight responses. Amazingly, teachers asked me to accept more students into my groups, as they reported students returning to the classroom calm and ready to work. Such experiences also suggest the usefulness of children's ability to artistically relieve themselves of stress. Of course, art may also include real clues of intent to harm others, and so it must be handled with caution.* Noah Hass-Cohen

The Long-Term Stress Response

The long-term stress response represents a state of endurance, reacting to events that are perceived as uncontrollable, and arousing feelings of helplessness and hopelessness. An example of this might be someone experiencing feelings of grief and loss and unconsciously giving up on gaining control. The way that our bodies adapt to this longer period of stress is by rallying our energy reserves, which involves the secretion of the hormone cortisol. Cortisol shuts down all functions that are not immediately needed, conserving energy to deal with the situation at hand. Cortisol is very efficient in coping with stress as it allows us to forget, and in so doing, ideally assists in turning off the stress response.

Cortisol also contributes to depressive symptoms such as numbness and the urge to sleep. Interestingly, these symptoms can actually be protective factors in the short term after a loss or a major stressor. Acting like guards, they protect us from dwelling on what happened until we have more energy to process what occurred. However, an unremitting secretion of cortisol or a failure to hinder the stress response can have detrimental effects. Chronic stress is potentially damaging to the body and the immune system, as it recruits all the individual's resources to adapt to the stressor (Sapolsky, 2004). It also negatively affects cognitive function by changing neurotransmission processes in the prefrontal cortex and the hippocampus (Popoli, Yan, McEwen, & Sanacora, 2011). Human stress responses also seem to be exacerbated when our coping resources are perceived as insufficient for the stressors we face (Lazarus, 1966).

An example is grief and bereavement. Long-term stress associated with bereavement has been linked to disruptions in memory (Rosnick, Small, & Burton, 2010; Xavier, Ferraz, Trentini, Freitas, & Moriguchi, 2002), decreased executive function (Ward, Mathias, & Hitchings, 2007), fertility problems (Sapolsky, 2004), a depressed immune system (Hall & Irwin, 2001; Sapolsky, 2004), exacerbation of existing medical conditions (Leserman et al., 2002), changes in mood and depression (Nuriddin, 2008; Onrust & Cuijpers, 2006; Sapolsky, 2004), increased health risks (Hall & Irwin, 2001; Cohen, Granger, & Fuller-Thomson, 2013), negative impact on cardiovascular health (Elwert & Christakis, 2008; Hall & Irwin, 2001), and even mortality (Elwert & Christakis, 2008). Most often, it is elderly populations who find themselves severely impacted by these factors when support systems or spouses pass away (Alexopoulos, 2005; Sapolsky, 1992). Specifically, studies show that bereaved spouses or partners are at higher risk for mortality in the first few months after the loss. Studies of bereaved parents show similar results (Stroebe, Schut, & Stroebe, 2007). However, grief itself is not a disease or a disorder. It is when integrating back into daily life becomes difficult, or when loss is compounded by extenuating circumstances, that grief can result in an enduring sense of loss of control.

The long-term stress response is mediated by the hypothalamic-pituitary-adrenal (HPA) axis (Kalat, 2012). Neurons in the hypothalamus secrete a corticotrophin-releasing hormone (CRH), which stimulates the pituitary to release adrenocorticotropin (ACTH) and arginine vasopressin into the blood stream. This process initiates the production of cortisol (glucocorticoids) in the adrenal gland. Cortisol, which is intended to stop the HPA stress response, travels through the vascular system back to the pituitary and hypothalamus. Next, it binds onto receptors there that stimulate reduction in ACTH and CRH secretion. This feedback loop can become dysregulated (Figure 9.8).

Cortisol also increases glucose metabolism, thereby producing additional energy and shifts in immune responses (Graham, Christian, & Kiecolt-Glaser, 2006). At the same time, the adrenal gland also discharges adrenaline

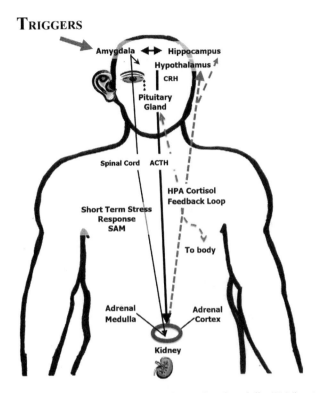

Figure 9.8 *The SAM and HPA Axis.* The sympathetic adrenal medulla (SAM) axis activates in response to the short-term stress response. Chronic stimulation of short-term stress response triggers the hypothalamus, pituitary adrenal (HPA) axis. This happens when the protective, SAM response gives way to the HPA response due to the experience and perception of a loss of control. Then the HPA loop is activated. The hypothalamus releases CRH into the bloodstream rapidly as the pituitary produces ACTH, which travels to the adrenal glands and stimulates the release of glucocorticoids or cortisol.

and norepinephrine (Lupien, McEwin, Gunner, & Heim 2009), which act as both hormones and neurotransmitters (Kalat, 2012). Once the stressor has abated, cortisol feedback loops signal the turning off of the HPA axis response and support the return of the body to homeostasis (Lupien et al., 2009). As indicated above, research suggests that excessive cortisol associated with long-term bereavement affects short-term and long-term memory, even when not associated with depression (Granic et al., 2007; Rosnick et al., 2010; Xavier et al., 2002). Studies with both animal and human subjects show that a deregulation of the HPA axis can negatively impact memory because high levels of cortisol cause damage to the hippocampus, which is the short-term memory storage center of our brains (Jameison & Dinan, 2001; de Kloet, 2012).

CREATE PRINCIPLES AND CLINICAL APPLICATIONS

This chapter focuses on the CREATE principle of Adaptive Responding. The benign, controlled environment of an art therapy relationship offers the opportunity to facilitate sensory experiences that bring on bodily stress responses (e.g., sweaty palms, increased heart rate) in clients. These bodily reactions are physical manifestations of psychoneurobiological interactions of the fight, flight, or freeze responses. Art therapists are able to use these in vivo reactions to help clients work through stressors and increase coping skills. Through carefully sequenced art interventions, difficult stress responses can be contained and stabilized. The sequence moves from the representation of a short-term stress reaction, complemented by the creation of an Adaptation Container, to the drawing of Safe Relationships. In other words, the drawing of turning or tending to others follows the simulation of an ongoing stress experience and efforts to cope with it.

In Turning Toward Others, the sequence of the art activities culminates in the depiction of a coping response to long-term stress. Providing the opportunity to imagine solutions, this is also a chance for clients to practice social coping and increase resiliency through imagery making. Given our relational understanding of the stress response, we invite a drawing of turning to others. Concretely creating, seeing, and exploring a coping response provides a tangible social solution that can stimulate and reinforce adaptability.

Resilient reactions to stress (fight, flight, freeze, or turning to others) can be mediated by Creative Embodiment. The Stressful Moment drawing complimented by the creation of the Adaptation Container allows for a concrete yet externalized embodiment of stress and its containment. For the experientials that we discuss, the opportunity exists to symbolically fight, flee, or turn to others during the recall of the stressful times, thus increasing resiliency. The symbolic or gestural arm movements of art making can be registered in the mind as if we are actually moving away from the sources of fear.

Relational Resonating is promoted by making images of safe relationships, or drawing representations of turning toward relational resources. Active strategies for reaching out to others for safety can be encouraged, as in the example of participants instinctively choosing to display their images of relational safety together as a group. Such a dynamic of support in groups is comforting. In addition, the unique human response to stress, seeking comfort and equilibrium through relationships with others, is a key focus of the ATR-N interventions. Relational resonance is an adaptive mechanism, which can foster a sense of comfort and control by imagining and drawing or painting images of safe relationships or protected places. Another resource conducive to achieving this balance is the Adaptation Container directive, which can increase awareness of one's relationship to the self as a coping resource.

Through Expressive Communicating, clients can access novel responses while grappling with a fundamental tendency to fight, flee, or freeze in reaction to stress. Such responses may occur via the creation of an emotional stress reaction image that is safely contained on the page, or by depicting the emotional comfort found in a secure relationship. Additionally, this is accomplished through art experiences, which provide an opportunity to control, tolerate, and safely experience dysregulated emotional states, to reflect upon their nature, and to practice emotional regulation.

The stress adaptation sequence supports several levels of Transformative Integrating. Implicit and explicit memories of stress are revealed and integrated throughout. Art exploration is also a foundation for clients' nonverbal (right hemisphere) and verbal (left hemisphere) processing of these experiences. Accordingly, the reflection and discussion of stressful times puts words to experiences, thereby supporting the integration of emotional-limbic and cognitive cortical processing. Last, creating the Adaptation Container supports communication and integration of the inside and outside selves. Therapists can share with studio participants how verbal processing of the artwork harnesses meta-cognitive functioning and resilient coping response. Titling and narrating the art while recognizing recurring visual themes or automatic thoughts organizes the experience and increases flexible mentalizing, approaching painful IWMs memories, and a felt sense of mastery. For example, Rachel named her short-term stress image *Don't Hide*, perhaps recognizing her tendency to freeze. In contrast, she reframed her long-term stress artwork as *Journey*. By giving such names to the images, she expanded their meaning and suggested that her obstacles can be overcome when the process is seen as a steady path (Figure 9.2). The visual depiction of a stressful experience permits new creative responses. For Rachel, the pathway may twist or turn but can be navigated with supported resilience. Furthermore, rumination can be interrupted by the positive sensory stimulation of the art expression, shifting repetitive thought-mood cycles. The positive limbic immersion in creative expression can curtail recurrent thoughts that perpetuate self-destructive anger, anxiety, and depression.

These art experiences not only bolster stress response expression and awareness but also encourage Empathizing and Compassion. As a result, under therapeutic conditions, a space is opened for empathic self-awareness. Additionally, an interpersonal neurobiological understanding of the client's stress response allows individuals to begin developing self-understanding as well as self-compassion.

CHAPTER 10

Adaptive Responding:
Secure Remembrance

I have been in Haiti since Wednesday, October 26, 2011. I so enjoy the crimson sun, the red earth, the lush Caribbean trees, the sound of my native tongue spoken loud in sing-song and loud everywhere and the aroma of tropical fruits and hibiscus in the warm October breeze. I came with a team of psychologists to train psychology students and those who work in the non-governmental organizations (Red Cross, World Vision, Médecins Sans Frontières, etc.). They treat the population in the camps and elsewhere. We are training them in how to survive in post-earthquake stressful environments. We taught them how traumatic events negatively impact a person's physical, emotional, or social well-being. We trained in English, French, and Creole (Kreyol). We heard many tragic stories of loss, death, assaults (rapes in the camps and elsewhere), sexual violence (preteens are giving birth in the camps), and separated, lost, or abandoned children (still unable to find parents). The mental health workers often feel helpless in helping their clients. The camp population lives in subhuman conditions. They are hungry, thirsty, no clothes, fearful, lacking in resources. These mental health workers are suffering from their own daily stress and their own losses. Some of the students knew a mental health worker/ psychology student who was murdered last month on his way back from working in the camps. Another just had a family member kidnapped. Four workers from one of the foreign institutions in Haiti were pulled out of their car, beaten, and were nearly killed until the other Haitian staff members pulled them out to safety just in time. Kidnapping is returning to Haiti. It is a huge traumatic event that Haitians are affected by daily. Our World Vision security chief forbade us to venture out. Period. But not all is bleak in Port-au-Prince. The mental workers are getting great training about different kinds of stress, how to identify their symptoms, and what they can personally do to care for themselves physically and emotionally (exercise 20 min-

utes a day until you perspire and have rapid heartbeat, as well as good social support, laughter, and downtime from the job . . . no thinking about work; turn off the e-mail and phones). Haiti has far to go . . . and the road has deep craters but they are surmountable. I love Pikliz (peekleez). . . . It is my favorite spicy condiment. I crave it everywhere I am in the world. I attempt to make it from scratch from time to time and I fail miserably to master the fiery sweetness of the ones made in Haiti. Since I arrived I have it morning, noon, and night, doesn't matter what I am having. It could be croissant and coffee—I must have my fix of Pikliz. So the meaningful work here is crucial and I am so honored to be able to serve my native land, but I find eating Pikliz with all my meals means that I am engaging in serious, meaningful, stress-reducing behavior. Bonne nuit. Good night. (Art therapist Marguerite Lathan lives in Los Angeles; she was born and raised in Haiti).

NATURAL DISASTERS, LIKE THE 2010 Haiti earthquake or Hurricane Katrina in 2005, can unleash a sequence of social traumas that contribute to a cycle of chronic and complex traumatization. Of course, chronic traumatization is not limited to experiencing wars or natural or large-scale social disasters. Experiencing existential threats to oneself or witnessing a threat to someone else's physical, sexual, or psychological integrity can generate a range of symptoms of post-traumatic stress disorder (PTSD; American Psychiatric Association, 1994). Depending on history and extent of trauma, a person may also experience a constellation of complex PTSD (C-PTSD) symptoms. In this chapter, we describe a sequence of art therapy strategies for dealing with complex responses to multiple traumatic assaults like those that Marguerite reports. We propose a Secure Remembrance trauma model that emphasizes the CREATE principle of Adaptive Responding. It includes five traumatology factors: Safety, Relationships, Remembrance, Reconnection, and Resiliency (SR-5).

Judith Herman coined the term C-PTSD in 1992 to denote the multiplicity of traumatic conditions that accompany sexual, physical, and emotional abuse. Herman suggested that one of the differences between PTSD and C-PTSD is an actual or perceived ongoing inability to flee from the abuse. Internal phenomena, like thoughts, memories, feelings, or flashbacks, may also be perceived as threatening and traumatic. A personal history of persistent trauma, such as abuse, furthers this vulnerability. The consequences are symptoms that are often difficult to resolve, have a tendency to reappear, and may overwhelm many areas of the person's life (van der Kolk, 2005). The formulation of further traumatology constructs, specifically disorders of extreme distress not otherwise specified (DESNOS, van der Kolk, 2005) and developmental trauma disorder (van der Kolk, 2005), have assisted in further understanding the cumulative effects of C-PTSD. DESNOS is associated with C-PTSD-associated cognitive and self-perceptual alterations such as dissociation, derealization, and depersonalization, while developmental trauma disorder focuses on the unique treatment required for children.

Moreover, it is likely that early and prolonged effects of interpersonal violence and repeated personhood violations contribute to significant and chronic neurobiological changes and complicated reactions to crisis (Vasterling & Brewin, 2005). This may partially explain why people with C-PTSD suffer from chronic and sometimes unexplained physical problems. C-PTSD is also associated with disturbances in impulsivity, avoidant behaviors, and intrusive symptoms. These effects invade the person's self-perception, relationship abilities, and systems of meaning making or sustaining beliefs (Herman, 1992), and they will frequently experience heightened stress reactivity to interpersonal cues that may seem very benign to others (Badenoch, 2008). Thus, reducing the reoccurrence of symptoms and minimizing their retraumatizing impacts requires establishing and maintaining a personal sense of safety before and throughout treatment (Baranowsky, Gentry, & Schultz, 2010; Herman, 1992).

Our approach to the art experiences is rooted in a broad framework of evidence, which suggests that the therapist-client relationship is critical for therapeutic success (Allen, 2012; APA Presidential Task Force on Evidence-Based Practice, 2006; Beutler, 2009). C-PTSD symptoms and experiences can also threaten the therapist-client relationship and, unbeknownst to the therapist, therapy may trigger and rekindle latent traumatic responses. Many clients with C-PTSD have histories of child abuse and have relationship issues associated with developmental or attachment deficits. Hence it is critical to establish an empathic relationship before commencing with the narrative trauma processing (Brier & Scott, 2012). Survivors of abuse report continuous painful experiences that include a lack of support and outright disbelief, devaluation, and betrayal from others. Subsequent to trauma, the person may also develop personality disorders, which present as pervasive difficulties in forming and maintaining healthy relationships (Linehan, 1993a, 1993b). Symptoms of such experiences can include a sense of mistrust, resignation, defeat, guilt, and shame that manifest in the therapy room. Hence, treatment goals include learning how to avoid the reenactment of abusive relationships, compassionate support, building healthy new relationships, and learning to reconnect to social networks. Both therapist and client should also take into account that C-PTSD treatment can take time and may be difficult.

From a neurobiological perspective, C-PTSD symptoms indicate a persistent perturbation of the stress response circuitry, which includes the sympathetic and endocrine axis, the brain's prefrontal lobe function, and its reward center, the locus coeruleus and the norepinephrine and dopamine circuitries. With developmental trauma disorder, trauma may have also generated some long-lasting structural brain deficits. Given the altered neurobiology of C-PTSD and the extensive traumatic influences on the individual's personhood and life skills, symptoms often reoccur under duress. The cumulative effect of early childhood trauma or interpersonal violence or violation may impose severe anguish and self-regulatory issues (Herman, 1992, 1997; van der Kolk, 2005). Examples include expressions of extreme rage, depressive symptoms, struggles in understanding and talking about feelings, and difficulty managing emotions (Linehan, 1993a, 1993b). Commonly, affect regulation is challenging. Many survivors of trauma report the reliving of memories as if they were taking place currently, rather than in the past. Additionally, intrusive and sudden symptoms may trigger memory lapses and depersonalization or dissociation experiences (Lanius et al., 2004; 2005).

The Neurosequential Model of Therapeutics (NMT) maps the neurobiological development of maltreated children (Perry, 2006). The premise is that the nervous system of children who are exposed to extreme cases of threat to self fails to develop as expected, resulting in heightened survival based responses to even benign interaction. Specifically, areas in the lower brain, the brain stem and the hypothalamus and thalamus (structures of the diencephalon) become kindled and strongly associated. As per our early review in Chapter 4, these areas are also strongly linked to the amygdala suggesting that that a fear response is dominant. Fear dominance results in severe behavioral emotional and cognitive impairments including a propensity towards interpersonal aggression that is not responsive to traditional therapeutic interventions. The child and later the adult are hyper-vigilant in their responses to external cues such as unexpected loud noises and internal cues such as hunger, which are experienced as intolerable. The NMT approach suggests that in this case it is important for interventions to first target lower brain areas responsible for basic human functions: body temperature, heart rate, blood pressure (brain stem); and sleep, appetite, sexual behavior, and processing of sensory information (diencephalon). These bodily-based interventions need to happen before or while attempting relational (limbic system) or cognitive (neocortex) based therapeutic work. Such interventions include, as reviewed earlier, multi modal efforts such as dance, music and touch. Most importantly, due to the neurobiological damage, it is necessary that the interventions are rhythmic and repetitive (Perry). From an ATR-N perspective, repetition is an important intervention principle that extends to the treatment of single trauma and psychopathology and includes a strong and available therapeutic presence. As in our SR-5 model, which is described below, this emphasizes the building of social supportive relationships as a critical task that must begin immediately in trauma treatment from the first session. It is also the therapist's responsibility to assist clients in figuring out and exploring where else can they have access to unconditional and safe support on a daily basis.

Contextual traumatic memory processing helps displace experiences stemming from reliving the trauma back into the past where they belong. Treatment goals include exposure to the re-traumatizing memories, desensitization, and verbal and cognitive processing and narration. Once memories are perceived as less threatening, remembrance can assist in mourning losses. Understanding how individuals process information is critical for effective treatment. As explained in Chapter 6, this is because of how episodic or intrusive memories are encoded and contextualized into long-term memory. Intrinsic memories can alternatively disrupt or enhance the individual's autobiographical sense of self and consequently their daily life, relationships, and future. Researchers and clinicians now know that when retrieving memories there is an opportunity to change them (Nader, Schafe, & LeDoux, 2000). In fact, as people recall memories some of the neurochemicals that bind them are loosened, making the old memories unstable and pliable (Schwabe, Nader & Preussner, 2014; a review). Current forms of therapy rely heavily on extinction, contextual and phasic trauma-based treatment for decreasing the impact of fear-based memories. However, many times functions of central areas of the amygdala, the brain's fear center, inhibits the long-term effectiveness of such change. More recently, findings from clinical neuroscience suggest that within a brief period of six hours, updating fear-based memories with non-fearful information leads to a permanent reduction in previously learned fear responding. This contributes to a lasting alteration in the original fear memory. Such memory reconsolidation may have significant implications for the treatment and perhaps prevention of PTSD.

Even with treatment, C-PTSD symptoms are so disturbing that people often resort to compromising, high-risk coping behaviors such as eating disorders, substance abuse, self-harm, sexual promiscuity, and violence. Lower economic and educational outcomes have also been further associated with C-PTSD. The complexity of symptoms may account for high treatment attrition rates and the lack of symptom remission. Overall, studies have shown that up to 50% of people who were successfully helped by exposure therapy may relapse (Gringage, 2003), and that there is a high relapse rate for all therapies (Benish, Imel, & Wampold, 2008).

It is incumbent upon the art therapist to include the development of relationships, resiliency skills, and relapse prevention interventions as part of any trauma treatment. This requires having basic familiarity with traumatology research and with trauma-informed treatment guidelines. Our model, SR-5 (Safety, Relationship, Remembrance, Reconnection, and Resiliency) is based on the empirically supported Tri-Phasic model, which has been informed by the International Society for Trauma Stress Studies (ISTSS) approved guidelines. Safety, Relationship, Remembrance, Reconnection, and Resiliency are not to be construed as fixed phases, as establishing safety and building relationships are ongoing tasks in trauma recovery. In particular, remembrance and memory processing may be contraindicated for some, while for others it may start the first day that the trauma is revealed (King-West & Hass-Cohen, 2008). Our suggestion is to include an ongoing focus on the compassionate exploration and development of relationships, informed by the literature on the efficacy of nonspecific therapeutic factors, such as trust and hope. The practice and application of relapse prevention strategies and development of resiliency meshes with the CREATE principle of Adaptive Responding. The other three factors, establishing perceived and actual personal safety, engaging in contextual remembrance, and supporting social reconnection, correspond to Herman's (1992, 1997) Tri-Phasic model. The art therapy directives suggested for each SR-5 factor are also informed by exposure therapy principles and empirically based PTSD treatments (Brady, Dansky, Back, Foa, & Carroll, 2001; Cohen, Mannarino, & Deblinger, 2006; Courtois & Ford, 2009; Friedman, Keane, & Resick, 2010; Foa, Keane, & Friedman, 2009). Our approach is further anchored in an ATR-N stress protocol that we use with individuals struggling with the short- and long-term stress of living with HIV or a cancer diagnosis (Bridgham & Hass-Cohen, 2008; Clyde Findlay, 2008; Hass-Cohen & Clyde Findlay, 2009).

In formulating the SR-5 model, we included information from the art therapy trauma literature. A number of art therapy models were reviewed, including Valerie Appleton's (2001) four-stage model, Savneet Talwar's (2007) Art Therapy Trauma Protocol, Anita Rankin and Lindsey Taucher's (2003) task-oriented approach, Cicione, Fontaine, and Williams's (2002) Trauma Relief Unlimited, Bonnie Meekums's (1999) creative model for recovery, and most recently, Chapman's, (2014) approach to working with children.

In terms of Safety (SR-1), art therapists have emphasized issues of perceived safety, underscoring helping the client gain a sense of internal and external control (Appleton, 2001; Backos & Pagon, 1999; Chapman, Morabito, Ladakakos, Schreier, & Knudson , 2001; Meekums, 1999; Pifalo, 2002; Rankin & Taucher, 2003; Sarid & Huss, 2010; Talwar, 2007). The main objective is to provide a traumatized person the opportunity to use the art as a way to safely express, process, and begin to make sense of traumatic experiences. Art therapy research suggested that perceived safety is directly correlated with positive outcomes, where the same interventions can result in client deterioration if perceived safety is not well established (Meekums, 1999). In terms of Relationships (SR-2), this literature presents interventions for building and maintaining strong therapeutic alliances and forming positive peer connections (Pifalo, 2002). In regards to Remembrance (SR-3), the literature cited above also highlights that art therapy is uniquely positioned to assist people with trauma due to its nonverbal methods. Gantt and Tinnin (2009) presented an argument for expanding the use of nonverbal therapy methods to treat trauma victims. Pizarro (2004) claimed that art therapy does not require literacy or verbal fluency, which facilitates applications to a wider population, and Talwar (2007) argued that the sensorimotor experience provided by art therapy taps into the nonverbal component of traumatic memories. We agree with these claims, and reiterate that unless structured therapeutically, nonverbal interventions have the potential to rekindle trauma (Allen, 2005). Trauma neurobiology, discussed later in this chapter, helps us understand the double-edged sword effect of nonverbal interventions. In terms of Reconnection (SR-4), Meekums (1999) explained that witnessing the art has profoundly therapeutic benefits for the client (Backos & Pagon, 1999). A group setting provides additional benefits, including decreased isolation and restoration of trust through repeated positive interactions with peers (Appleton, 2001). The therapist assists the client in fostering connections with friends and family. Art therapy interventions can be implemented in a group format, as repeated positive peer interactions can decrease isolation and restore trust (Backos & Pagon, 1999; Howie, Burch, Conrad, & Shambaugh, 2002; Pifalo, 2002). Sarid and Huss (2011) and Hass-Cohen and Clyde Findlay (2009) provide valuable insights as to how Resiliency can be supported through the transformation of the imagery through added resources.

Most art therapy techniques utilize short-term interventions that range from two to 10 weeks (Backos & Pagon, 1999; Kalmanowitz & Lloyd, 1999; Pifalo, 2002). Populations include victims and survivors of child sexual abuse (Backos & Pagon, 1999; Meekums, 1999; Pifalo, 2002), female child and adolescent victims of sexual abuse (Pifalo, 2002; Chapman, 2014), and adolescent burn victims (Appleton, 2001). Additional examples include art therapy with children of the 9/11 Pentagon attack victims (Howie et al., 2002), refugees of the former Yugoslavia (Kalmanowitz & Lloyd, 1999), adult survivors of child sexual abuse (Meekums, 1999), children and adolescents hospitalized for trauma-related injuries (Chapman et al., 2001), and adult trauma victims (Rankin & Taucher, 2003).

This chapter expands on the CREATE principle of Adaptive Responding.

As in Chapter 9, the art directives are sequential but can also be used as stand-alone experientials. Generally, we propose that stress and trauma treatment includes building sequences of art directives that link to each other. For example, in Chapter 9, we suggest experientials to adapt to stressors and cope with stress. Those activities started with portraying a short-term stress response and using images of internal and external resources to concretize the struggle to maintain control. Then we asked the artists to explore antidotes to stress by seeking a safe relationship and reaching out to others. A cycle of directives provides a progressive learning experience and transforms the image on implicit and explicit levels. Accordingly, in this chapter we further develop the idea that it is helpful to pair a representation of stress and trauma with a representation of support and resiliency. We also advance the idea of reworking the image as an antidote to the effects of trauma (Hass-Cohen, Clyde Findlay, Carr & Vanderlan, 2014; Sarid & Huss, 2011).

ATR-N TRAUMATOLOGY: OVERVIEW OF SR-5 FACTORS AND EXPERIENTIALS

This chapter's art therapy sequential directives incorporate principles from evidence-based treatment interventions (Baranowsky et al., 2010; Herman, 1997). The SR-5 approach and the directives are provided here as an introduction to working with adults. Space does not permit full description of the approach and the related directives for children.

The starting point of the Safety art directives is to choose an object that promotes perceived safety, and then to experiment with approaching safe relationships. One example of a Relationship-based directive is the manipulation of a hand silhouette. Once safety is accessible and some trust is established, traumatic issues and memories can be represented and processed. The Remembrance directive leans toward imagery transformation, reconsolidation of memories, and contextual processing. The latter focuses on how the narrative is processed, rather than on its content. Contextual processing is what allows memories to be repressed or placed in the past. As this process occurs, actively reconnecting with trusted others and building a repertoire of interpersonal and intrapersonal resources is encouraged. This cycle of Reconnecting- and Resiliency-based directives culminates with self-care strategies and a vision of future well-being. Furthermore, corresponding art directives increase in complexity; they start with simple object manipulation, progress to drawing and painting, and conclude with complex cutting, gluing, and changing of the artwork. Such manipulation of the imagery contributes to contextual trauma processing, encourages cognitive and emotional flexibility, and contributes to a felt sense of change and hope.

Safety (SR-1)

Affirmation of initial physical safety, tending to ongoing emotional safety, and establishing a felt sense of stability are critical ingredients for therapeutic success. The overall purpose during the stabilization period is for individuals to first accommodate to the therapy setting and then learn how to contain fear, manage body-based symptoms and behaviors, cope with intrusive memories, and reduce such occurrences. These reoccurring and threatening phenomena are most likely a result of conditioned neural circuitry responses and neurobiological alterations, which must be taken into consideration. Polyvagal clues to such responding could include clients' frozen facial expressions, sensitivity to low sounds, and jitteriness (Hass-Cohen, 2015a). We reiterate that the main concern is that the repetitive reoccurrence of trauma memories can be retraumatizing. Therefore, the art therapist is also mindful that the sensory qualities of ATR-N directives may also activate traumatic triggers, which are often encoded as sensory images. Practicing grounding, relaxation, and mindfulness-compassionate techniques lays the groundwork for safe contextual memory processing. In addition, the ATR-N studio experientials include sensory directives that assist in the containment of fear and dissociation, reduce experiences of freeze-based helplessness, and aspire to establish therapeutic safety in the room. The safety-directed experientials in this chapter are the SURF Tracking Device, Anchor, Safe Place and Loving-Kindness, and Walking Meditations.

Relationships (SR-2)

Establishing a therapeutic relationship during treatment is as critical as establishing safety. As discussed above, individuals with C-PTSD may often feel a keen fear and mistrust of others (Herman, 1992; van der Kolk, Roth, Pelcovitz, Sunday, & Spinazzola, 2005). These deep mistrusts may explicitly and implicitly extend to include the therapist. Thereby they have the potential to contribute to negative therapy outcomes. In trauma treatment, establishing transparent relational trust is critical in preventing the traumatized individual from prematurely terminating treatment due to fear. Similar to our comment about sensory triggers, the client may be quick to interpret nonverbal information as threatening, such as the hand gesture that accompanies the invitation to draw, or perceiving a lack of care from the therapist's neutrality. Therefore, the directives focus on the therapeutic relationship, interpersonal security, and hope. The purpose is to establish an empathic therapeutic relationship to enable progress, which requires the capacity to tolerate and feel the emotions that this process evokes (Allen, 2005). Directed art experientials attempting to elicit the here-and-now experiences of actual and perceived social support include Musical Chairs, the Hand Silhouette, the Color Check-In, Draw Yourself With a Safe Person, or Draw a Safe Relationship.

Remembrance (SR-3)

Contextualized remembrance of art experiences can facilitate the purposeful visiting of painful or disturbing autobiographical memories. Autobiographical memory is a mental representation of the self in time and space that, among other things, strings together our most unforgettable personal memories. For the majority, these episodic memories are safely held in the past. For others, some memories seem to escape, leak, and take over the present. Traumatic remembrance is easily triggered because it is not integrated into the person's autobiographical memory or knowledge base (Ehlers & Clark, 2000). As mentioned earlier, autobiographical memory reflection can improve affect regulation within the safety of the therapeutic relationship (Allen, 2005). The purpose of Remembrance is not to ascertain the truth or the complete picture of what has happened, but rather to contextually integrate autobiographical memories, appropriately placing them in the past. The distinction between autobiographical memory and traumatic memory informs the goals of narrative trauma processing and allows for mourning of loss and death (Table 10.1).

As stated, the main purpose of the directive experiential is to contextually place upsetting memories in the past, while at the same time facilitating emotional expression and mourning. The content of the memory is less important than the ability to create, refine, and narrate the story in a secure attachment relationship over time (Allen, 2005). A highlight of contextual processing is transforming implicit imagery, supporting reflexive mentalizing, making the implicit explicit and attaining a sense of coherency. The goals are to make the most painful memories tolerable to speak about, to maintain a sense of self-regulation and self-control as well as to be able to coherently narrate what happened in the past and what is happening right now. Visual memory processing can aid in building such a secure trauma narrative and experience. Stimulating these processes are the following ATR-N protocols, which are intended to change and transform the meaning of the image: "(a) If you were to paint the problem, what would it look like? (b) If you could change one aspect of the memory or keep one aspect of it, what would you choose? (c) Select the parts of the image you want to rescue and cut them out. (d) Draw yourself, or draw yourself with someone from your past. (e) Now draw yourself or draw an image of yourself or self-portrait" (Hass-Cohen et al., 2014; Bridgham & Hass-Cohen, 2008). Requesting to alter the original

Table 10.1 Autobiographical Memories and Traumatic Memories Processing

Autobiographical Memory	Traumatic Memories	Emotional and Cognitive Processing of Complex Trauma
• a contained sense of the past history • organized by themes and personal episodes • coherent temporal dimensions, "when" associations • connected with visual and spatial, "where" connotations • integrated and associated with other memories • retrieved through association with other memories • cognitively held • inhibits sensory memories that feel as if they are happening right now • allows for mourning of losses related to the self and the loss of others to gradually take place over time	• missing contextual information appearing as flashbacks • are sensory-based and perpetuate PTSD symptoms • lack information and are not well elaborated, can be fragmented • give a sense of here and now • are as if the trauma is in the present • threat is perceived as current • lead to or strengthen danger-based appraisals • disturb autobiographical memory • increase negative appraisals and rumination • increase bonding with the deceased • strong attachment to a lost sense of self	• place disturbing memories in the past and deny access to the present • stipulate that avoiding the past is only helpful in the short term • assert that avoiding the past is unhelpful in the long term as it does not resolve the fear • assist in accessing only necessary upsetting past memories • seek coherent and contextual narration of the memory rather than focusing on the content of the memory • done at a very slow pace together with the therapist • support a letting go of deceased significant others • instill acceptance of a new self • allows that initially there may be an increase in symptoms

image, we not only ask for a representation of the stated problem but also allow for the inclusion of a variety of issues that may cluster under the C-PTSD umbrella. The next sequence supports inclusion of resources and empowers the person to make changes. Then the self-portrait pulls for the mental image of the self and can be an invitation to explore how to undo the effects of the trauma on the development and maintenance of selfhood. In addition, this kind of autobiographical portrait often includes clues to the participant's attachment style (Hass-Cohen & Clyde Findlay, 2009).

Reconnection (SR-4)

The experience of chronic trauma can constrict a person's functional engagement with the world. Therefore, once the person with C-PTSD is able to experience safety and forms a therapeutic relationship, the difficult task of remembrance continues with reconnecting to social and personal resources.

The reconnection art strategies described in this section assist individuals in reaching out to family members with whom they feel safe, approaching supportive friends, and looking for healthy work relationships. For people with C-PTSD, the reconnecting and coping process may need to be actively managed and maintained by the therapist. With explicit support, the individual with C-PTSD can better tolerate the risks and rewards of connecting with others and face the demands of daily life. In contrast, individuals who are managing defined or time limited stressors may benefit from being more independent in these endeavors. Both types of strategies assist individuals with envisioning a different future and redefining self-identity. These kinds of activities and social reconnections can in turn continue to nourish intrapersonal resources. In the art therapy studio, the reconnection process can be activated and concretized by a two-stage directive. First is the Resource Collage, a collage of intrapersonal and interpersonal resources for reconnecting. It is followed by an art change request to "Amplify each one of your resources," which further transforms the image and process.

Resiliency (SR-5)

Working with clients on relapse prevention strategies is a critical component of trauma work. The ability to prevent relapses or to quickly recover from recurring symptoms requires avoiding isolation and developing autonomy through self-care. Relatedness, which we label as actively reaching out to others and asking for help, is encouraged (Allen, 2005). The therapist can help the client become aware of, and control, his or her own personal warning signs of relapse, which could include changes in thinking, behavior, and mood. Moreover, setting achievable short-term goals for self-maintenance and connection supports hope and long-term resiliency. The art directives we propose are as follows: "Represent yourself with your resources today, in the future, and reaching out to others. We also request "Represent your relapse prevention strategies." As part of this work the client and therapist also plan termination. The therapist's office and the memory of compassionate support become part of these resources.

General Guidelines

A well-thought-out and reflective pace of therapy is critical for trauma treatment. It is often necessary to revisit all five factors throughout the different phases of therapy. In ordinary therapy, the therapist and client can indulge in the presentation and exploration of new directives for each session. Moreover, the novelty of each session is a joy that stimulates growth. In contrast, for C-PTSD patients, novelty can be perceived as a threat. In traumatology, requests that are perceived as demanding can immediately stimulate a felt sense of loss of control and fear. Therefore, we suggest the use of familiar and repeated directives. We end each activity with an outcome tracking directive, as we ask clients to reflect on and rate the experience. The repetition forms a connection to a soothing anchor, and the ritual can nurture the therapeutic relationship by fostering control and predictability. Similarly, altering existing images of previously made art supports an experience of control. Each group of directives may be practiced together or separately. We want to reiterate that we do not limit the time and sessions spent on each factor.

EXPERIENTIAL PRACTICES AND DIRECTIVES

Experience I: Safety, Anchoring, and Grounding (SR-1)

Attention to safety is an ongoing focus of the SR-5 model. Once physical safety is assessed and clearly ascertained, it is critical to develop self-soothing and supporting strategies that can help contain the intrusion of post-traumatic images, feelings, thoughts, and numbing. For group work we are sensitive to the possibility that some of the members may present with differing levels of traumatic history. We explain that for the art experiential in this section, individuals' self or their personhood may be called upon in ways that may be more challenging. Therefore, we ask the group members to sit across from each other in pairs or in groups of three. We suggest that they sit with peers that they feel close to in order to maximize relational support and minimize negativity or conflict.

In these small groups, we discuss how people with C-PTSD are often overwhelmed by bodily, emotional, behavioral, cognitive, and psychological reactions to the memories of the traumatic experiences. Moreover, their symptoms frequently become the source of recycled triggers. This cycle of trauma can result in re-traumatization through continued experiences of perceived unpredictability and endangerment. We encourage the studio artists to make this conversation personal. Those that do not wish to disclose are welcome to role-play a movie or a story character. This kind of role-play is a safe way to begin gaining stability through a narrative.

The purpose is not to process memories, but rather to capture and contain them as they resurface or intrude. In trauma treatment, reactions are usually measured with a rating system known as subjective units of distress (Wolpe & Lazarus, 1966). For this reason, sometimes the group members will be asked to rate their current reactions to their memories. We utilize this rating system in an art form by using a folded paper fortune-teller device. The paper fortune-teller functions as a Subjective Units Rating Form (SURF) device. In order to create a SURF device, we use a square sheet of paper that is folded diagonally and then flattened. Each corner is then folded into the center to achieve a smaller square with four flaps. Each flap is once again folded into the center. The square is now turned over and on the smooth side the corners are folded to the middle for the last time. Once this is folded along the perpendicular seams, the tips can be folded and pushed in and out (see appendix to this chapter). Either we let the individuals choose a trigger for each quadrant, or we make a suggestion to: "Place the who, what, where, or when of your experience on the upper visible flap." By opening up the two hidden layers underneath the studio experiential, the studio participants can rate the changing impact of the trigger up to four different times in each folded triangle. We ask them to: "Rate the amount of stress that each quadrant contains by labeling it (with either colored markers or pencils) with a number from one to 10." The visual rating provides a concrete container for the traumatic experiences, which can be revisited and reevaluated over time. In this way, the closing and opening of the SURF promotes a sense of control (Figure 10.1).

I chose to put the who, what, where, and when triggers of my memory on the outer flaps. Finding symbols to represent these triggers felt like I was making a secret code that was comforting as no one else could tell what they meant to me. It felt like I could disguise the content, but at the same time it made me focus very clearly on these four aspects of my memory. I was startled at how powerful this experience of rat-

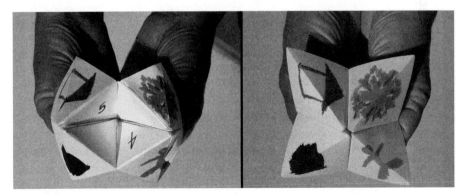

Figure 10.1 *The SURF Tracking Device.* On the left, the folded paper SURF device when held with the fingers pinched together with symbols for the triggers. On the right, the device held with fingers open reveals the inside surfaces with numbers written in color corresponding to the intensity of the trigger. Joanna Clyde Findlay

ing each aspect of my experience was. Having to describe my response via a number made me focus on the essential reality of my memories and confront their impact. Rating the triggers underlined that the who and what elements are still very powerful for me, rated at way over five out of 10. This indicated to me that although I think about this memory less and less, it is still very emotionally loaded. It also allowed me to get a sense of control as I can see how I could possibly move the numbers and, with them, the experience down a notch, meaning maybe downregulate them to a lower number. Joanna Clyde Findlay

In addition to this quickly constructed SURF object, we also ask group members to bring to the studio a small personal object of choice, which represents security and/or the memory of a safe place or situation. We call these objects empathic anchors. In the middle of each table we also place a community anchor box with sensory-based objects or manipulatives. The box will often include magical and fantasy creatures. We are careful to avoid including objects such as shells, pebbles, string, cloth, or ribbon in the anchor boxes, as these may often trigger traumatic memories. For example, shells or pebbles may trigger a rape survivor if he or she was raped at the beach or outdoors. Alternatively, the smooth feel of a satin ribbon may evoke the memory of a nightgown or a bedroom (Figure 10.2).

We then ask group members, "Choose an anchor that provides you with a felt sense of security and comfort." The purpose is to use these objects for sensory grounding and containment purposes. We aim to use sight, touch, and smell to stabilize the person in the present moment while he or she is talking. We emphasize that the object chosen needs to be perceived as safe, and ask members to describe the object, including its texture, color, and asso-

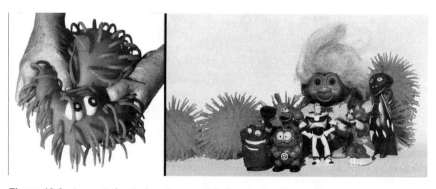

Figure 10.2 *Sensory Safety Anchors.* Commercially found soft or fantasy objects.

ciated reactions. For example, we ask, "What do you like about how it feels in your hand?" Subsequently, we invite group members to place the object in their pocket or purse and to share the feeling, knowing they can keep the preferred object with them when they leave the meeting. This kind of intervention is intended to encourage using the found object as a transitional object that can be taken home and integrated into daily life after the session. It is a modified form of grounding techniques (Baranowsky et al., 2010). Nonetheless, we advise group members to treat themselves with kindness as they touch and select the objects. As aforementioned, at this early stage, a directive to establish safety is of paramount importance and caution is needed for those with dissociative tendencies. We ask that attention be paid to the nonverbal signs by asking questions such as, "Do you or your peers report feeling distracted? Are you hearing each other? Do you find yourself staring off into space? Are you aware of the passage of time? Do your peers' expressions alter or glaze over? Do they recall what you have been discussing? Do they seem to find the requests unclear?" We ask that group members check in with each other, simply noticing out loud what they have observed, and checking out each other's sense of safety.

If the group members prefer to do so, they make a small anchor item out of self-hardening polymer clay instead of choosing an object. This object can be left to dry or, if necessary, baked in a portable toaster oven during the next session: "Make an anchor that evokes safety, comfort, and self-soothing feelings through form and texture." It is important that the object be small enough to hold as it increases an internal locus of control. As mentioned earlier, the anchor is a broad metaphor that lends itself to more specific client-driven symbols, such as a rock, a power animal, or a representation of a safe place. The directive is similar to an experiential in Chapter 5 about interpersonal touch. There the studio participants make three personal art pieces in small, medium, and large sizes from three different clays. We suggest choosing an object that they associate with a time when they had a strong sense of wellbeing. Sometimes, the process of making an object allows beneficial reinforcement of its value. Creating the anchor supports its soothing symbolic meaning as it is intentionally and repeatedly considered, inspected, touched, and held.

> *I had brought in a Star of David necklace pendant that was given to me as a child. This pendant, along with my other childhood jewelry, was kept in a jewelry box in the safety of my mom's home until a month ago, when the contents of the jewelry box, along with my mom's precious jewelry, were stolen during a home robbery. This pendant was the only remaining piece of jewelry from my childhood that*

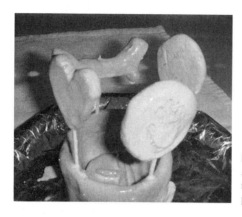

Figure 10.3 *Wet Clay: Love, Spirituality, Family, and Self.* A small, smoothed coil pot supports four wooden sticks with personal clay symbols painted in white glue. Channie Thal

was mistakenly left behind. To replicate that emotional feeling, I made a container and the Star of David symbol. Along with that symbol I created other symbols to represent myself, my identity. I created a heart for love, a bone for my puppy, a Hamsa for protection and well-being, and finally an "F" for family. My original idea of a pendant and a jewelry box became multiple symbols to represent love, spirituality, family and self. Channie Thal *(Figure 10.3)*

In choosing to depict myself as a precious pearl, I referred back to the meaning that I carry in wearing a pearl daily around my neck: discovered significance. Pearls are created through intense circumstances and, much like the ugly duckling becoming a swan, an irritating grain of sand emerges from a clam in the shape of a molded and worked shiny pearl, resonating with white clarity. Likewise, I consider myself to be a found beauty, emerging only in the awareness of my own lack. I delight to consider myself fallible and imperfect and yet, in that raw condition, as an emerging form of polished beauty. That is where I feel most safe. Moreover, through the analogy of being hidden in a comforting bed of soft feathers, covered in protection, I can envision a place of peaceful calm. So as that pearl, I sit peacefully in a wing, "hidden." Robin Shanon *(Figure 10. 4)*

The anchor directive is informed by a set of self-help batteries that include empirically based interventions for emotional stabilization and containment (Baranowsky et al., 2010). Alternative directives could be to: "Draw your anchor or a safe place."

When we notice that the group members revert to triggered behaviors and reactions or seem distracted, we ask them to identify the reaction. We

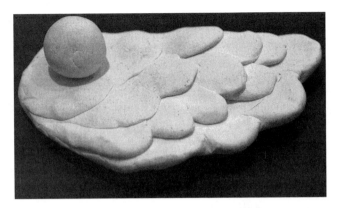

Figure 10.4 *Hidden.* A small golden wing-like shape supports a small pearl. Robin Shanon

discuss that these reactions could signal lack of safety. We also share some bodily signs of emotional expression, which may include eyes reddening, a change in skin tone or color, psychomotor agitation, or a constricted position. For example, clients may curl up into a semi-fetal positions or suddenly become quite agitated and want to leave the room. We then ask clients if they would like to work together and receive help in moving away from these reactions, or in adjusting to uncomfortable images, thoughts, and feelings. Similarly, the group discusses how drawn images of an anchor or a safe place may transmit stress indicators. They ask themselves and explore: "Do the marks indicate a sense of being in control, a striving for control, or a feeling of being out of control?" Other questions are, "How do the marks help me understand what kind of reaction this is? Could there be other indicators of short-term or long-term stress responses, PTSD or complex trauma, or responses such as dissociation?" Colleagues Barry Cohen and Carol Thayer Cox (1995) provide an extensive typology of art forms that provide insight into clients' world of trauma.

In the context of this discussion, and consistent with Chapter 12 mindfulness-inspired approaches, we may also invite the small groups to walk together mindfully (Kabat-Zinn, 2005). This is another technique that can be used as a stabilization resource. By paying close attention to the four options of Walking Meditation, the movement anchors the individual in the here and now and offers embodied awareness. The intentional motions of lifting, moving forward, putting down, and pressing or touching provide the realization that an intention can precede automatic movement. For the person with trauma, this can be freeing, as it suggests the possibility of controlling automatic intrusive behaviors. Sometimes we suggest that this be a loving-kindness meditation where studio participants walk between the tables, and as each foot comes up and down, we whisper, "Secure, happy, well, free" (Hanh, 1976). We suggest such loving-kindness meditation techniques for group members who are experiencing strong negative emotions such as anger, hate, blaming, and shame toward themselves and others. One of the very lovely and exciting things about this technique is that it contributes to community building. Everyone walks together, which supports group cohesiveness.

Finally, during the stabilization period we also offer information on the stress response (see Chapter 9), as well as information on the neurobiology of the trauma, discussed later in this chapter. Learning that idiosyncratic symptoms are known attempts of the mind, brain, and body to adapt to trauma increases the experience of feeling heard, contributes to a better understanding of reactions, and reduces feelings of guilt and isolation.

Experience II: Relationships with People and Places (SR-2)

The experientials in the next meeting are about trauma and relationships (SR-2). As group members find their places at the wide studio tables, they are asked to notice if they choose the same place each time. We invite those who are amenable to try switching places and talk about how it feels to make this change and how they feel about those who did not move. Symbolically, willingness or unwillingness to move can be paired with flexibility or restlessness, as opposed to stability, resistance to change, or insecurity. Sometimes the studio facilitators, will pick up their art supplies and books and move to the back or side of the room, generating a discussion on how it feels to be displaced. Naming this intervention Musical Chairs, we talk about how it requires us to build different relationships with those who are now the farthest away from us and those that are closest. This directive was inspired by one of Noah's clients with a history of developmental trauma, who could not find a "good enough" place at the art therapy table.

> At that time, my office had a very large square art therapy table that could easily and spaciously seat eight people. It was very spacious, perhaps too much so, and most of my individual clients preferred to sit kitty-corner from me, to my right, and they pretty much preferred the same seat every time. In fact, if the chairs—which had different colors—moved around, they often asked for the same blue chair. Over time, many of the art materials shifted to that particular area of the table and new clients usually interpreted this as an invitation. This client was different. Coming in for the first time, she chose the seat

that was farthest from me. Coming in the second time, she shifted to the left and then to the right and so on, trying each of the eight chairs positioned around the table, sometimes close to me, sometimes far. I accepted her movement in the room, acting as a third hand, moving the media to wherever she was seated and accommodating to her pace. A short time after trying all of the chairs, she terminated therapy, and I recall a keen sense of failure and sorrow. One is reminded of Goldilocks trying out the bears' chairs, porridge, and beds; except my client never found the right chair and the safe enough degree of distance or closeness to my seat. In retrospect, I wondered if my nonverbal responses were sufficient. Should I have brought the therapeutic relationship to the table by also speaking about it? Was she ready for that? At birth, my client was at risk, so she was not touched, an incubator holding her rather than a loving parent. A cutter by choice, she reported additional traumas that resulted in social isolation, which she enacted at my table. To return to my Goldilocks metaphor, we were not told much about Goldilocks, but we can hypothesize that she had good enough attachment strategies, as she was able to leave the forest and for a short time find a good enough fit for her needs in another home. For this client, that did not happen, and she left, going back to her forest. Years later, working with a different client with a severe history of complex trauma, we accommodated her pace and distance by coming and going within the same session. After coming in and working together with me for 10 to 15 minutes, she then left the room for a break of 5 to 10 minutes. Sometimes I joined her, and we returned to the room together. Most times, I needed to accompany her when she came back to the room. She spent many sessions talking about how much she distrusted therapists until she was finally ready to leave the "forest" and enter the creative space. Noah Hass-Cohen

After discussing the impact of studio seating choice on intimacy and relational resonance, we gather in two- or three-person groups and experience unique ways in which to chart the therapeutic relationship. First, we are reminded of the implicit practice of setting up the media on the therapy table, suggesting support and nurturance. The therapist's steadying hand, the "third hand" (Kramer, 2000), is an implicit yet clear indicator of support (Figure 10.5).

During the course of the experientials, we have had many opportunities to engage in such third-hand relational support. Group members have held bits and ends of others' art pieces, and we, have also helped hold, mend, and carry artwork. When this kind of nearness was unwarranted or contraindi-

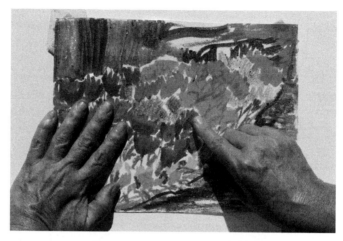

Figure 10.5 *Holding the Page.* Building the therapeutic relationship. Flowers surround and support a central aching red spot. Noah Hass-Cohen

cated, we engaged in other implicit ways of conveying our support. Examples include taping the paper to the table while one of our studio participants was working, providing soft towels to catch clay scraps, and wrapping up the art. These examples demonstrate active gestures of caring and support. Joanna recalls a time while working with children when the ritual of packing precious art creations in soft tissue and then securing them for storage or transport was part of the relational closure of the session. Many of our studio art therapy clinicians talk about similar opportunities that they have had. For trauma work, it is critical that these gestures are perceived as supportive and not as intrusive. We discuss how social support is perceived through the eye of the beholder, meaning that it is perceived positive support rather than actual support that is critical.

To build the therapeutic alliance, we propose the Hand Silhouette cutout as a means of making the relationship overt. As described in earlier chapters, our late colleague, Shirley Riley, who was masterful at building relationships, introduced the Hand Silhouette experiential. Intended to contain and convey emerging feelings, the first step is to place both hands on a piece of paper, palms down. Studio participants then trace each hand with the other; the right hand traces the left and the left hand traces the right. Then we ask them to: "In one hand outline draw what kind of different things you bring with you today. Include sensations, emotions, feelings, and thoughts." In the other hand outline, we ask them to: "Draw what you hope we will achieve together." Inclusion of the word *together* is an explicit reference to the therapeutic relationship and suggests security and support. Similarly, the inclusion of the

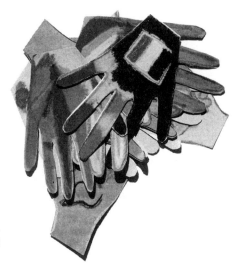

Figure 10.6 *Building Relationships.* Personally decorated hand silhouettes, touch and overlap each other in support. Anonymous.

word *today* provides a time-based container for any difficulties brought into the studio. This kind of request continues to be safety oriented as we include an emphasis on their hands or your hands. This is necessary because people with trauma may have experienced other people's hands as abusive and hurtful, where touch inflicts pain and suffering. In addition, the combination of the two requests with the directive's present and future time framework evokes a message of hope and stability. After hand drawings are completed, studio participants are asked to: "Cut out your hands from the paper and place them on a shared piece of paper, working either in pairs or in small groups" (Figure 10.6).

Once the hand silhouettes are placed, similarities, differences in colors and designs, and shapes and spaces created between the two hands can be noticed. Group members may muse about how it would feel if the proximity of the hands changed or, as in the image above, overlapped. Sometimes they put their hands on top of each other, like a couple would, and sometimes they place their hands far away from each other.

We occasionally role-play a therapeutic scenario with the hand cutouts. In the role-play, the role-therapist makes a hand silhouette alongside the role-client. They then choose a colored paper on which they will both place their decorated hands and discuss who places their hand down first. In case the therapist goes first, he or she should choose a non-dominating spot, such as the side of the page. The therapist then invites the role-play client to place their own hand cutouts at the most comfortable distance. Once the hands are placed, the therapist and client can talk about the process and its particular

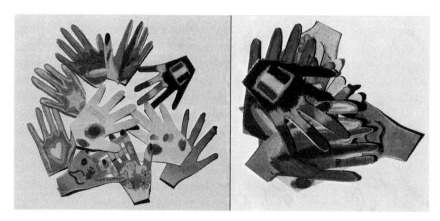

Figure 10.7 *A Group of Friends Were at a Party During Which Someone Got Hurt.* The image on the left represents the time when everyone was doing well. The image on the right shows how they came together to support the hurt person.

meaning. This representation of the therapeutic relationship can also be repeated throughout treatment, allowing a valuable visual tracking. The hand directive can be a concrete and symbolic representation of interpersonal communication and trust, and provide an easy way to reflect on relationships (Figure 10.7).

Many other art therapy directives, such as "Draw yourself with a safe person" or "Draw a safe relationship," elaborated on in Chapter 9, can be modified for trauma work so long as they include a relational aspect. Following the chosen directives, we invite our studio participants to reflect on and track the relationship that they have just experienced.

For this purpose, each person receives a roll of paper. The idea is for the tracking-based drawings to unroll after each session. As each section is exposed, a saucer-sized circle is drawn in pencil. Offering a selection of at least 24 soft pastels, which permits varied dark, saturated, and pastel tones, the facilitator asks the participants for a Color Check In: "Use a color to represent how the session was for you today inside the circle. On a scale of warm to cold colors, please show if we worked on what you wanted to work today and if you feel closer to your goals." Responses can range from a quick squiggle of color to densely filling in the circle. We encourage rapid process art, which can become a color barometer of the pulse of the relationship (Figure 10.8).

Irit Ivey depicted the therapeutic relationship. Representing herself in warm yellows, hot oranges, and fiery, painful red squiggles, she showed what she called her true colors and was pleased that she was able to do so. She used a cool green mesh at the bottom, to convey the therapist as a safety net.

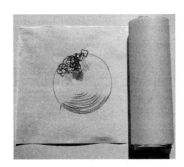

Figure 10.8 *Week 4 Color Check In.* A blue outlined circle is partially filled with lower green lines and upper red squiggles, orange hatches, and yellow shading. Irit Ivey

The Color Check In directive can help visually track the therapeutic relationship. Each circle provides valuable feedback to the therapist. In clinical trials and practice settings, the individual therapist has been shown to have a substantial impact on outcomes (APA Presidential Task Force on Evidence-Based Practice, 2006; Beutler, 2009). Central to clinical expertise is the therapist's interpersonal skill, which manifests in forming a therapeutic relationship, encoding and decoding verbal and nonverbal responses, creating realistic but positive expectations, and responding empathically to the patient's explicit and implicit experiences and concerns. Feedback from the Color Check In provides the therapist opportunities to address therapeutic impasses and problems in the therapeutic relationship. Similarly, clients can directly communicate their experience of the therapist's interpersonal skills, allowing them to consciously participate in building the relationship. Research supports the contribution of an active and motivated patient to successful treatment (e.g., Bohart & Tallman, 1999; Clarkin & Levy, 2004; Miller & Rollnick, 2002; Prochaska, Norcross, & DiClemente, 1994; Figure 10.9).

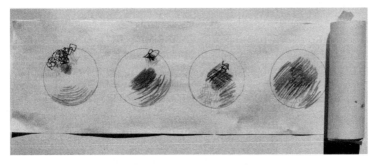

Figure 10.9 *Four Sessions of the Color Check In.* Looking from left to right, the patches of red and green colors change positions. The green-lined patch continues to provide support. The orange-red patch diminishes in the second circle and yellow appears. By the final circle, red-orange is no longer present and the center of the circle is yellow. Irit Ivey

These kinds of Color Check Ins can be done either each session or periodically. We suggest ending each session with some kind of similar monitoring. Other than devising art-based check-ins, psychometrically normed options are available (the Outcome Rating Scale and the Session Rating Scale—Bringhurst, Watson, Miller, & Duncan, 2006; Miller, Duncan, Sparks, & Claud, 2003; Smith, Crocker, Staton, Gillaspy, & Charlton, 2010).

Experience III: Contextualized Remembrance and Visual Narrative Processing of Trauma (SR-3)

As we begin this experiential, we are reminded that a felt sense of personal, interpersonal, and environmental safety must still be maintained during memory processing (Herman, 1992). For this third factor (SR-3), groups of two or three members form. The creative space facilitator asks each person to think of a personal traumatic experience. The request is to find a challenging but not overwhelming event that they feel comfortable sharing with the group. Alternatively, we suggest that they consider picking an event that they have rated as five or lower on the SURF device. We ask them to depict an aspect of a traumatizing event, rather than drawing a reaction to a stressor. In preparation for the directive, we also reiterate the difference between a stressor and a traumatic event.

For this experiential, we use a large and heavyweight piece of colored paper and ask each person to paint the trauma: (a) "If you were to paint what happened, or an aspect of what happened that you feel comfortable painting, what would it look like?" As the images dry, we ask (b) that the "painting be titled" and then we (c) share the titles and paintings in small groups. We also inform everyone that since we will be asking them to continue to work with their paintings, they can choose to preserve paintings in their current form by (d) "taking a digital image." We then ask, (e) "If you could change or keep one aspect of the painting, which aspect would you choose and what does it look like?" We suggest that: (f) "Either take out the traumatic aspect by cutting it out, or paint over it using the color of your paper." Then, (g), "you may want to paint or glue on the necessary images that can satisfactorily alter the trauma." A derivative of this sequence is when we ask the artists to: "Select the parts of the trauma image that you want to preserve." In this alternative sequence, we similarly encourage painting over, cutting out, and possibly gluing the rescued parts on a fresh page to create a new image. The focus of the directive always has the following sequence: first depicting the memory of the trauma, then altering the image of the trauma, and then creating a new experience, that is, a transformed image and reconsolidated memory (Figure 10.10).

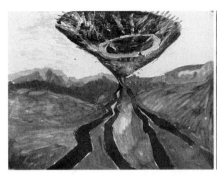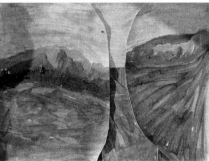

Figure 10.10 *The Traumatic Event and the Released Landscape.* A black tornado shape representing associated harsh truths that has a broken circle inside funnels into a peaceful landscape. Two jagged chasms of red and black cut into the green hills (left). On the right is a released landscape. A landscape is made with a blue sky made from recovered green and blue painted paper. Joanna Clyde Findlay

The making of these images was intense and conjured difficult material. I chose a green sheet of paper on which to represent the traumatic event, thus envisioning some support for myself. I showed it as a tornado with a broken yellow circle. It has a nasty swirling type of energy. My landscape is torn, with jagged red pathways. A fundamental breaking of trust is embodied in the broken circle in the hurricane of dark memories and emotions that splits an innocent landscape and shatters a dream. I felt the need to symbolize the trauma. Symbolizing such a personal experience felt difficult and forced me into using cartoon-like strokes, which I did not like. So I then cut out the tornado with the broken yellow circle and the jagged pathways. Cutting out the trauma and releasing the beautiful setting from its contamination was a relief. I was left with scraps of green, earth, and sky that I rescued and put together again. I did this by fitting the pieces of green together like a jigsaw until I found a version of the landscape that came together well. I did not have to add any more green as it was all there. I was eager to re-create a whole image from the rescued parts and used every last scrap to restore the environment to its blameless beauty. I believe it was valuable to do this artwork and that more work could be done. I felt that the altered image shows me a new open horizon that I can move towards. It also changed my memories of the event, as they now include the altered image. Noah added that perhaps additional reworking could be done by firmly gluing down the bits and continuing to rework the second image with more paint and specificity. The space is now there for new things to be created in.
Joanna Clyde Findlay

Many group members report that they experienced discomfort and tension as they created the trauma painting. We explain that some emotional arousal is a necessary first step for memory processing and may reuse the SURF Tracking Device or other safety interventions. Drawing an aspect of what happened provides an exposure to the trauma, which can help in desensitization. However, there is always the possibility that revisiting the memory may re-traumatize the individual, because episodic memories are very resilient (LeDoux, 2000) and can easily reoccur. One way to avoid such reoccurrences is by inviting the use of symbols and abstractions in the same way that Joanna did in her art and her reflection (Figure 10.10).

Sometimes group members also say that while acting upon the original image brings a real felt sense of moving on, the experience is still anxiety provoking. The sense of moving on is facilitated by actively cutting into the trauma image, removing some of the parts, and choosing what to do with the removed parts. The parts can be torn up and thrown away, safely burned, or kept by the therapist in an envelope. Promoting a sense of control, this can assist with self-regulating the difficult emotions that may occur. Repainting, regluing, and reorganizing the trauma image support a deliberate experience of self-regulation. These two main states need to occur simultaneously for contextual memory processing to be successful. First, emotional arousal needs to be paired with self-regulation, and second, the internal backdrop for this experience requires the perception of a supportive therapeutic relationship and felt sense of safety.

Another goal of this work is to cognitively restructure any negative schemas evoked by the image and contribute to memory reconsolidation. An example would include pervasive thoughts such as, "I will never amount to much." Verbally processing this two-part directive of painting and repainting reveals the ability to shift such negative constructs. It also provides the opportunity to update participants' autobiographical memory, which now includes their artwork. Thus, altering the painted image leaves a lasting take-home image of new possibilities.

A follow-up directive would be, "Draw yourself, or draw yourself with someone from your past." We build upon former skills as we suggest the use of paper cutouts for this portrait. Here, artists are asked to build an image from scratch, which requires higher levels of attention and cognitive function. "Draw an image of yourself, or create a self-portrait," is taken from our original ATR-N protocol (Bridgham & Hass-Cohen, 2008; Clyde Findlay, 2008; Hass-Cohen & Clyde Findlay, 2009). This directive pulls forth the mental image of the self and can be "an invitation to explore how the pain affects the development and maintenance of selfhood. The autobiographical portrait often includes clues to the participant's attachment style" (Hass-

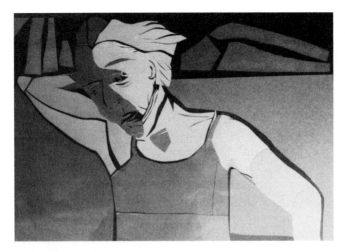

Figure 10.11 *Leaning into Shadows.* Using black, white, and people-colored papers. A figure with right arm raised behind its head leans backward. Noah Hass-Cohen

Cohen & Clyde Findlay, 2009, p. 182). Traumatic experiences can impact a person's sense of wholeness and efficacy. Therefore, exploring a person's view of himself or herself is an important part of processing traumatic memories. Paper cutouts can be useful for making this portrait because the technique can intensify the image making (Figure 10.11).

> *My shadows seem to always be there. They are my familiar strengths and my known vulnerabilities. I am attached to both these sources of comfort, as they are both reliable. In this image I agree with Joanna that it is not clear if I am relaxing comfortably or leaning forwards. What is clear to me is that my vulnerabilities are as much part of myself as are my strengths, hence the title.* Noah Hass-Cohen

Noah's image shows how trauma can cast long shadows into the person's present, and this could be a clue to the therapist to take a slower, measured pace. Any scribbles, scratches, repetitive images, or symbolic shadows are all possible indicators of intrusive flashbulb memories. Could a paucity of expression, unexpected disconnections between the drawn head and body, a peculiar placement of objects on the page, a lack of any people, or a seemingly arbitrary shifting between artistic styles point to dissociative responses? Such signs may indicate a need to refocus on establishing safety. As the group discusses the self-portraits, the participants are also invited to be mindful of how working with trauma can stir their own experiences. Issues of therapist compassion fatigue, secondary trauma, burnout, and personal risk signal the need for support and self-care. We therefore highlight that the next two experientials can also be valuable tools for the therapist, as they call for the mobilization of social and professional support and coping skills.

Experience IV: Reconnection to Others and to Meaningful Activities (SR-4)

In preparation for directives based on the fourth factor, Reconnection, we ask the studio participants to put together a personal stock of cutout magazine images and to: "Make a collage of your intrapersonal and interpersonal resources." If we are not using collage materials, we may ask, "Draw an image or symbol for internal and external resources that help with the problem" (Hass-Cohen & Clyde Findlay, 2009). Intentionally specifying intrapersonal and interpersonal resources helps focus on relational support, rather than the more general request for the person to explore internal and external resources. Sometimes the terms are interchangeable. For example, through the image of a place of worship, a client may depict all four resources: internal, external, intrapersonal, and interpersonal. Thus, this directive, the Resource Collage, assists in identifying interpersonal support, social support systems, and meaningful relational activities. It allows behavioral and emotional goals to be visualized, personalized, and imagined. We ask the group members to title their collages so as to anchor the meaning of the images cognitively (Figure 10.12).

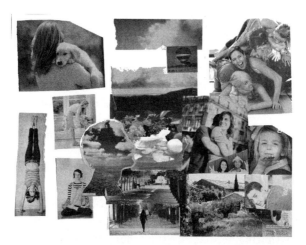

Figure 10.12 *My Resource Collage.* Maintaining balance in my life by nourishing connections; my intrapersonal and interpersonal resources. The collage shows images of a female figure on the left side doing various activities on her own. On the right side there are images of a couple, family, and children. The central part of the collage shows natural images of the sky and avenues of trees. A profile of a head filled with sky and fields overlaps these parts. Joanna Clyde Findlay

I found using collage to represent my relational resources was an easy way to simplify a complex topic. The image has three parts: on the left, my intrapersonal resources of yoga, meditation, and simple family activities; on the right, my core connection in my personal relationship, family, children, and friends. In the center, I placed concrete anchors for my well-being in nature and my environment. When I see this image as a whole, I am grateful for all the richness and possibilities in my life. Joanna Clyde Findlay

Listening to participant reflections on this directive, it became clear that turning toward others, either concretely or symbolically, was a source of succor. As mentioned, intrapersonal and interpersonal resources may frequently blend. In this case, the relationships may be depicted as either external or internal. For example, family, friends, community, memories of loved ones, or spiritual teachings are all evocable as important supports.

We follow up by asking to: "Choose one or two resources and amplify them." This second part of the directive offers a means to deepen the experience of the resources in the present. It is an aid when there has been difficulty identifying internal or external resources, or when the collage is sparse. Either on the same page, or on a new page, the studio participants use bold color media to explore their resources in depth. Once completed, we sometimes ask them to talk about their gut reaction to the activity. Sometimes seen as the location of what we call the sixth sense, the gut has many neurotransmitter receptors. Participants can then use this gut reaction to expand their exploration. Once each person has had a chance to embellish and expand at least one element of their original resources, the group gathers to reflect on what they have discovered (Figure 10.13).

I decided to focus on the head contour from my intrapersonal and interpersonal collage. I realized that a central element in being able to benefit from my resources is to maintain a connection between my mind and my body. This was visually evident in the head's place in my collage and represents a literal center point of managing and benefitting from my resources. I copied a photograph of the original collage, then cut out and enlarged the head contour. I was pleased I did not have to actually change my original image, as I don't want to permanently alter its overall structure. I decided to define the outline with a marker and to add a simple symbol, an arrow, to express my body-mind connection. I am at my most centered when I remain tuned into my bodily responses, which are represented by the earth in the lower part of the head contour. I then do not get lost in the chatter

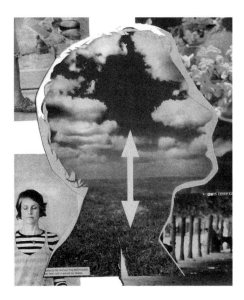

Figure 10.13 *My Amplified Resource: My Body-Mind Connection.* A black-and-white photocopy of the head outline from the previous image is boldly outlined in blue marker. A bidirectional arrow in blue marker crosses across the horizon inside the head. Joanna Clyde Findlay

of my brain, represented in the sky or top part of the head contour. The zooming in on my previous image was a powerful visual reminder of my ability to affect my well-being. My profile also represents looking outwards to other people and connecting with them, so I am at the same time looking inwards and towards others. Joanna Clyde Findlay

This directive provides a glimpse of hope and change and places the individual as an agent in establishing and promoting self-care. It optimally evokes positive expectations and a sense of agency. Aiming to provide this experience in real time, we ask that the artists change their group membership or share in the large group.

Experience V: Resiliency and Relapse Prevention (SR-5)

The relapse prevention directives build upon artwork from the previous experientials. Here we ask people to make a copy of their paper cutout Self-Portrait (Figure 10.11) and of their Resource Collage (Figures 10.12 and 10.13). These can be either black-and-white or color copies. We then suggest that participants add to their self-portraits or resource collage by using one of the following directives: "Represent yourself with your resources today, reaching out to others, and in the future or represent your relapse prevention strategies." The group is asked to use simple shapes and lines to alter and transform

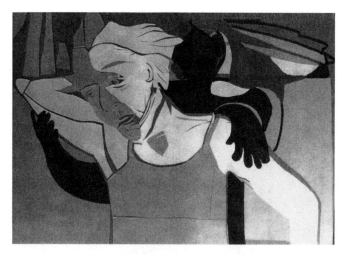

Figure 10.14 *Draw Yourself with your Resources: Being Held.* The earlier figure made of collage paper now has a dark shape behind it with one arm holding the raised upper arm from below and one hand on the left shoulder. Noah Hass-Cohen

one of their scanned pictures. Options available are cutting into the scanned image, gluing images or shapes on top, or drawing on it (Figure 10.14).

> For this image of myself reaching out to others today, I first photo-
> copied my original cutout art. Then I drew in black marker to show
> someone supporting and holding me from the shadows. I wanted to
> convert the shadows into a human holding me and myself reaching
> out to them. The process felt comforting and positive. However, Joanna
> commented that there was an ambiguity where it could also appear
> that I was being taken by the shadows. I also noted that I had frag-
> mented the background behind the image. I understand Joanna's com-
> ment, but I felt good about doing this. I particularly loved the soft
> scratching and screeching of the black marker. I also like the softness of
> the black hands. Their roundness is an antidote to my sharp elbows
> . . . if that makes sense. Two years later, updating the image feels just
> right. Yet I agree with Joanna that the image continues to express the
> common tension in relapse prevention between tendencies to ambiva-
> lence and helplessness and a healthier lifestyle and hope. Noah Hass-
> Cohen

Most often, our studio participants add simple symbols of support to their portraits. Heart shapes, religious symbols, and figures representing friends and loved ones are often placed next to or behind the image of them-

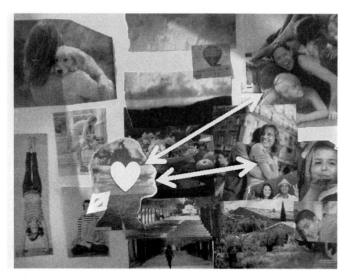

Figure 10.15 *Me Reaching out to My Resources.* A black-and-white photocopy of the original resources collage is now focused on a white heart in the center of the head profile with two bidirectional arrows reaching from the head to an image of a couple and of a group of laughing women. Joanna Clyde Findlay

selves. Words such as "my spiritual life," "love," "creativity," "health," and "growth" are often drawn or created from magazine collage letters. The images of the resources are sometimes rearranged or clarified by simple lines or arrows (Figure 10.15).

> *The resources I most wanted to emphasize as currently important were my close friendships, my personal relationship, and my spiritual practice. At first, I wanted to add a contour of white around the head shape to make it stand out, but did not find this easy, so I simply added a heart shape to the center. I chose a heart as it would be clearly visible and would show that my focus was on relationships. I then added clear arrows connecting the heart to images of my friendships, my personal relationship, and my meditation practice. In so doing, it felt like a confirmation of what I already knew but needed to remind myself; I need to nurture my relationships to nurture myself.* Joanna Clyde Findlay

Group discussion reveals that the members appreciate the safety of working with copied images because it entails no risk of damaging their previous work. Therefore, the copies liberate members for experimentation and bold alteration. Group members often reflect on the simplicity of adding lines and shapes, the ease of trying different versions, and the ability to restart when making a mistake.

In trauma treatment, the emphasis is on the present tense or immediate future, not an ideal distant future that can lead to frustration and failure. The goal is to help clients think about what they have experienced throughout their therapy work and how that might affect their perception of self. To ascertain the potential for change, it is useful to discuss and compare the two self-portraits and together decide how to proceed in therapy. During this process, higher-cortex structures are privileged to update meanings and experience. Thus, the final image can jump-start a different entrainment of the past, present, and future. This entrainment may diminish or interrupt a preexisting mesh of sensory triggers, specifically those associated with trauma, mental perceptions, and psychosocial function. Therefore, these directives deliberately reinforce and reemphasize the notion of a self who is not solely defined by the trauma experience.

Similarly, the directive to: "Draw your relapse prevention strategies" concretely addresses the means to maintain gains and continue to make progress. These strategies are specific and achievable. For example, group members can explore interventions regarding when, where, and how the strategies can be implemented. We solicit approachable goals and resources rather than elusive ones. It is better to envision managing anxiety by showing oneself going for a walk than to represent oneself as being anxiety free. These goals can be revisited and updated, as can self-images. We strongly suggest that, especially in the context of relapse prevention, the directives be used repeatedly. Such repetition may free the client and the therapist to deepen their preventive work and to reconsolidate and shift memories to a new more adaptive direction.

RELATIONAL NEUROSCIENCE: COMPLEX TRAUMA

As mentioned earlier in this chapter, we use C-PTSD as an umbrella term to describe a continuum of trauma-based symptoms. C-PTSD symptoms range from isolated or repetitive flashbacks to fear-inducing response. Multiple, repetitive symptoms that evolve into a chronic condition are usually experienced. Furthermore, the symptoms can generalize to dysfunctional states of mind, struggles with day-to-day living, and personality traits such as avoidance and mistrust. These enduring states contribute to a persistent relational and emotional instability as well as to vulnerability to substance abuse disorders and violence. In addition, people with C-PTSD may be at greater risk of frequent and significant health issues (Cyders, Burris, & Carlson, 2011). To promote insight and awareness of symptoms and of relapse prevention, we offer the following neurobiologically-based educational information:

1. From a neurobiological perspective, the all-encompassing symptoms of C-PTSD reflect an altered functionality in neural circuitry related to trauma. The understanding of PTSD as a disease can help reduce trauma survivors' feelings of shame and guilt.
2. It is critical to attempt to reduce the reoccurrence of fear-based symptoms, as fear responses condition further fear responses. This information may support the construction of an active therapeutic alliance around a concrete goal.
3. Pharmacological treatment with selective serotonin reuptake inhibitors (SSRIs) is an empirically approved treatment for C-PTSD. Medication provides stabilization, which allows treatment to proceed. This understanding mitigates the stigma associated with medication. However, it is critical to work with a psychiatrist who is an expert in trauma treatment (Steckler & Risbrough, 2012), as medication can have irreversible effects on the changed neurobiology of the trauma victim. This is particularly important for trauma clients who are also experiencing pain disorders.

Below we first provide brief information regarding three major neurological systems involved in the processing of trauma: the stress response or cortisol system, the reward or catecholamine system, and the good feeling or serotonergic system.

The stress response or cortisol system involves the long-term stress response, which is stopped by the release of cortisol. For people with C-PTSD who experience both frequent bursts of short-term stress responses and long-term stress, this regulatory system seems to be out of kilter and loses optimal function. In other words, too much or too little cortisol might be released by the body. Too little cortisol may contribute to a flood of memories, whereas too much cortisol results in difficulties in retaining and remembering new information while also reducing immune function.

The reward or catecholamine system works in concert with the cortisol system. Catecholamines are a family of neurotransmitters that include dopamine (DA), norepinephrine (NE) also called noradrenaline, and epinephrine (E) also called adrenaline. DA circuitry in the brain's reward center motivates and inspires pleasure. (As a side note, almost all addictive substances influence the brain's reward system by flooding it with excessive DA, which, over time, creates tolerance and dependence). NE and E stimulate organs such as the heart to pump more blood into larger muscles, and prime the flight, fight, or freeze stress response (see Chapter 9). This catecholamine system also engages the brain's fear and higher thinking regions. The frequent bursts of short-term stress responses or long-term stressors contribute to on-and-off catecholamine responses. Frequent or enduring responses help to consolidate anxiety and fear while decreasing the ability of the thinking brain to regulate these fears. Regardless of gender, individuals with a history of sexual abuse are particularity susceptible to these problems. In addition to fear, other related symptoms include dissociation, substance abuse, and chemical dependency.

The good feeling, serotonergic-based system function is also altered by fear responses. In fact, increased fear responses associated with C-PTSD contribute to a depletion of serotonin. These decreased serotonin levels may contribute to depression and misinterpretation of emotional stimuli. In fact, two of the antidepressant and anti-anxiety medications approved for trauma treatment, sertraline and paroxetine, reduce symptoms of arousal, avoidance, and the reexperiencing of symptoms. In other words, pharmacological treatment with SSRIs can be very helpful in the treatment of C-PTSD.

The Stress Response-Cortisol System

The cortisol system involves the neurobiology of the short- and long-term stress responses (see Chapter 9; Kravits, 2008b). They continue to be of interest in C-PTSD. The cortisol system is an endocrine neurotransmitter system that involves the short-term sympathetic adrenomedullary (SAM) axis stress response, as well as the long-term hypothalamic-pituitary-adrenal (HPA) axis response. The SAM and the HPA axes work together to create cortisol. Although the structures and neurohormones involved in C-PTSD are the same as those involved in stress responses, their functions differ due to impacts of trauma. These impacts chronically dysregulate neurochemical responses, which results in brain structure changes and increased vulnerability to damage. In this case, HPA axis synaptic connections may be permanently transformed (Vermetten & Bremner, 2002), resulting in dysregulated cortisol baseline responses and altered regulatory feedback loops.

Some at-risk populations, such as Holocaust survivors, women with PTSD, and those with a history of childhood sexual abuse (Kaufman, Plotsky, Nemeroff, & Charney, 2000; de Kloet, Joels, & Holsboer, 2005), are subject to decreased cortisol levels. Lower cortisol levels are also implicated in dissociative symptoms and the experience of fragmented memories (Schelling et al., 2006). In contrast, high cortisol levels have been found in people who experience immune system problems (Sapolsky, 2004) and difficulties with affect regulation (Yehuda, Halligan, & Grossman, 2001). The complexity and idiosyncrasies of cortisol function suggest that it may be specific to certain PTSD situations or secondary to comorbid preexisting psychiatric conditions (Shin, Rauch, & Pitman, 2006). It has also been suggested that the amount of cortisol is related to the size of the hippocampus, as women with a history of childhood sexual abuse have often been found to have a smaller hippocampus (Newport, Heim, Bonsall, Miller, & Nemeroff, 2004; Teicher et al., 2006). Hippocampal differences may be attributed to childhood trauma or depression, genetic vulnerability, or cognitive constraints (Shea, Walsh, MacMillan, & Steiner, 2005). In addition, it has been hypothesized that amygdala hyperreactivity exacerbates fear responses in clients with a history of childhood sexual abuse (Bremner, 2003). Specifically, the anterior cingulate cortex's (ACC) failure to help suppress the amygdala (AMY) and HPA responses during posttrauma recall (Lanius, Hopper, & Menon, 2003) has been associated with chronically impaired emotional processing of trauma. According to neuroimaging studies, ACC volumes appear to be smaller in abuse-related PTSD (Bremner, 2003; Kitayama, Quinn, & Bremner, 2006; Lanius et al., 2002), again underscoring childhood abuse as heightening PTSD risk factors (Brewin, Andrews, & Valentine, 2000). Dysfunctions of the ACC have been implicated in numerous psychiatric disorders (Yucel et al., 2003), which may account for the correlation of PTSD with psychiatric problems.

Therefore, memory, learning, fear, and stress are associated with one another. For individuals with complex trauma, these kinds of persistent cognitive and emotional processing deficits are largely due to neurobiological deficits (Scaer, 2001). They constrain the pace of therapy and the person's availability for therapeutic change. In other words, the traumatized person's ability to control the stress response and rebalance the capacity to contain or access memories is driven by neurobiological changes.

The Reward-Catecholamine System

The catecholamine system works in concert with the cortisol system and with the brain's reward center, specifically a region called the nucleus accumbens. Catecholamines are a family of amine-based neurotransmitters that include DA, E, and NE. DA, which regulates motivation, pleasure, and reward, is released in the ventral tegmental area to the nucleus accumbens and to the substantia nigra. The DA's mesocortical circuit is served by the nucleus accumbens, which is the main reward circuit linking the midbrain and the prefrontal cortex (PFC) together in learning and consolidating potential gains from our actions (Carr, 2008a). The catecholamine system also engages the AMY and the limbic functions in the brain. E and NE are released by the SAM axis to create the flight-or-fight response. The locus coeruleus produces the majority of the norepinephrine and, in combination with the SAM axis, arouses the prefrontal cortex (PFC) and the limbic-based fear center connected to our flight, fight, or freeze response.

Because of frequent stress responses, the on-and-off dosages of E, NE, and cortisol further consolidate fear-based memories in the AMY (Vasterling & Brewin, 2005). Anxiety and fear are aroused by traumatic stimuli and traumatic memories, and, most importantly for the trauma survivor, by fear of the symptoms associated with the onset of these memories. These amygdala-generated reactions are assumed to be modulated or extinguished by the medial prefrontal cortex (mPFC). In other words, mPFC activity is inversely related to the activity in the amygdala (Shin et al., 2006).

Unfortunately, catecholamine cascades have an opposite effect on the MPFC, as they effectively shut off PFC cognitive functions, barring it from regulating stress and emotion. Thus, the AMY, in concert with the catecholamine system, captures rational thoughts, leaving a person vulnerable to impulsive and risky behaviors (Vasterling & Brewin, 2005). Furthermore, high levels of NE and cortisol greatly impair PFC functioning, specifically as it relates to memory. This is in contrast to moderate levels of NE or cortisol, which enhance memory as well as alertness in the reward system. Therefore, it is likely that this phenomenon is survival based, as it inhibits the content of working memory to allow an automatic response to threats. As a result, it is critical that the client and therapist understand how this vicious catecholamine cycle of enhanced AMY function and decreased PFC function act to reduce reoccurring fear and unremitting stress states.

While the fearful and anxious responses described above are significantly correlated with decreased activation of the mPFC, it has been suggested that, in contrast, dissociation presents with greater activation in the mPFC (Lanius et al., 2004, 2005). Dissociation is thus conceptualized as an extreme response of the mPFC attempting to overregulate fear. These findings assist in understanding how trauma can present with either an overexpression of affect or an extreme shutdown and inhibition of affect (Vermetten & Bremner, 2002). Overexpression reflects right-hemisphere functioning, while inhibition reflects a stronger left hemisphere (Shin et al., 2006).

Similarly, exposure to childhood sexual abuse activates a pattern of unremitting amygdala fear-based responses to others. The ensuing neurochemical cascade can alter the child's developing brain, inhibit neurogenesis, and contribute to neurochemical alterations (Perry, 2001; Schore, 2001b). Child sexual abuse contributes to changed corpus callosum size, significant bilateral reduction in hippocampal volume, and greater than average nonverbal right-hemisphere dominance (Teicher et al., 2006). Exposed to violence, the child with a predominately hyperarousal response will eventually become vulnerable to persistent hyperarousal-related symptoms and disorders within the spectrum of anxiety and fear disorders (Perry, Pollard, Blakley, Baker, & Vigilante, 1995; Perry, 2001). Prominent related symptoms include somatic complaints, dissociation, anxiety, helplessness, dependence, and isolation.

The Good Feeling-Serotonergic System

The serotonergic system is complex and is found in multiple brain areas. However, it is in the reward circuitry, specifically in the dorsal raphe nucleus, that serotonin is mostly synthesized and released. Prominently, the reward system has many projections to the PFC, affecting cognitive function. Furthermore, serotonin plays an important part in neuroplasticity and the regulation of the AMY and the hippocampus, as well as during orbitofrontal cortex–mediated tasks, which filter and evaluate social information. Decreased serotonin contributes to the misinterpretation of emotional stimuli. Specifically, reduced levels of serotonin are associated with decreased thresholds of amygdala firing, whereas increased 5-HTP, which is a serotonin precursor, increases the threshold of amygdala firing, decreasing vigilance and fear. In other words, pharmacological treatment with SSRIs can inhibit the locus coeruleus's NE neuronal firing as 5-HTP modulates NE production. Again, it is critical that the therapist and the client be aware of this information as the two medications approved for treatment, sertraline and paroxetine, are helpful in reducing arousal, avoidance, and the re-experiencing of symptoms.

Finally, it is also important to note that creativity may be negatively impacted as there seem to be changes in the default mode of the resting brain. Because people with PTSD tend to be vigilant, they are constantly operating outward. Therefore, the functions of the default mode network, which are associated with introspection or self-referential thought and the generation of varied responses, may activate less or in a different way. This is because default neural network activation is negatively correlated with brain systems that focus on external visual and sensory cueing. In fact, lower connectivity was found across this network for people who have chronic trauma, such as childhood abuse (Sripada et al., 2012). It is possible that as a consequence of default network disruptions, traumatized children and adults may find it difficult to engage with an inner creative world, demonstrating concrete rather than symbolic play. This understanding contributes to better understanding of the kind of clinical interventions needed.

CREATE PRINCIPLES AND CLINICAL APPLICATIONS

As this chapter has focused on the phenomena and treatment of trauma, we provided the clinician with an overview on the ATR-N trauma model called Secure Remembrance (SR-5). To recap, the five factors of Safety, Relationships, Remembrance, Reconnection, and Resiliency act as a framework for navigating trauma work. The starting point is to choose an object that promotes safety, then experiment with approaching safe relationships though the manipulation of a hand silhouette. Once safety is accessible, then traumatic issues and memories can be remembered, represented, processed, transformed, and reconsolidated. We advocate contextual processing of remembering, which focuses on how the narrative is processed, rather than on the content of the narrative. As this process occurs, actively reconnecting with trusted others and building a repertoire of interpersonal and intrapersonal resources and personal resiliency is encouraged. We have described a sequence of directives for the SR-5 factors. This sequence will usually take more than one hour. It is suggested to either extend the therapeutic hour, or to engage clients with the sequence of directives within a period of six hours; as from a neurobiological perspective this seems to provide an optimal window of opportunity. The primary focus of the CREATE Adaptive Responding–based art therapy directives are linked to the SR-5 factors:

- Safety: the SURF Tracking Device, the Anchor, and the Safe Place and Loving-Kindness Walking Meditation
- Relationship: the Hand Silhouette, Color Check-In, Draw Yourself With a Safe Person, or Draw a Safe Relationship
- Contextual Remembrance: "If you were to paint the problem, what would it look like? If you could change one aspect of the memory or keep one aspect of it, what would you choose? Select the parts of the image you want to rescue and cut them out. Draw yourself, or draw yourself with someone from your past."
- Reconnection: "Make a collage of your intrapersonal and interpersonal resources." This is followed by the request to amplify each one.
- Resiliency: "Represent or make a collage of yourself with your resources today, yourself in the future, or reaching out to others; represent or draw your relapse prevention strategies."

The principle of Adaptive Responding informs the sequencing of the SR-5 directives. This is represented by a simple manipulation of an object, which may then progress experiences of mastery and control involved in the use of drawing and painting, and the manipulation of complex cutting, gluing, and changing of the artwork. The empathic manipulation of the artwork contributes to clients' contextual trauma processing, encourages cognitive and emotional flexibility, and contributes to a felt sense of change and hope. This cycle of directives concludes with self-care strategies and a vision of future well-being. A sense of safety, new attempts at control, and coping efforts are all supported by the safety-based directives. The building complexity of the art directives lays a foundation for clients' adaptive coping as well as resiliency and relapse prevention. Thus, when working with clients to support resiliency, therapists are encouraged to use self-compassion, coping and safety-oriented directives from across all five factors:

- The SURF Tracking origami device offers self-rating of the intensity of triggers, assisting clients to self-gauge their readiness to progress with processing trauma memories.
- The Color Check-In provides immediate weekly feedback, increasing clients' perceived sense of control and their striving for control.
- Choosing which part of a memory to process and whether to rework or discard it supports the client's experience of being in control.
- Creating, reflecting upon, and amplifying images of personal coping resources and relapse prevention promote resiliency and hope.
- Starting to do the art with small manipulatives (objects) supports control and safety.

Movement is an innate function of the CREATE principle of Creative Embodiment. Because implied or explicit threat of movement may easily trigger traumatic memories, therapists are encouraged to initially avoid the use of images with implied or explicit motion. It is necessary to carefully work toward the symbolic and actual use of motion in trauma-informed therapy. The pace of therapy will depend upon the severity and complexity of the person's trauma. As trauma is an embodiment of emotional dysregulation, the introduction of movement-based art directives, and general movements in the studio, seek to support clients' experiences of tolerable disequilibrium and of novel emotionally meaningful events. A sample of such directives in this chapter includes:

- The Musical Chairs directive, which allows studio participants to move away from perceived stressors.
- The Loving-Kindness Walking Meditation, which encourages mindful and aware movement.

Relational safety and support is a foundational interpersonal context, which is threaded throughout the SR-5 framework. Examples of the CREATE Relational Resonating directives include the following:

- The Hand Silhouette directive allows for a concrete experience of safety in the room.
- Draw Yourself With a Safe Person or Draw a Safe Relationship directives support the emotional and cognitive exploration of relationships.
- The reconnection and relapse prevention experiential offers an opportunity to explicitly focus on connecting to others via images of reaching out to others or interpersonal resources.

- The therapeutic alliance is directly evaluated and communicated each session via the Color Check In directive, which gives a visual trace of the relationship.
- With time, within the safe relationship with the therapist, the SR-5 directives build a safe therapeutic relationship.

Four of the Secure Remembrance art directives request clients' active, expressive representation of emotions. Examples of Expressive Communicating include:

- The SURF Tracking origami device and the Color Check In directive provide an ongoing opportunity to track sensitivity to emotional triggers, including interpersonal safety.
- The creation and use of the safety Anchor and mindful walking directives serve as immediately accessible sensory means to regulate emotion and self-soothe.
- Using the fluid, expressive, and colorful medium of paint for the memory processing work intentionally fosters the arousal of painful emotional information and allows dynamic expression of emotions, inviting affect regulation via the translation of implicit emotional states to explicit images.
- The media of choice and collage used for the reconnection and remembrance phases exploits the emotionally expressive impact of found images, but in a contained way.
- In the reconnection and relapse prevention art experiences, symbolic movement toward others is explored.
- Approaching others brings on left-hemisphere connections.

The neuroscience of C-PTSD and trauma warns us of the altered structure and functionality of trauma-related neurobiological circuits. Yet our ability to support client stabilization techniques, affect regulation, and safe memory processing supports the possibility of more integrated functioning. The CREATE principle of Transformative Integrating and SR-5 directives provide support as follows:

- Contextual memory processing directives allow unacknowledged traumatic memories to be included in a visual and verbal narrative.
- Actively cutting out, removing, and gluing pieces of an image of trauma memories, within the safety of the art room and therapeutic relationship, begins the movement toward integrating the traumatic past.
- Reworking images of reaching out to others or seeing oneself in the future makes those images more deeply explored, elaborated, and cohesive. The art directives and products mirror the more stable assimilated states of mind that are desired.
- Hemispheric integration is facilitated by the sequence of making the hand silhouettes, when the right hand traces the left and the left traces the right.
- Hemispheric integration is supported when clients make verbally mediated, left-hemisphere sense out of their right-hemisphere autobiographical representations.

- Vertical integration is sustained via the linking of implicit limbic memories to explicit verbal narratives of client trauma history and identity.

Paying attention to one's bodily reactions, triggers, impulses, behaviors, emotions, and thoughts supports the cultivation of a compassionate inward focus that also encourages mentalizing and updating of attachment-based internal working models. The methodology of introducing the SR-5 factors via studio art directives also allows therapists to reduce their compassion fatigue. Moreover, the tangible art directives allow therapists to work on their empathy for client processes in addition to working on their own material, cultivating empathy for themselves. The directives focusing on reconnection and relapse prevention are important experientials for therapist self-regulation and care. The principle of Empathizing and Compassion is embedded throughout all of the SR-5 directives. It is a compassionate stance promoted by:

- Introducing simple breathing tools from mindful awareness practices as a way to effectively manage stress, promote stabilization, and increase attuned responses in both client and therapist.
- Paying attention to automatic movement in the Loving-Kindness Walking Meditation.
- Bringing awareness to trauma triggers by rating them in the SURF Tracking experiential.
- Offering opportunities to visibly see the process of change, to narrate the change, and control the pace and extent of change in contextual memory processing.

APPENDIX: SURF DEVICE

Materials: construction paper, pencil, and scissors (Figure 10.16)

1. The corners of a sheet of paper are folded up to meet the opposite sides and (if the paper is not already square) the top is cut off, making a square sheet with diagonal creases.
2. The four corners of the square are folded into the center, forming a shape known in origami terminology as a blintz base or cushion fold.
3. The resulting smaller square is turned over, and the four corners are folded in a second time.
4. All four corners are folded up so that the points meet in the middle.
5. Working fingers into the pockets of paper in each of the four corners completes the SURF.

CHAPTER 11

Transformative Integrating:
Creating, Mentalizing, and Connecting

Building my dream house was something that felt deserving of careful planning, deliberation, and execution. Once I had an idea of what I wanted to make and I started constructing, my anxiety dampened. The creating process was very calming for me and became very enjoyable, and I moved along and started adding details to my creation. I thought about what I wanted others to know about me, what I was willing to share with them, and how what I displayed would be perceived. Along with those thoughts came concern with the final product, and questions arose, such as: Is my house well constructed? Is my house as attractive as the other homes? How innovative are my ideas? Since this experience, I assume that that which streams through my mind may be similar to what my clients might be thinking. Veronica Avalos

MENTALIZING, A CORE INTERPERSONAL NEUROBIOLOGY and ATR-N process, is involved in the function of several affective, cognitive, and social domains that are discussed throughout this book. Mentalizing is essential for creative and mental imagining, visual-spatial manipulating of sensory information, and forming and maintaining internal working models of attachment; ascertaining the minds of others; and developing and maintaining a sense of autobiographical and social self. Mentalizing is a form of imaginative mental activity about others or oneself, namely, perceiving and interpreting human behavior in terms of intentional mental states. Meaning intuiting the needs, desires, feelings, beliefs, goals, purposes, and reasons of others (Fonagy & Bateman, 2004). Beginning in early childhood it develops and is amendable to change throughout the life span (Allen, 2012; Harel, Kaplan, Avimeir-Patt, & Ben-Aaron, 2006).

We contend that mentalizing is involved in every aspect of therapeutic art making. Art-making is a reiterative process that oscillates between mentalizing and executive decision making. This involves going back and forth between imagining the art product and making it, as well as mentalizing about, and engaging with, the therapist's perceived internal world and words. In other words, the client–art therapist relationship is infused with implicit mentalizing, decision making, and actions (Gavron, 2014a; Sholt & Gavron, 2006). Contingent and coherent self and social mentalizing is a foundational ATR-N concept of Transformative Integrating. Together, the information provided in Chapters 11 through 14 which are devoted to mentalizing, mindfulness, and empathizing, embody the ATR-N approach.

Our ability to recognize our own mental states, as well as understand the intentions and mental states of others, based on their covert and overt behaviors, are at the core of mentalizing (Bateman & Fonagy, 2011). Mentalization and reflection are metacognitive processes that require linking knowledge of the past with the present moment. Both processes are necessary for the formation and updating of autobiographical memory. When accompanied by mindfulness and empathy, mentalizing can transform our relationships with others. This kind of imaginative and cognitive activity allows us to perceive and interpret others' behaviors in terms of their needs, desires, feelings, beliefs, goals, and motivation. In order to do so, we rework existing mental images of people and their behaviors that are stored in our memory (Siegel, 2010). Active mentalizing takes into account other people's perspectives, simulates their experiences in our imagination, and constructs imaginary social scenarios. This critical process evokes theory of mind (ToM, Premack & Woodruff, 1978), which is a reference to the act of experiencing other people's minds indirectly. People learn this early on in joint dyadic and familial constellations through reiterative mentalizing feedback loops (Asen & Fonagy, 2012). Without this capacity, we lack the ability to understand other people's actions and perspectives. ToM mind impairments are associated with neurodevelopmental disorders, such as autism spectrum disorders. A turbulent attachment history is also associated with a tendency for non-relational and concrete thinking which is lacking in complex judgment about social behaviors and other viewpoints (Allen, 2012).

Thus, unsuccessful mentalizing contributes to disorders of self- experience, which are a central phenomenon in many psychiatric disorders (Bateson & Fonagy, 2011). There can be a range of mentalizing difficulties, from an overall failure to comprehend the feelings of self or others; to the inability to see others as having any psychological complexity (Wallin, 2007). Depending on the situation, there can be a significant mentalizing failure. When the person simply cannot hold the relationships between thoughts, feelings and actions there is usually also a lack of reflective ability. Other difficulties with mentalizing include pseudo mentalizing subtypes, intrusive or other misuses of mentalizing (Allen, Fonagy, & Bateman, 2008). Both intrusive-accurate mentalizing, and overactive-inaccurate mentalizing lack considerate and supportive attunement. Destructive and inaccurate pseudo mentalizing involve a denial of objective reality and an inference of unlikely mental states that can be very damaging to child development. For the most part misuses of mentalizing are less about mentalizing impairments and more about distortions in the service of a self-serving agenda. In a mild expression, they have a coercive influence, humiliating or manipulating others, and in a severe form the person is using knowledge of others feelings or wishes to knowingly confuse and control the other (Bateman & Fonagy, 2011).

So mentalizing functions directly and indirectly inform how we pay attention to others and understand their thoughts, actions, and intentions. While mentalizing is usually an unconscious and implicit process (Kampe, Frith, & Frith, 2003), it can also be conscious and explicit (Allen, 2006). In an everyday context, both emotive and higher-order cognitive functions determine our responses to mentalizing questions such as, How do I see myself? How do I see others? How do others see me and perceive my art and art making? In this regard, active mentalizing estimates in real time how others may perceive us. Processing implicit mentalizing experiences into explicit mentalizing communication assists in gaining interpersonal awareness. One way to achieve such insight is by purposefully slowing down our thought processes and focusing on the here and now in order to reflect upon implicit mentalizing experiences (Allen, Fonagy, & Bateman, 2008). Kabat-Zinn, 2005). In the mentalization-based treatment approach, one's perceptions, emotions, feelings, and actions are examined, questioned and narrated (Fonagy & Bateman, 2004; Fonagy & Target, 1998). Thus, self-awareness extends to the intentional awareness of what others have in mind (Allen, 2006). As stated in earlier chapters, the individual's ability to remain self-aware and empathic while negotiating interpersonal relationships has thus been linked to attachment styles (Coates, 2006). Disrupted and traumatic attachment experiences not only impact the capacity for affect regulation and reflective function (Fonagy & Target, 1997; Fonagy & Bateman, 2004) but also skew cognitive ability to approximate how others perceive them, thereby limiting creativity (Cozolino, 2010). This state has been termed, "mindblindness," meaning an awareness of physical things but a blindness to mental functions that for most humans underlies social emotional interactions (Baron-Cohen, Leslie, & Frith, 1985).

The mind is continuously mentalizing. Most of this activity has been linked to functions of the medial prefrontal lobe (Frith & Frith, 2003). Exciting and very pertinent to art therapy is that the mPFC is also associated with attention to perceptual stimuli (Gilbert, Williamson, Dumontheil, Simons,

Frith, & Burgess, 2007). Reflective mentalizing also includes daydreaming, imagining the future, and generating thoughts, which have been associated with creativity. These creative activities take place in the brain's default resting state (Raichle et al., 2001). The default cognitive network is also stimulated when imagining or simulating future events (Buckner, Andrews & Schacter, 2008). In other words, we can be open to understanding others' new ideas and creative solutions when the mind focuses on others, and when it wanders. Periods of time when we have fleeting thoughts about life events is another way of characterizing resting states (Qin & Northoff, 2011). Furthermore, the default system is likely involved not only in autobiographical musing but also in social cognition (Mars, Neubert, Noonan, Sallet, & Rushworth, 2012). Training the mind-brain to self-reflect and mentalize may serve as an antidote to the influences of traumatic experiences. Mentalizing can be a prelude to denying the influence of impulses and fears and instead engage with decisive executive functions. Overall, research suggests a shared neural network for daydreaming, mentalizing and executive function, which is found in the default mode network (DMN). This finding "contributes to the overall endeavor of an exciting, integrative, cross-disciplinary approach to cognitive neuroscience" (Spreng, Mar, & Kim, 2009, p. 506). As reviewed in Chapter 7, our interests in the DMN stem from emerging research, which suggests that the DMN is also implicated in creativity (Jung, Mead, Carrasco & Flores, 2013) and seems to be emerging as the core of human functioning and connectivity (Hagmann et al., 2008).

In this chapter, we describe individual and interpersonal art based experientials that deliberately call for active and interactive reflective mentalizing, as well as creative mind wandering. We evoke this process by pairing two experiences: Each of the creative milieu participants creates an individual three-dimensional paper artwork, My Home, which puts creativity in action and requires oscillation between DMN and executive functions. My Home is then brought into a Community of Homes, activating mentalizing. Thus, an ATR-N skills sequence is put into operation requiring the activation of several implicit and explicit neuropathways, and mentalizing feedback loops such as imagining, problem solving, checking in with others in the milieu, and self-reflection.

To create the paper homes, group members engage in an intricate art task that involves the construction of a three-dimensional structure from two-dimensional paper. Requiring reflection and purposeful attention, this task activates creative musing and executive functions. Emotions, self-awareness, attention, and concentration are called upon in order to conceptualize, plan, and execute the creation of three-dimensional forms.

Next, studio participants imagine and inhabit their home with personal imagery. This activity calls for reflection on family of origin and current family mental representations and cognitive processing of the directive, as well as on the metaphorical meaning of *home.* Such metaphorical exploration calls attention to the individual's personal, familial, and environmental history, as well as to his or her personal belief system. It may also engage the creators of such homes in an imaginative state, involving future hopes and aspirations.

We then bring the paper homes into a community, highlighting the social-interactive aspect of mentalizing. Sharing the art product and engaging in the process involves estimating and negotiating how other group members regard each other's creations. Furthermore, sharing requires a complex engagement of interpersonal and personal mind states as self-reflection. One reason that we chose the topics of home and community was to evoke interactive mentalizing and prosocial connectivity. This is in contrast to other art therapy group directives, such as "imagine yourselves on an island and draw on one sheet the resources that you need," which can arouse competitiveness due to the limited availability of imagined resources.

Such intricate individual and group art therapy tasks are also likely to activate prefrontal functions, such as attention, concentration, and multi-tasking. These are informed by limbic-medial parietal neural circuitry that is implicated in mentalization and self-awareness. As mentioned, these brain regions have been implicated in intrinsic self-referential states, or an organized mode of a predetermined brain function, also called the default mode (Gusnard, Akbudak, Shulman, & Raichle, 2001). The default mode refers to semi-reflective states that the brain relies on when we are inactive yet awake.

We hypothesize that semi-reflective states may be implicated in pre-contemplative stages of art making. Developing the capacity for mentalizing and for reflective awareness is a foundational ATR-N skill. Although the field lacks the neuroimaging research to support these claims, we strive to show how ATR-N based directives can contribute to the development of mentalizing. The overall learning methodology described in this book, specifically the narration and reflections on the art, are intended to contribute to the development of an active mentalizing habit.

EXPERIENTIAL PRACTICES AND DIRECTIVES

Experience I: Paper Home Sculptures

Group art therapy and client-therapist dyad processes provide opportunities to hone implicit and explicit therapeutic mentalizing experiences. This is a form of mind-brain training. We contend that under therapeutic conditions, such as the studio environment, executing a complex task and sharing it in a group setting creates insight and changes the capacity for mentalizing. It

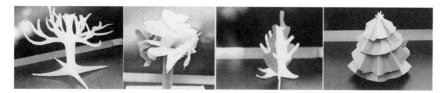

Figure 11.1 *Paper Tree Examples.* Simple tree sculptures made from intersecting cutout and folded paper in green, brown, and white construction and tissue paper. Joanna Clyde Findlay

leads to an experience of mentalizing that allows studio participants to gain awareness regarding interpersonal behaviors and intentions.

The first suggestion is to: "Create a three-dimensional home or house environment out of two-dimensional materials," such as multicolored craft paper and card stock. Additional craft accessories, including feathers, ribbons, wrapping papers, and stickers, are intended to stimulate reflection on clients' associations and promote mentalizing. To begin, we demonstrate key techniques for folding and attaching paper so that they can form three-dimensional structures. Because it is easier to work with smaller structures, we start with small environmental elements that might surround the home, such as trees, fences, and gates, all of which can be created by folding, cutting, and gluing together construction and tissue paper (Figure 11.1).

To form the house, sturdy poster board can be folded into four sides; the roof can be a triangular elongated tunnel; and masking tape lines can join the house together. Cylinders and triangular forms become building blocks for a structure, and stability can be further ensured by cutting small flaps at the ends of a cylinder, which are then folded and secured to a cardboard base with glue. Masking tape holds glued seams until they dry, and swatches of folded paper adhere to interiors in order to secure rafters, roofs, and beams (Figure 11.2).

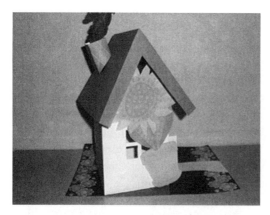

Figure 11.2 *My House (Home).* A base decorated with flower stickers supports a four-sided structure. A neatly cutout window is on one side of the house, over which a large flower in a pot is pasted. There is a red chimney with dark smoke protruding from the pointed roof made of gray paper. Veronica Avalos

To invite spaciousness, we suggest that the home be as large, tall, or wide as the participants desire. Although couched in visuospatial and perceptual terms, these terms also evoke the kind of symbolic spaciousness that is needed for slowing down and mentalizing.

The sculptors reflect on what kind of home and house they would like to create for their selfhood. Such thoughts occur in a period of inactivity or when people alternate between periods of activity such as cutting and preparing, and quiet contemplation. These are contemplative precursory states that stimulate creativity and an opportunity to let the mind linger and daydream. Creativity is further supported when infused with both intention and kindness. Kindness supports the emergence of nonreactive states that reduce defensiveness, leaving room for introspection.

Creating the three-dimensional structure then shifts to conscious and deliberate expression. Constructing a sturdy house from two-dimensional paper requires executive function. Multitasking, planning, and concentrating all entail prefrontal skills. An exploration of the spatial dimensions and orientation options is also required, which involves parietal function. For example, structures are rotated 360 degrees to consider all sides as external settings for paths, foliage, and trees. Constructions generally reach upward and outward in space as intricate details are continuously added. Assimilating technical guidelines, imagining form, and executing successive steps require the complex orchestration of thoughts and actions. Furthermore, our participants report that they also assess and reflect upon how others will see their self-representation of a home. As demonstrated by Veronica's quote at the beginning of this chapter, this kind of mentalizing requires a balancing act that involves the self and others (Allen, 2006).

Experience II: Inhabiting the Home

A brief introduction to mentalizing constructs calls for ideas about how to represent internal and external states. In this vein, we ask each person to: "Inhabit the inside of your home with images of your thoughts, perceptions, and beliefs by painting the interior or using collage images." These can be pasted inside or outside the home. Inhabiting the home with a collage or painting of one's thoughts, perceptions, and beliefs requires both inner reflection and active self-awareness. For some, the task of self-mentalizing through images and symbols is easily accessible and enhances meaning making. For others, this metaphoric work is challenging. It may provoke a strong reaction, triggering unwanted memories. Most will slow down their work processes considerably, taking the time to figure out exactly what they want to include, while others will work rapidly to plaster the interior space with intention and meaning. As part of this process, some participants will spread out other

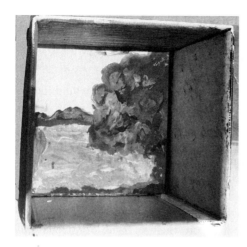

Figure 11.3 *Inner Home.* Photographed from above, the interior of the home is decorated with a mixture of paint and collage. The bottom of the home portrays a tranquil green field and tree. The four sides are decorated with different textured and colored papers. Norma Y. Guerrero-Lewis

materials around themselves and share the media, scissors, glue, and images. As they translate abstract beliefs or perceptions into images, they also interact socially and imagine themselves interacting in person.

> *I realized that I saw the home as a representation of me (Figure 11.2). I am a person that does not share my personal information with anyone unless I feel safe. My home had all these beautiful colored papers inside, which are rich with experience and knowledge from my past and present, but the outside walls were white and dirty only to be left for interpretation. Although the doors are wide open for people to come in, still the outside could be scary for someone to come close enough in order to be invited in.* Veronica Avalos

> *You see part of the inner house, which represents four different aspects of my life: the personal, mind, family/community, and love for myself (Figure 11.3). The personal is represented by purple cosmos-like paper; mind is the horizontal lavender lines with geometric shapes; family and community is represented by a textured ocean-color paper that represents the ocean's ups and downs, but always having a constant experience; and the beige color with wording on it about love is the area in which I have to love myself in order for me to open the door to love others.* Norma Y. Guerrero-Lewis

Experience III: A Community of Homes

The joining of individual sculptures allows the relational context of one's home to become evident. Arranging the community of homes is also an implicit reflection of the unspoken social relationships of the group. There-fore, as the individual homes are nearing completion, we ask the creators to: "Bring your homes together into a community." There is often a period of milling around and an increase in volume of social chatter as the homes are maneuvered. Group members may choose their neighbors and dwell next to them. Sometimes the community organizes coherently as a particular locality with an ocean to the left, or mountains to the right. Other times there is more of a struggle where some homes remain on the periphery unable to connect. In Figure 11.4, the group chose to arrange in a circular community.

This interactive mentalization experience calls upon the ability to reflect on one's own thoughts and feelings while empathically considering the goals and desires of others. Higher-order consciousness and theory of mind (Frith & Frith, 1999) are thus concretely manifested. The experience of seeing one's home in a crowd of homes or positioned on the outside of a semicircle may also evoke interpersonal related feelings of attachment-based security or inse-curity, as expressed in Figure 11.4.

> *When we were all finished and all structures were put together, I noticed that many of them were decorated on the outside. The symbol-ism of the structures being put together was very eye opening. I felt happy to see everyone's structures together because for that moment I saw harmony and togetherness from all of these people in the room. It did not matter that all these homes were different and unique; they all became as one.* Lisa Kandaros

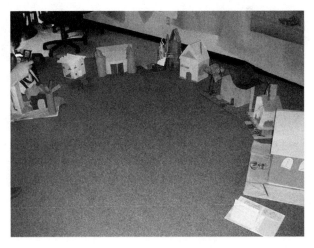

Figure 11.4 *Homes.* The group decided to make a semicircular community with each home evenly spaced, facing inward. Most homes are positioned on a base and are made of a variety of colored papers.

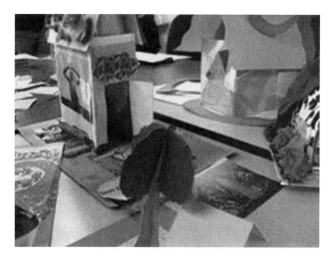

Figure 11.5 *Happy Home in Community.* This close-up photograph shows a section of a community of paper sculpture homes. A paper tree is visible in the foreground, and the homes nearby are made with a mix of brightly colored construction paper and tissue paper. Robin Shanon

For other group members, the community directive touches upon a relational nerve as it stirs autobiographical memory and brings awareness of attachment issues (Figures 11.5 and 11.6).

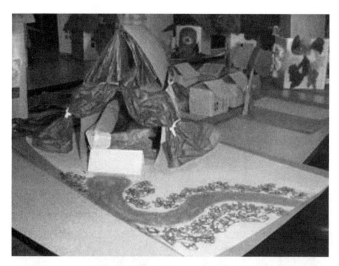

Figure 11.6 *Happy Surface and Hidden Injury.* This home is made rather like a traditional camping tent, with an open end partially concealed by dark blue tissue paper curtains. One can see a small part of the interior, which seems to show some type of furniture covered in dark pink tissue paper. Kazuko Numato

My Asian cultural background has ingrained in me the importance of showing a positive front to society and it does not allow the external expression of inner suffering. Therefore, I put a damaged wall under the roof where it could not be seen. In addition, the curtains also concealed a damaged part of the house. Many of the group members mentioned the feeling of connection that arose from seeing the houses grouped like a small town. For me, this emphasized isolation because I often try to hide my vulnerable feelings and prefer to keep my distance from others. My culture respects harmony and tries to avoid disturbing the structure of any situation. Therefore, I followed the direction to put my house next to that of my colleague; however, physical closeness required patience in order to show I had normal feelings. I had to numb my pain and pretend that I was fine. Kazuko Numato

Once the sculptures are placed in a group, the facilitator guides an ATR-N mentalizing discussion. Helpful questions include: Where did you think so-and-so would put down her home? How did you decide where to put down yours? What would you have liked to be different? Additional questions are: Did the actions of others fit what you expected them to do? Were there any surprises? What have you learned about others and your expectations of them? This observation and discussion of the paper homes enables group members to identify representations of a variety of abilities for reflective functioning. Three of them are openness to discovery, perspective taking, reflection and contemplation (Asen & Fonagy, 2012). There are several levels of perspective taking (Selman, 1980). The most evolved is level three, the ability to mentalize the other, and negotiate. Most importantly dyads, families, and communities can come together to create a new "we" in which needs of the individual are included. There is an ability to analyze the perspectives of several people involved in a situation from the viewpoint of an objective bystander, and it is possible to imagine how different cultural or social values would influence the perceptions of the bystander. This kind of perspective taking is associated with a secure self. Level two represents the ability to mentalize self and the other, and negotiate co-constructing an environment of compromise. This could be the highest level of perspective taking that people who are insecurely attached can arrive at during times of stress. Level one is a state where there are difficulties and/or inabilities to see the perspective of an other, which are indicative of general struggling with mentalizing during stressful moments. In the table below, we have associated perspective-taking factors with attachment-based interactions as they might express during the art making of the Paper Homes (Table 11.1).

Table 11.1 Art Therapy Relational Neuroscience Mentalizing Factors: Connecting Attachment Security, Mentalization, and the Paper Home Sculptures

	Secure Mentalizing States	Insecure Mentalizing States	Non Mentalizing States
Openness to discovery	• appreciation of changes as they occur during sculpting • ability to repair and adapt sculpture when difficulties encountered • ability to use color, symbol, and form in the paper sculpture to represent one's story	• an explicit anti-reflective stance toward any change • unwillingness to join the community of homes • evasive, nonverbal reactions to moving the sculptures from self-space to interpersonal space	• no openness to discovery • preoccupation with the rules of making the sculptures; how to glue and roll paper correctly, etc. • unawareness of the social aspects of therapeutic art-making
Perspective taking (Levels III to I)	• a perception of self and other's mental function; making explicit connections between self and other's homes • taking a developmental perspective on one's life; the ability to see change in one's own creative skills • forgiveness of self and others; ability to be vulnerable about the creative process • creating a new "we"	• lack of elaboration inside of home • lack of explanation for meaning of home and its construction • with or without discomfort able to negotiate a space to join a community of homes yet maintaining a separate sense of self at all times • worried about disclosure and discussion regarding self, creative process, and the sculpture	• denial of difficulty with technical aspects of construction • an inability to reflect upon inner meaning of group members' homes • a preoccupation with the material while avoiding self and other considerations • not available for negotiation
Reflection and contemplation	• genuine interest in others' internal and external worlds and homes • awareness of the impact of affect—one's own and other's—on making process • tentative and moderate commentary on others' work	• inappropriate social interaction • intrusive commentaries on others' sculptures • insensitive moving of others' sculptures • gross assumptions regarding meaning of others' colors and symbols	• expression of certainty about the thoughts and feelings relating to others' homes in the group • difficulty and discomfort in tolerating others' sharing of their process of creativity • literal meaning of words and colors, for example, "my garden is green"

Group discourse and self-reflection not only engage the uniquely human cortical functions that require meta-reasoning, but also attach significance to relational experiences. The paper sculptures and collages concretely demonstrate how mentalization, working memory, and autobiographical memory all work together. This meta-representation is an amalgam of implicit and explicit mentalizing experiences. Mentalizing includes both implicit art making and active sharing, as well as explicit discussion. Most interactive mentalizing is implicit, which in verbal therapy may remain hidden. However, in-group art therapy activities, it can be revealed and available for reflection and change.

> *The experiential had me focus on certain aspects of my inner self-awareness in which I was studying my emotions, which were felt physically, and later I was able to better analyze the feelings subjectively. Consciousness is thought to emerge from the cerebral cortex, more precisely the prefrontal cortex. This area is also believed to contain conscious perception of emotion and our ability to attend and focus. More importantly, this area contributes to the sense of purpose in our lives. Lisa Kandaros*

RELATIONAL NEUROSCIENCE: MENTALIZING, REFLECTION, THE DEFAULT MODE NETWORK, AND EXECUTIVE FUNCTION

Intrinsic, non-explicit mentalizing states can be characterized by inactivity, reflection, daydreaming, and overall mind wandering (Buckner et al., 2008). Such intrinsic mind states are a systematic way of brain function that is present in the brain as a baseline activity. They are states of mind that are informed by the accumulation of our life experiences (Raichle & Snyder, 2007). Intrinsic, implicit mentalizing states involve self-reflection, projection, and story processing. These activities contribute to the capacity of theory of mind, the integrity of autobiographical memory, and the ability to imagine the future (Mar, 2011).

In the last decade, researchers have started investigating what brain activity happens during intrinsic states, operationalized as times when no specific goal-oriented task is presented (Raichle et al., 2001). They have found that intrinsic states share a core mentalizing neural network, the DMN. Also known as the default resting system, the DMN interfaces with frontal brain region areas that are needed for active mentalizing and executive function.

The default resting system has also been associated with creativity (Andreasen, 2011). Mind wandering is akin to contemplation and can be a precursor to art making. Subsequently, art making requires a shift to active executive functions. As stated, it is likely that successful ATR-N interventions activate a shared and linked mentalizing, creativity, and executive neural network. Thus, the ATR-N hypothesis is that, under the right conditions, combined effects of group art making, storytelling, executive planning, and reflective sharing promote interactive mentalization, social cognition, and enhanced executive functioning. Moreover, it is likely that the neurological pathways activated by complex, social art making contribute to these functions and support a sense of mastery and control. A sense of control and coping both have long been associated with positive mental health (Peterson, Maier, & Seligman, 1993; Sapolsky, 2005). Below, we first review the brain regions associated with mentalizing, the default system, and those which are associated with executive function and mastery.

Mentalizing and Default Mode Network Circuitry

The shared neurobiology of mentalizing involves the activation of midline and surface fronto-parietal brain regions and structures. These are the medial prefrontal cortex (mPFC), posterior superior temporal sulcus (PSTS), temporoparietal junction (TPJ), anterior temporal lobe areas, posterior cingulate cortex (PCC) and precuneus, most likely the left inferior frontal gyrus (IFG), and Broca's language area. It is likely that the amygdala (AMY) and the occipital cortex are also involved in the mentalizing neural network (Mar, 2011). As described in earlier chapters, the AMY contributes to a threat evaluation of social stimuli, and the occipital cortex function likely supports visual simulation or imagining scenes (Mar, 2011; Figure 11.7).

The Medial Prefrontal Cortex
As discussed earlier, mentalizing is correlated with specific regions of the prefrontal cortex (PFC), specifically the mPFC. As a reminder, the PFC is the most forward part of the frontal lobe, located in front of the motor and premotor areas. Responsible for assessing future events, it also distinguishes between mental and physical states. The mPFC plays a central role in the mentalizing neural network (Frith & Frith, 2003; Mar, 2011; Spreng et al., 2009). One of seven discrete brain regions in the PFC, it is responsible for monitoring self and emotional states (Saxe, 2006). The suggestion is that the most ventral mPFC region is concerned with monitoring emotions of the self and of others, and that its dorsal region is concerned with monitoring actions of the self and of others (Amodio & Frith, 2006). More specifically, the frontal area of the mPFC (anterior rostral) is activated as we consider what people similar to us are doing or intending to communicate (Frith & Frith, 2006). Neuroimaging studies have further implicated a designated back (caudal)

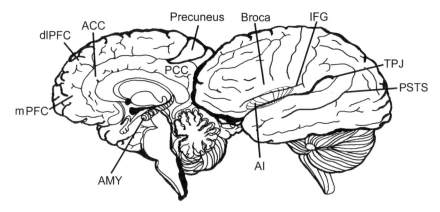

Figure 11.7 *Midline and Surface Brain Regions and Structures.* Midline fronto-parietal brain regions that are involved in mentalizing include the medial prefrontal cortex (mPFC), the posterior cingulate cortex (PCC), and the precuneus. Surface areas include the posterior superior temporal sulcus (PSTS), which is activated by perceived or anticipated biological motion, the observation of faces, and the interpretation of goals; the temporoparietal junction (TPJ), which is involved in thinking about mental states; and the left inferior frontal gyrus (IFG). Also shown are the amygdala, anterior cingulate cortex (ACC), Broca's area, and the anterior insula (AI), which are involved in social cognition (Blakemore, 2008; Modinos, Ormel, & Aleman, 2009).

area in the mPFC as involved in paying attention toward external perceptual stimuli, suggesting a functional organization within the mPFC that corresponds to reactions to both internal and external generated information (Gilbert et al., 2007). Thus, as group members make art, the mPFC function most likely promotes monitoring: How am I feeling, and how are others feelings? Is there a problem I'm sensing or becoming aware of? What are others doing in relationship to me? And what sense do I make of the colors, textures, and forms?

The Posterior Superior Temporal Sulcus and Temporoparietal Junction
The PSTS and TPJ are involved in cooperative efforts between people who are not genetically associated (Suzuki, Niki, Fujisaki, & Akiyama, 2011). The TPJ is also involved in reasoning about mental states. It is an area where the temporal and parietal lobes meet and is considered critical for distinguishing between self and others (Saxe & Kanwisher, 2003). Located about halfway between two visual information-processing streams, the TPJ interfaces the *how* and *where* visual processing streams with the *what* visual processing stream (Frith, 2001). The *how* and *where* streams process visual spatial inputs and guide action. The *what* stream processes object recognition and texture. Integrated *how, where,* and *what* information assists in the recognition of individuals or objects and their actions and intentions. From the TPJ, pro-

cessing is forwarded to the corresponding *how, where,* and *what* PFC brain regions that orchestrate attention, concentration, and planning. Also involved in the perception of movements, the PSTS/TPJ junction is likely to be critically involved in art therapy practices (for a review of its role as well as a review of the visual streams, see Hass-Cohen & Loya, 2008).

Anterior Temporal Lobe
The anterior tip of the temporal lobe is implicated in both story- and non-story-based theory of mind studies (Mar, 2011). This bilateral area, which includes the temporal pole, is involved in the processing of emotions, music, facial expressions, and insight. Moreover, the left tip of the temporal lobe helps in processing language.

Posterior Cingulate Cortex and Precuneus
Located in the posterior of the cingulate cortex is the PCC. Just above it, between the two hemispheres in an area of the parietal lobe, lies the precuneus. The PCC and the precuneus have been identified as a hub of human awareness. A central node in the default mode, the PCC is involved in the capacity to understand what other people believe. Furthermore, the precuneus is implicated in self-referential processing, imagery, and memory:

> *The precuneus belongs to a medial prefrontal-mid-parietal neural network supporting the mental representation of the self. Some of the visuo-spatial imagery studies suggest involvement in internally guided attention and manipulation of mental images, whilst those directed at mental imagery more directly draw upon internal self-representation, which is also implicated in most episodic memory retrieval and first-person perspective taking tasks. All of this seems compatible with a hypothesis that the precuneus plays a central role in the modulation of conscious processes. (Cavanna & Trimble, 2006, p. 579)*

Left IFG-Broca's Area
As described in Chapter 4, Broca's area is the language production center of the brain. While this area is involved in mentalizing activities that involve storytelling and processing, it is unclear whether it has a more general mentalizing role (Mar, 2011). In Chapter 13, we discuss that this region has also been associated with the function of empathic mirror neuron responses.

While mentalizing is informed by previous knowledge (Frith, 2001; Frith & Frith, 2003), executive function requires higher-level cognitive functions such as attention, concentration, and the ability to multitask. An important question is whether task-oriented activity, mediated by prefrontal areas (primarily the dorsal areas), can coexist with mentalizing and reflective-default states mediated by core neural structures. However, given the participation of the AMY fear center as well as the visual center, it is evident that task-oriented prefrontal activation is likely mediated by explicit or implicit knowledge of security and safety embedded in imagery.

Emerging research points to this integrative interface. In one study, the DMN was associated with activity related to solving a set of problems in the future: "This goal-directed task involves introspective, self-referential processing, and also requires formulating a plan to solve the problem, integrating and sustaining relevant information, and maintaining an abstract sequence of steps leading to the problem's solution" (Gerlach, Spreng, Gilmore, & Schacter, 2011, p. 1821). The default system and executive brain areas, including the DLPFC, were found to be activated in this study. They also suggested involvement of the PCC areas above the hippocampus. According to Spreng and colleagues (2009), these same areas are involved in imagining familiar spatial situations, perhaps such as those depicted by our neighborhood scenario. The art experientials described may also recruit and integrate functioning of many more brain and bodily regions. These findings are promising as they support the benefits of group or dyadic therapy. Although it may not be necessary to understand all the neuroimaging details at this time, this information holds exciting clinical implications as it provides "a cognitive neuroscience account of how mental simulation contributes to solving future problems" (Gerlach et al., 2011, p. 1823).

Mentalizing, Executive, and Higher-Order Cognitive Function Networks

The mPFC, implicated in mentalizing and self-functions, interacts with seven other areas in the PFC that are recruited for multitasking, executive function, and directing attention (Goldberg, 2009). Typically considered to be the executive center of the brain, the PFC orchestrates thoughts and actions to achieve goals. These executive functions allow for the differentiation between conflicting thoughts and the assessment of future consequences. Also supported by PFC function is the ability to work toward defined goals, as well as outcome prediction and evaluation. Executive functioning also relates to the determination of good or bad, better or best, and same or different. It allows us to manage expectations based on actions and gives us the ability to suppress urges that, if unsuppressed, could lead to socially unacceptable or personally adverse outcomes. We contend that the brain capacity required for complex, social art making contributes to interactive mentalizing, to social cognition, and to enhancing executive function and a sense of control.

Mentalizing and higher cognitive functions start developing as early as three months of age (Frith & Frith, 2003) and continue to evolve during adolescence and young adulthood (Blakemore & Choudhury, 2006). Tremendous growth in limbic gray matter takes place during the first few years of life (Elliot, 1999). By the third year, synaptic density in the PFC likely reaches its peak, at up to 200 percent of its adult level, as this region continues to create and strengthen networks with other areas (Bunge & Zelado, 2006). While the ability to mentalize begins in infancy, it evolves to be reliably testable closer to the age of four (Baron-Cohen, Leslie, & Frith, 1985).

As myelin rapidly covers limbic area neurons, the PFC develops more slowly and reorganizes during teenage years and into young adulthood. Interestingly, some of the synaptic density, reflected in gray-matter volume in MRI scans, decreases over time. This synaptic reorganization in the PFC might underlie the functional changes that are seen in the social brain during adolescence.

During this period, difficulties managing emotions, social exchanges, and interactive mentalization arise. Overall, PFC activity is dependent on extremely high input from the other cortical and limbic regions in the lower brain. This is one way in which it integrates affective and cognitive information. However, too much information from the lower regions can overwhelm frontal lobe activity, while too little information will not yield any frontal lobe activity. The early adolescent brain can be overwhelmed with emotional impulses from the limbic area and will most likely lack the full capacity to inhibit such impulses until the PFC develops further in adolescence and young adulthood (Yaxley et al., 2011). Other observed changes in the social brain may further explain the erratic behavior of adolescents (Siegel, 2013). For example, research suggests that PFC activity associated with social tasks, such as processing faces, increases from childhood to adolescence, yet, surprisingly, it decreases from adolescence to young adulthood (Cohen Kadosh, Johnson, Cohen Kadosh, & Blakemore, 2013). Consistent with this finding, activity in the MPFC during mentalizing tasks decreases between adolescence and adulthood (Blakemore et al., 2007).

As previously mentioned, one way to examine PFC function is through its connection with subcortical limbic structures. Another option entails dividing it by top/side and bottom functions. This suggests the division of labor that occurs between the dorsal and the ventral/lateral areas of the PFC, and further clarifies understanding of the PFC's cognitive and emotional integrative purposes (Longe, Senior, & Rippon, 2009).

Several main discrete brain regions influence PFC top/side and bottom function. One of these areas, the anterior cingulate cortex (ACC), borders the PFC, while the remaining are within the PFC. They include the dorsolateral prefrontal cortex (dlPFC), the lateral prefrontal cortex (lPFC), the ventrolateral prefrontal cortex (vlPFC), the orbitofrontal cortex (OFC), the mPFC, and the ventromedial prefrontal cortex (vmPFC; Figure 11.8).

PREFRONTAL CORTEX- PFC

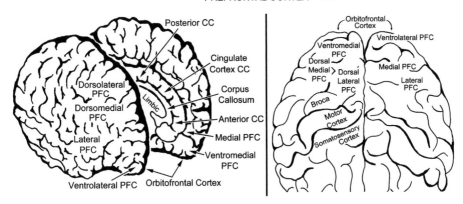

Figure 11.8 *The Prefrontal Regions.* The dorsolateral PFC, the lateral PFC, the ventrolateral PFC, the OFC, the medial and ventromedial PFC. Also shown are the cingulate and anterior cingulate cortex. The image on the right provides a bird's-eye view of the PFC areas and includes Broca's area and the motor and somatosensory cortices or strips. Please note that besides Broca's area, the PFC regions and strips are found in both hemispheres. For clarity, they are shown only on one hemisphere or the other.

It is proposed that the integrated function of the lPFC and the vmPFC significantly contribute to the PFC's cognitive and emotional integrative function (O'Reilly, 2010). The suggestion is that cognitive function is associated with dorsal or higher areas, which are concerned with how to organize, plan, and implement. Conversely, content-based information and emotional processing, such as empathy, is associated with ventral areas that pay attention to the qualities of information (Saxe, 2006). Accordingly, the association between the lPFC and the vmPFC provides ATR-N insights into an integrative task: How do I want to plan for and make my art, and what do I want it to express? The top-bottom division also highlights the role of visual information processing in cognitive function and contribution to mentalizing. The what-temporal and how-parietal visual processing streams extend from the occipital lobe and terminate in the vlPFC. The vlPFC sorts out specific information qualities, while the dorsal areas process complex rules as they relay the relationships between information sources and stimuli (O'Reilly, 2010).

The Dorsolateral Prefrontal Cortex
In charge of cognitive organization and affect regulation, the dlPFC is the uppermost cortical region. Developmentally, it is the last area in the cerebrum to be myelinated, usually between late adolescence and early adulthood (Blakemore & Choudhury, 2006). The dlPFC is especially crucial for judgment, decision making, and anticipation of consequences. In addition, it is key in planning, rational problem solving, and working memory. The dlPFC is central to the integration of complex mental activity, and particularly to

working memory, as well as the regulation of intellectual function and action. As described earlier, it is likely that the later myelination of this area may account for the unpredictable tempers of adolescents (Giedd et al., 1999). Damage to the dlPFC results in widespread emotional and social judgment problems, due to impairments in the ability to plan ahead, resulting in deficits across executive memory, abstract thinking, and intentionality (Bell, 2001). It is likely that dlPFC functioning significantly contributes to conscious awareness, which is created by meaningfully linking internal imagery to external sensory or visual stimuli and with affective material. These connections facilitate the ability to integrate emotions, engage in meaningful relationships, change one's behavior, engage in future planning, and consider one's own or others' emotions (Wood & Grafman, 2003). It is critical for encoding action sequence tasks, internal goal coordinating, and abstract sequential movement maintenance (Badre & D'Esposito, 2009; Badre, Hoffman, Cooney, & D'Esposito, 2009). Therefore, the dlPFC likely is engaged during ATR-N problem-solving simulations, such as planning for art making. Most importantly, the dlPFC looks for options and possibilities and acts as an analytical hub, connecting with other cortical and subcortical areas (Zelazo & Muller, 2002). As hypothesized in ATR-N, explicit planning, organization, and art making, involving higher executive functions, most likely assist in integrating emotional, social, and higher functions.

The Lateral and Ventrolateral PFC
Located below the dlPFC, both the lPFC and vlPFC play a central role in paying attention to selected goals and unexpected events. As stated earlier, the main differences in function between the dlPFC and the vlPFC are similar to the differences between the *what* and *how* visual streams (O'Reilly, 2010). In a nutshell, this distinguishes between attention to the content of the stimuli (*what*) and the attention to the relationships between stimuli (*how*). From an ATR-N perspective, this is a question such as, "How does what I planned to do fit in with the message that is coming across from what I did in my art? Are there any unexpected results, and should I adjust for them?"

Most unexpected events and information are processed ventrally, whereas selected and thus expected goals are processed dorsally. The integration of this information most likely occurs in the lPFC. Thus, coherent behaviors and awareness emerge when attention to unplanned occurrences and planned events comes together (Asplund, Todd, Snyder, & Marois, 2010). In this regard, the lPFC is involved in mentalizing (Spreng et al., 2009).

The Orbitofrontal Cortex
The OFC is positioned just behind the eyes and is also extensively connected to subcortical areas and other prefrontal regions (Cavada, Company, Tejedor,

Cruz-Rizzolo, & Reinoso-Suarez, 2000). The OFC is the primary inhibitor of the amygdala and is directly related to emotional regulation and organization. The OFC helps establish intuitive judgments and rewards, and aids in decision making.

Emotional regulation, as well as empathic and collaborative engagement, make up some of the OFC's functions. Both functions are influenced by relational-social experiences and early childhood history of emotionally meaningful interpersonal attachment (Siegel, 1999). Regulation of emotional arousal abilities is formed by the coherence and consistency of a caregiver's attunement. OFC integrative functions include the ability to infer from significant others' interpersonal social behavior, to deduce from reward and punishment experiences, and to interpret complex emotions (Grafman & Litvan, 1999). The OFC is also responsible for the retrieval of autonoetic representations—an autobiographical consciousness that provides a sense of self in the past, present, and future, as well as an ability to mediate perceptions of others.

Accordingly, the following ATR-N questions can sharpen self-awareness: "What art-based choices have inspired me in the past and why? How does this art strike me or move me now? How does the activity speak to my personal history, and where I am going in the future?" Mental representations are part of autobiographical memory, providing a sense of self in the past, present, and future (Frey & Petrides, 2002). Research suggests that dysregulated OFC decision making, emotion regulation, and reward expectation is implicated in attention-deficit/hyperactivity disorder, substance dependence (Brown, Robertson, & Fibiger, 1992), obsessive-compulsive disorder, and some dementias, including the later stages of Alzheimer's disease.

The Ventromedial Prefrontal Cortex

Located in the lower (ventral) central (medial) region of the PFC, the vmPFC is more associated with pure emotional regulation than with social regulation (Decety & Michalska, 2010). Involved in the reactivation of past emotional associations and events, the vmPFC's functions are likely linked to the neural circuitry associated with PTSD (Koenigs et al., 2008). The vmPFC is also likely to play a central role in moderating associations between mental objects and visceral, bodily feedback: "Which emotions do the art images bring up in my body? And how can I manage that?"

The Anterior Cingulate Cortex

The ACC is an area of cingulate cortex that is found in front of, above, and behind the corpus callosum (Bechara, Tranel, & Damasio, 2000). It connects to the brain stem and spinal cord, which control basic gut reactions and movements. This contributes to the speed of nervous system connectivity and can explain adolescent impulsive emotional reactivity, as well as the importance of social evaluation during adolescence (Crone, 2009). The ACC is the front part of the CC and borders the PFC, the motor system, and the parietal cortex. Assisting in processing top-down and bottom-up stimuli, it also delegates control to other areas in the brain. In addition, the ACC activates in response to psychosocial conflicts via involvement in emotional regulation and impulse control (Sohn, Albert, Jung, Carter, & Anderson, 2007). Furthermore, the ACC contributes to rational cognitive functions, such as reward anticipation, decision-making, empathy, and emotion (Decety & Jackson, 2004). Playing a role in the registering of both emotional and physical pain (Hass-Cohen & Clyde Findlay, 2009), it is related to assessing the salience of emotion, error, and conflict detection processes, as well as intrapersonal conscious awareness (Lane et al., 1998). The ACC assists in focusing on and filtering internal thoughts, thereby producing an ease of processing and sense of "going with the flow," a state that is often reported by artists and writers when they feel that they are, so to speak, in a coherent state.

Integration!

Art therapy tasks provide the opportunity to concretely represent inner mental landscapes and to act upon such representations with imagery and words. Such skills can promote a receptive mental state and integration in the PFC favoring flexible, adaptive, coherent, energized, and stable states of mind (Siegel, 2006). According to Siegel (2006), these states comprise the goals of interpersonal neurobiology. Such skills also give us the ability to identify and capitalize on the emotions we experience, rather than be overwhelmed by them (Siegel, 2007). Such focused attention integrates the brain, bringing clarity to the understanding of our inner lives and enhancing our relationships with others.

CREATE PRINCIPLES AND CLINICAL APPLICATIONS

This chapter focuses on mentalizing, reflecting, and creating. As described in the introduction, mentalizing describes our imaginative and cognitive ability to recognize our own and others' mental states. It speaks to our understanding of clients' intentions in terms of their needs, desires, feelings, beliefs, goals, and reasons. The primary focus of the art therapy activities in this chapter is the CREATE principle of Transformative Integrating.

We contend that group art therapy and the execution of complex and self-referential art tasks provide the opportunity to integrate inactive default and active mentalizing. This claim is based on the relational neurobiology that we have reviewed, that of a shared executive, mentalizing, and default neural network. This mentalizing network is responsible for executive functions, higher-order thinking, and associated limbic and cortical integration. It supports our claims that art making provides clients, therapists, and artists with the opportunity for integrative function.

The evolution of this chapter's directives offers a meeting place for the therapeutic knowing of minds on emotional, cognitive, interpersonal dyadic, and social levels. Therapeutically supported art experientials such as making and inhabiting a three-dimensional home, and then bringing these paper homes into a community evoke integrative executive and revisiting of mentalizing functions. As group members create and share art, they assign mental states, beliefs, intents, and desires to themselves and to others. Skills in perspective taking are necessary for sensitive understanding of socially constructed exchanges such as narratives of "He made and said," "She made and said," or "They made and said." As exemplified by our participants' reflections, clients will continually self-evaluate while taking into consideration the others who observe their behaviors. The experientals and discussions request an elaboration on actual experience and reflection on a reconstructed past, as they narrate their creative process as related to themselves and others. Through the cumulative effect of the guided directives, there is a possibility for individuals to gain executive planning experiences, self-awareness, and self-regulation. This ability to mentalize continues to evolve over the person's life and plays a critical role in self-growth, self-confidence, and social exchanges. This chapter also focuses on higher cognitive processes that engage the PFC circuitry. This emphasis aligns closely with the fact that many therapies consider cognition work as key to change. Art therapy elicits and integrates cognitive processes, which are needed in order for clients to engage in quick mark-making, complex manipulation of materials, choosing titles, and verbal processing of artwork. Overall, the ATR-N tasks ask clients to assign meta-cognitions to executive art making rules and to the content of the art making.

With regard to Transformative Integrating, we hypothesize that various experiences of neurological integration are facilitated through the ATR-N directives. Soliciting theory-of-mind representations associated with mental states of self and others stimulates the right hemisphere in analogic, holistic forms of thinking. On the other hand, interpreting and explaining situations requires left-hemisphere analytic processing. For example, the construction of homes requires the activation of right-hemisphere visuospatial perception and nonverbal imagery along with left-hemisphere linear processing of verbal and written reflections. This supports the conscious attention necessary for the development of socially constructed narratives. Written reflections and narrations of the art concretize integrative functions of self and social mentalizing processes. They are an integrated personal record of events, facts, thoughts, and understandings and each individual can integrate and come to his or her own conclusion. Intrinsic midline brain pathways give rise to further self-refection. When bringing the paper houses into the community, these integrative processes reoccur with a cognitive focus on social activities. Central to this unifying process is vertical brain integration, which is promoted by coping with the arousal of self-exposure to others and negotiating space with others. This contributes to an integration of limbic emotions with cortical higher-order directing and thinking. Another key function involves the embracing of subcortical emotional arousal, which is stimulated by accessing autobiographical attachment memories. This takes place while simultaneously employing higher cortical faculties to conceptualize, plan, and execute complex tasks. Furthermore, cognitive processes and coping are supported via activation of the cerebellum, sparked by moving the paper home around and shifting the sculptures, and oneself, from one's table to the communal interpersonal space. Driving these integrative processes is a coherent, integrated personal narrative, which is supported by creatively sorting, ordering, and reflecting upon how one is perceived by others.

Creative Embodiment occurs as group members make a three-dimensional object from two-dimensional paper (the paper home), move their sculptures, cut, glue, and explore interior and exterior surfaces. In so doing, they actively symbolize what they want to reveal to others. In contrast to creating smaller two-dimensional art, this task's size and content exposes participants to others' artwork and mentalizing processes. Moving the paper homes into a shared community activates mentalizing, requiring conscious perception and interpretation of other people's needs, goals, and purposes. This is a social and creative embodiment.

Relational Resonating is expressed through the paper home-making process, creating a home from two-dimensional paper and moving it into the community, which moves participants into a reflection and active engagement with the mental state of the self and others. Paying attention to oneself and one's thoughts while building a paper house and then placing it in a community stimulates attachment behaviors, as group members contemplate the mental models of others. Building the art structures and then inhabiting them with content that is informed by attachment histories creates an accepting climate. Accordingly, the group setting expands opportunities for prosocial interactive mentalizing as group members make room for everyone's home in the community.

The principle of Expressive Communicating involves emoting. Emoting processes enrich mentalizing and meaning making by: (1) using color, texture, and symbols; (2) providing emotionally arousing family-related art directives, such as "Make your home"; and (3) inviting arousal from interacting with others in the community of homes.

Sequencing the art directives in such a way as to support a crescendo and fluctuation of feelings supports Adaptive Responding. Related to attachment security, stress also compromises mentalizing ability triggering procedural memory and automatic behaviors. Hence the opportunity to adapt to the potential stress of the creation and sharing of one's paper home, within a safe group setting, and promote continued reflection, supports adaptive responding.

Beginning with the initial executive task of creating a three-dimensional home, and then negotiating where the home will be placed in the community, requires adaptation and mentalizing. Following this directive calls for coping with potential negative stressors associated with moving from individual client to group interpersonal work. The relocation of the homes, for symbolic or technical reasons, can also stimulate stress responses. Interacting with others, group members are required to understand and be aware of their own mental state as well as that of those around them. For some, positive coping adaptive responses are supported by the invitation to contribute an existing three-dimensional home to the community. Others may experience conflicted feelings, such as feeling unprepared for such a move. Both reactions provide the opportunity to share, enhance, or mend the perceived experience, inspiring self-control, social mentalizing, and acceptance. Accordingly, group members can learn to shift in their relationship to stressors when the self and other mental states are taken into consideration and tolerated. In turning outward for resolution, control, and relief, transformation happens, which both supports and depends upon mentalizing.

The cumulative integrative processes contribute to Empathizing and Compassion. Exploring the experientials from this principle's lens exemplifies support for the self and other. The communication and acceptance of self-other emotions can open doors to seeing others and increase the capacity for mentalizing. Softening reactions toward others decreases defensive positions and assists in shifting to reflective, default creative states. The directives encourage the development of resonant empathy as clients can shift attention to others, perhaps cultivating a desire to relieve the suffering of others. As an example, the placing of homes in a community manifests compassion and intensifies self-awareness, as thoughts and feelings are shifted against a collective backdrop. With a simultaneous inner and outward focus, empathic association balances the self-other dialectic transformation.

CHAPTER 12

Transformative Integrating: Mindful Awareness

Next, we went through the magazines that we'd brought with us . . .
ripping out the pages that we wanted to keep, and those not to keep,
placing the pages into different piles. I found this exercise to be cathar-
tic. It was fascinating how I got a rhythm to what I was doing, and
started to use both hands towards the end. The synchronicity of my
mind and body seemed to develop strongly over a period of just a few
minutes, and I felt as though I'd temporarily integrated my mind and
body. I loved the sound of the ripping and had the feeling that I was
really, physically doing something. Kara Wahlin

THIS CHAPTER INTRODUCES THE THERAPEUTIC philoso-
phy of mindful awareness and the acceptance of moment-to-moment
living, as well as some formal and informal mindfulness practices. Mindfulness practices promote intentional awareness of present experiences, as well
as an intentional departure from negative thinking, critical judgment, and
desire for change (Germer, Siegel, & Fulton, 2005). A tranquil and compassionate attention to one's bodily functions, sensations, feelings, objects, and
insights of consciousness, thoughts, and perceptions are practiced (Wynne,
2007). Based in the ATR-N approach, compassionate practices support
functional integration of emotions, cognitions, and thoughts with sensory
perception (Hass-Cohen, 2007). Thus this chapter contributes to the CRE-
ATE principles of Transformative Integrating and Empathizing and Compassion.

According to Buddhist teachings, mindfulness leads to liberating psychological discernment (Kang & Whittingham, 2010). Thus, both formal and
informal mindfulness practices support such attention and are available for
therapists' use and clients' benefits. Specifically there is strong support for
mindfulness based stress reduction (MBSR), which improves mental health
and for mindfulness based cognitive therapy, which prevents depressive

relapse (Baer, 2006; Fjorback, Arendt, Ornbol, Fink, & Walach, 2011). Pioneered by MBSR (Kabat-Zinn, 2005), additional models have evolved in order to address specific problems. Mindfulness based models have been found to be beneficial to those suffering from pain, anxiety, depression, substance abuse, smoking cessation, and eating disorders (Brewer, Mallik, et al., 2011; Hofmann, Sawyer, Witt, & Oh, 2010; Williams, Teasdale, Segal, & Soulsby, 2000). Neurobiology studies have helped explain the benefits of mindfulness (Lazar et al., 2005), suggesting that mindfulness meditation primarily activates the prefrontal cortices and the insula, thus stimulating an integration of mind-body function. It is also established that meditation affects brain plasticity (Hölzel et al., 2010, 2011). More specifically, meditation may deactivate the posterior cingulate cortex, which has been implicated in anxiety, addiction, and other psychiatric disorders. Therefore, it is most probable that mindfulness may help change neural activation patterns of these disorders (Brewer et al., 2011; Hofmann, Sawyer, Witt, & Oh, 2010).

There are four Buddhist foundations for insight meditation practices: mindfulness of the body, of feelings and sensations, of the mind and consciousness, and of mental experiences (Silananda, 2002). The first practice, mindfulness of body and breath, is directly experienced through meditation practices. This here-and-now practice works well with the present experience of art making. Art therapists may choose to incorporate both informal and formal mindfulness practices in session and advocate for their use outside of the therapy room. Informal practices include pausing in session and breathing, mindfully walking with clients, cultivating focused attention on art making, and helping clients develop their own everyday mindful awareness outside of session.

Art directives can also be bookended by traditional mindful practice, such as a breath awareness exercise, a walking meditation, or a body scan. Art therapy directives can be built in accordance with the four foundations of mindfulness. The second foundation of mindfulness, feelings and sensations, is usually cultivated by developing awareness of pleasant, neutral, or unpleasant feelings and recognizing how feelings are experienced in the body. For the untrained mind, feelings and sensations are usually linked to wanting more or less of something. These mind states are associated with stress and suffering. How we experience our senses and interpret our perceptions influences our well-being. The third foundation of mindfulness arises from the awareness of the body and develops further insight into mind states. Often, confused, distracted, or scattered mind states are encountered, which can be soothed by the art making. Finally, the last foundation, which involves the contemplation of mind objects, can be roughly translated as the contemplation of the obstacles and pathways to a contingent and clear self. From a Buddhist perspective, these are usually desires that result in clinging to fixed ideas or avoidance.

Buddhism, from which mindfulness-based psychotherapy approaches derive, offers several meditative and daily life practices to work with these mind states (Moffitt, 2012). From meditation, which is an essential way to train the mind, joy, equanimity, and concentration arise. Efforts and intentions are also made to follow what is called the eightfold path: right view, intention, speech, action, livelihood, effort, mindfulness, and concentration. Loving-kindness meditation and self-compassion practices provide another gateway to, in essence, become a better and happier, more fulfilled person (Germer, 2009). In loving-kindness meditation, individuals are called upon to experience the support of someone who has cared deeply for them and also to experience deep caring for those they love and care for, as well as for humankind. Accordingly, four Buddhist tenets called the immeasurables—loving-kindness, compassion, joy, and equanimity or balance—are therapeutic goals. These inform not only the therapeutic relationship but also how we regard the client's psychotherapy progress and mental health. Within ourselves and for each client, we uphold respect and create space for their truth, what Buddhist psychology conceptualizes as sanity (Bradford, 2012). From a Westernized perspective, loving-kindness meditation can be conceptualized as training for the development of secure attachment. For example, participants who were asked to practice and recall comforting attachment words demonstrated more accepting attitudes and altruistic behaviors toward others (Mikulincer, Shaver, Gillath, & Nitzberg, 2005). These supportive interpersonal behaviors are associated with earned attachment security (Thompson et al., 2000).

Practicing mindfulness offers an art therapist the theoretical framework and the skills needed to develop an attuned relational presence. The client-therapist relationship, the key determinant of positive therapeutic outcomes, is rooted in the therapist's attuned self-presence as well as presence to the client (Norcross, Beutler, & Levant, 2005; Siegel, 2010). Such skills increase psychological flexibility, adaptability, empathy, and a sense of well-being that is vital for successful relational therapy (Siegel, 2010). Via a creative space informed by mindfulness, our intention is for participants to access a sense of well-being with a continued cultivation of their own therapist selfhood.

Both art making and mindfulness practices are about doing and practicing. A distinction can be drawn between two styles of meditation practices: Vipassana, which is known as insight meditation, and Samatha, or concentration meditation (Germer et al., 2005). For concentration meditation, any object, whether internal or external, may be the focus of concentration. Practical actions involve meditating on a word, one's breath, sounds, or sights to help direct attention. Conversely, insight meditation involves a focus on bodily awareness, intended to promote clarity about the function of the mind. ATR-N mindfulness directives can be aligned with either style. In this chapter, four experiential art therapy directives cultivate mindfulness: the collage collection, media exploration, a body silhouette, and the creation of a mandala. For example, a mandala experience is typically more aligned with concentration meditation whereas art therapy meaning-making approaches are more aligned with using the senses to aid awareness.

Regular formal mindfulness requires a daily commitment to sitting, lying, or walking meditation, which takes place outside of the therapy room. Empirically proven, we highly recommend formal practices as adjunctive therapies to art therapy. However, for these models to be advantageous, producing long-lasting change, a consistent and committed practice is strongly suggested (Lazar et al., 2005). Informal mindfulness practices, such as those described by the Zen Buddhist Thich Nhat Hanh (1976), include breath awareness and mindful eating or performing everyday tasks. The invitation is to cultivate mindfulness by integrating alertness with acceptance, gentleness, and kindness into daily life. Moreover, these practices are accessible at all skill levels. Informal practices can be used as an extension of formal practices, or they can complement therapeutic endeavors.

MINDFULNESS AND PSYCHOTHERAPY

Contemplative practices of examining the mind, of being fully awake, and of conscious moment-to-moment living have been a staple of religious and cultural teachings for thousands of years (Hanh, 1976; Kabat-Zinn, 2005; Siegel, 2007). Buddhist psychology offers practical means to know, influence, and free the mind (Germer et al., 2005). It describes the psychological process of being mindful as systematically and intentionally paying attention to current experience in an open and discerning way via specific practices, such as meditation. This approach recognizes human suffering as a source of pain, yet also identifies that the desire for things to be different is the ultimate cause of conflict. Accordingly, change is seen as inevitable and necessary, whereas people's attachment to impermanent outcomes results in suffering. Generally, problems lie in our relationship to an experience rather than in the experience itself. The key idea, therefore, is that suffering can be mediated by changing our attitudes toward unpleasant experiences. Also, pain can be mitigated by cultivating compassion, kindness, and joy (Hanh, 2012).

Westernized approaches such as MBSR (Kabat-Zinn, 2005) provide an active learning process that uses mindfulness meditation techniques influenced by Buddhism. MBSR meditation includes a wide range of meditation foci: bodies, thoughts, and the nature of our minds (Erricker, 2011). It is a structured, time-limited group approach that provides specific training in formal mindfulness meditative techniques. MBSR consists of eight weekly group meetings lasting two and a half hours each, with a full day of practice during the sixth week of the course. Change is supported by a regular meditation practice and the incorporation of mindful awareness into everyday life (Kabat-Zinn, 2005). Interestingly, MBSR was originally intended for patients suffering from chronic pain disorders (Baer, 2003; Carmody, Baer, Lykins, & Olendzki, 2009; Hofmann et al., 2010; Kabat-Zinn, 2005; Praissman, 2008) but has since been expanded to a variety of problems. Via meditation at home and in-group exercises, participants employ mindfulness and acceptance as a means to self-regulate, as well as increase psychological flexibility and reduce stress and increase well being (Carmody et al., 2009).

Fostering awareness, compassion, and acceptance is also a core value of a third wave of such behavioral therapies. Dialectical behavioral therapy (DBT; Linehan, 1993a), acceptance and commitment therapy (ACT; Hayes et al., 2012), MBCT (Segal et al., 2002), and mindfulness-based relapse prevention (Bowen et al., 2014) employ various formal and informal mindfulness practices (Baer, 2003). Mindfulness-based relapse prevention has shown positive effects of mindfulness and meditation for substance use and relapse.

DBT focuses on fostering affect regulation and distress tolerance for clients pulled between extremes of thoughts and emotions. This theory conceives of emotional conflict as the primary source of psychopathology and, therefore, that emotions are at the core of therapy. Furthermore, DBT involves simultaneously balancing change and acceptance to counter the vicious, emotionally rooted cycles of avoidance or escape strategies. As such, individual psychotherapy includes skills training in mindful awareness, distress tolerance, emotional regulation, strategic behavior, and meaning making. DBT pinpoints a distinction between content skills and process skills. Content skills orient to a consideration of what is happening in order to observe, describe, and fully participate in present experience. In contrast, process skills concentrate on the cultivation of a nonjudgmental stance, focusing on one thing at a time and in the moment (Linehan, 1993b). In other words, process skills provide a mechanism that directs us on how to attend to what is being experienced.

ACT is based on behavioral therapy and conceptualizes clinical problems as a result of emotional avoidance and cognitive entanglement (Hayes et al., 2006). These mental patterns result in psychological rigidity that can cause failure to take the necessary behavioral steps in accordance with one's essential values. Therefore, the goal of ACT is to increase psychological flexibility through acceptance techniques, behavioral commitment, and conduct strategies. Acceptance of unwanted personal experiences is supported by various cognitive techniques. They include diffusing the stranglehold of thoughts, engaging fully with the present moment, and witnessing oneself day to day. In addition, the suggestion is to commit to a more valued life, promoted by clarifying values and setting goals. ACT does not typically include any meditation practices.

Psychologists Segal, Williams and Teasdale (2002) developed MBCT to decrease the remission rate of major depression disorders. Its primary goal is to help depressed clients refrain from ruminating and from other habit-driven patterns of thinking, feeling, and behaving that sustain depression (Carmody et al., 2009; Foley et al., 2010; Hofmann et al., 2010). Formal mindfulness strategies target the negative cognitive triad regarding the self, the world, and the future (Beck, Rush, Shaw, & Emery, 1979). In addition, MBCT offers a mini meditation tool to use when one's mood starts to spiral, known as the three-minute breathing space. This exercise anchors awareness of one's thoughts, feelings, and bodily sensations to the present moment in the breath, and emphasizes the power of such immediate tools. Research suggests that this approach may also be beneficial for individuals suffering from current depression (Kenny & Williams, 2007), chronic depression (Barnhofer et al., 2009), and residual depression (Kingston, Dooley, Bates, Lawlor, & Malone, 2007). Finally, mindfulness training for Attention Deficit Hyperactivity Disorder (ADHD) for teens and adults with ADHD has also emerged as a promising treatment approach over the last decade (Zylowska et al., 2008). Based on MBSR and MBCT, this program also includes education on ADHD throughout.

ART THERAPY MINDFULNESS PRACTICES

Art therapist Caroline Peterson developed a mindfulness-based art therapy approach (MBAT). Her randomized controlled clinical trial yielded promising initial data regarding its ability to reduce distress symptoms and improve quality of life in women with cancer (Monti et al., 2006). One aim of the approach is to promote bilateral brain integration; right-hemisphere stimulation is promoted through sensory art experientials while the left hemisphere is activated during verbal group discussion. In this way, balancing verbal and nonverbal processes supports neural integration and stress reduction.

The MBAT eight-week course closely models the MBSR course. It also includes a protocol of mindfulness-based art tasks used to understand the physiology of stress and expand receptive attention. Moreover, it explores the impact of the disease and the experiences of physical and emotional pain, considering self-care, and representing the self and the disease.

Specific art materials, which match fine art media with textured professional art paper, are used. The art making accompanies each of the MBSR course topics over eight weeks. The sequence begins and concludes with a request to draw a complete picture of oneself. During the intervening weeks, after a mindful exploration of art materials, participants engage various directives related to their bodies and illness. They make pre- and post-images of the mind-body relationship before and after engaging in mindful activities. These activities include yoga, meditation. Peterson's participants also make art about specific topics: pain, body image, stress, and kindness. The last week is an open studio experience, which allows for an exploration of clay.

Art therapists may reap the benefits of mindfulness self-practice and reduce their stress and increase clinical attunement. Thus, mindful awareness practices may protect against the burnout of clinical work, serving as a way to manage stress. It is necessary that the art therapist also engages with meditation practice and possesses the education or training to provide it to others.

EXPERIENTIAL PRACTICES AND DIRECTIVES

We introduce mindfulness-based art experiences by beginning each experiential with an informal or formal mindfulness practice. In this manner, our group members can experience the different practices for themselves and identify those with which they feel most comfortable, or those that they wish to learn more about. Before starting the first art activity, the mindful collage collection, we guide everyone through a brief mindfulness breath awareness exercise informed by MBSR practices (Kabat-Zinn, 2005). Likewise, before the media awareness task, we practice a formal walking meditation, and before the body silhouette drawing or painting we practice a formal body scan. For the last experiential, a concentration meditation precedes a mandala drawing. Each of the experientials targets specific mindfulness constructs: the collage collection brings attention to the phenomenon of impermanence, and the media awareness tasks focuses alertness on the present moment. Additionally, the body scan helps access relaxation, and the mandala making favors concentration. Such art experientials promote acceptance, regulation, insight, awareness, and integration.

Experience I: Mindful Breathing and Mindful Collage Collection

We begin by inviting our group to settle themselves comfortably with their collage materials nearby, either on a chair or on the floor with a wall behind them to support their backs. They then participate in a 10- to 15-minute breath awareness meditation. An abbreviated version of a breathing meditation is provided below. The purpose is to create a safe pause and to begin processing insight by directing attention to the breath.

> *Find a seated posture that is comfortable for you. It is best to sit erect and not lean against the wall or the back of your chair. Once you are comfortable, either close your eyes or keep them open and take a few moments to bring your attention to where you can most vividly feel your breath. This may be at the nostrils, during the outbreath, or in the rise and fall of your belly. Keep noticing the gentle movement of your breath. There is no need to breathe in any special way [quiet pause with additional directions to notice the breath]. You may notice that your mind very quickly wanders. This is to be expected. Gently return your attention to the breath [quiet pause, followed by additional redirection]. Instead of fighting whatever might occur during meditation, attempt to accept that this is how things are right now. As best you can, have patience with yourself or observe that reaction. You can always return your attention to the movement of your breath . . . your breath that is always there to remind you of this moment [quiet pause followed by an invitation to gently stop meditation and return to the room].*

Without getting up or talking, studio participants are then invited to go through a pile of their magazines and to select pages that they want to keep. As part of this process, they are asked to take the magazines apart, page after page. A rhythm of movement and sound develops with the removal of each page. They put the images that they want to keep on one side, and unwanted images are placed on the other side. Just as they paid attention to their breath, studio participants are asked to pay attention to the bodily sensations, emotions, and thoughts aroused by the activity and by the image. In the same vein, cultivating openness to the images in whatever way works for them is suggested. The rhythmic sound of ripping pages orients the listener to the here and now. As this happens, a palpable shift in mood seems to take place; no one talks as the sound rises and falls like a wave. Each person dwells in individual motion and personal space, yet a group momentum seems to evolve.

> *I personally chose to sit on the floor. I like the feeling of freedom and comfort the floor gives me rather than being constrained in a chair. While tearing out the magazine pages, I became very aware of the noise of tearing paper, and at one point the noise became soothing, something like the constant sound of waves crashing rhythmically.*

When choosing images I wanted to keep, I looked for a wide variety of feelings the images could provoke. I also looked for images that most people could relate to, such as houses, families, cars, pets, and travel destinations. I decided to categorize my images by size into my boxes and folder. I used images and text to decorate my boxes, based on things I liked. For the most part, everyone else chose to sit on the floor. It made me feel as though we were all connected even though we were not talking. Patti Russell

When the work time comes to a close, we invite the group to give the facilitators all of their unwanted or disagreeable images. We place them in a collective pile in the middle of the studio floor and invite the group members to take those that appeal to them, despite having been rejected by others. Then they gently move the images into a large file folder or any other container that they have. This kind of acceptance and gentleness signals an empathic response to the discarded images, which are considered a symbolic part of the self (Figure 12.1).

We were to make a pile of "yeses" and "nos." I sat on the floor and started ripping. There was a definite rhythm to the motion of ripping and turning the page, ripping and turning. There were also times when the sound of all the ripping became rhythmic. I found it easy to decide between the images I liked and the ones I did not, although I did not know why I liked or disliked them. People had put the "nos" into a collective pile in the middle of the space and discussed briefly what that pile represented—essentially they were images that evoked

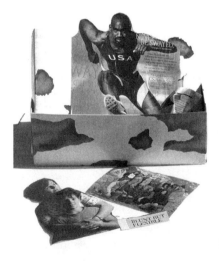

Figure 12.1 *My Yes and No Pile.* Anonymous

> *adverse responses in us. But we also discussed how the images that had*
> *a negative association to one person might be pleasing to another.*
> Tamara Cates

Together, we explore how the process of mindfully seeing images, and noticing whether we like them or not, draws attention to noticing present experience without reactivity. As we view each image, responding with a yes or a no, tearing out the page and placing it in a pile, we can witness how our reactions are allowed to be fleeting. Thus, the collage collection exercise encourages us to see our thoughts as mental events. We witness that while we may like an image and someone else may reject it, the image remains the same. This concept is reminiscent of the content and process model tenets used in DBT (Linehan, 1993a). The images serve as content while the process facilitates full and nonjudgmental attendance to the images for what they are. In that regard, this is a dialectical continuum exercise. Each time we select or do not select an image, we oscillate between wanting and not wanting, acceptance and non-acceptance, or rejection and empathy. We are also reminded by this practice of the Buddhist impermanence principles. The collage selection reveals the human tendency to hold onto experiences, objects, and status. Many studio participants remark on the awareness of the sound of the tearing and the synchronizing of the group, the lost sense of time, and the stepping back from engagement in the images. One group member remarked that while she began by reading all the eye-catching text, shortly she was able to notice her hand tearing, lifting, and placing the pages. Others talk about a genuine relief, need, or satisfaction felt when uncomfortable or unwanted images are taken away, and their surprise that others may desire their unwanted images. The symbolic and relational impact of the facilitator containing the unwanted imagery, holding it, and removing it emphasizes the importance of attuned responses. Such containing and confirming foster acceptance and compassion.

We conclude by discussing how this practice supports the therapist's self. First, the collage selection can be used as a time to self-soothe, relax, and sit in silence. Second, if we see the collage images as a representation of our likes and dislikes, we can extrapolate other uses for the activity. For example, we can realize that our emotional responses are in fact reactions. Such awareness can become more attuned to fluctuations in our liking or disliking of a client, supervisor, or clinical team. In this regard, the practice serves to support nonreactive attuned attention. Such consideration and genuine acceptance can generate secure attachments and trust. In preparing for clinical work, moreover, the therapist must spend time replenishing collage stocks by going through magazines and other media. This practice takes time and could potentially be interpreted as a chore. However, treating it as a mindfulness practice that heightens the awareness of breath, body, emotions, and thoughts can become part of a practical and beneficial self-care ritual. As demonstrated here, mindfulness can therefore be applied and embodied in a variety of ways in daily life for both client and therapist.

Experience II: Alert and Mindful

For this activity, we group two or three tables together into stations, with wide spaces between each station. Placed in the center of each station is a very large sheet of drawing paper and one type of media. The media are selected to represent a spectrum of easily controllable to less controllable characteristics: charcoal, soft lead pencils, soft dry pastels, oil pastels, colored markers, and acrylic paints. For this experiential, we end the art activity with mindful walking. Studio participants are asked to identify an area between two media-laden tables in which they can walk. We explain that while we are not going anywhere, some may want a smaller distance and others a longer one. As studio participants go back and forth, they are also asked to stop at a table and look at, as well as take in, the media laid upon it. The intent of the walking meditation is to be in the present moment and to appreciate each step. We walk all the time, but usually it is more like running. Here, we suggest taking one step at a time. Some prefer to breathe in and out with each step; some practice conscious counting of steps; and others may use a mantra, assigning a word for each step such as secure, happy, healthy, or free. The details of the mindfulness walking meditation technique may vary. For example, in a self-talk approach, where each step can be coupled with an internal dialogue, "I am *shifting*, I am *lifting* one foot, I am *moving* it forward, and I am *placing* my foot." Or for each step they may focus on: "I am *secure*," "I am *happy*," "I am *well*," and "I am *free*" (Hanh, 1976). It is important not to control the breathing or the stepping: "Allow the lungs as much time and air as they need, and simply notice how many steps you take as your lungs fill up, and how many you take as they empty, mindful of both your breath and your steps. As you approach a table, stop for a minute before you turn, and take in the media that are there. The key is mindfulness." Aware walking can be an indoor or outdoor activity: "Each step: Through the deserted gate, full of ripened leaves, I follow the small path. Earth as red as a child's lips. Suddenly I am aware of each step I make" (Hanh, 2011, p. 64). Outdoor mindful walking can transform ordinary stressful environments such as the noise of traffic filtering through the windows of the studio into a lullaby of rising oceanic waves. Reframing the noise as just noise rather than "traffic" provides this relief.

After 10 minutes or so of walking, we invite the studio participants to stop at whichever table is closest and pick up the marker, pastel, or one of the

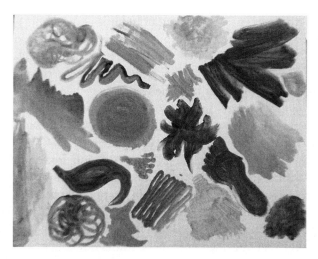

Figure 12.2 *The Painting Page.* From the exploration of mindful walking with media.

various paintbrushes. While keeping close attention on their movements, participants make a mark on the paper, exploring the specific table media on the shared central page. For example, they can feel the contact of soft pastel as it is gently rubbed on the paper, then touch the dusty traces directly with their fingers and feel its texture, and notice its residue on their skin, its odor, and density of color. Or, as in the case of the group art described below, group members can explore painting. In a similar way, they mindfully move to another table and again experiment with the media. This interspersed walking and mark-making continues until each person has visited all the different media laid out on the tables (Figure 12.2).

> *I loved the walking and art making. I could not believe how much everything slowed down. It was odd at first and I was getting annoyed, thinking it was a waste of time. Then, the more I paid attention to each part of my foot, I became more absorbed and tranquil. When I got to each table, I found the process of drawing really different from the regular way that I draw. I was acutely aware of how my fingers held the pastel and what the contact with the page was like—and could let go of judgment and performance anxiety.* Lisa Kandaros

As we discuss the walking and art making experiences, the studio participants report how each one allowed them to be more alert and attentive to automatic movements and gestures. They also comment on the increase in attention to the qualities of the art and of working together on one page. Influenced by MBAT (Monti et al., 2006), the slowing down of attention to the component experiences of walking or holding and drawing with a familiar medium contributes to living minute by minute. For her cancer survival group, Peterson led the research participants through a clearly defined sequence of exploring various media, which matched with specific papers. Studio participants talk about how the walking practice slows time to allow insights to gently emerge. They discover their bodily reactions and some express how it reminds them of tai chi or yoga practice, allowing a letting go of the activity in their minds and becoming more focused. Often the walking meditation is appealing since it is an active meditation process that feels safer than sitting meditation. We discuss how such a formal mindfulness practice can become informal, when used at the beginning of a session or during a session when needed, as recounted by Noah. When one of her clients was creating imagery of a distressing event, which was upsetting her, Noah suggested that they walk together around the studio office, just as they did during our media practice. This mutual activity was stabilizing and allowed the client to process her memory at that moment. A clinician who engages in this practice can also benefit from walking meditation by taking a few moments while setting up the room to walk mindfully. The clinician may test materials and set up the media while remaining alert to what is happening within and around him or her as this is occurring. These practices allow the time between sessions to become a space for personal alertness. Similar to MBCT protocols, these mindful awareness practices suggest bringing intentional awareness to everyday activities (Hayes et al., 2006).

In many ways this activity reminds me how a new client might explore my studio office. We walk around and I introduce them to the space, tables and easels, the painting supply cabinets, and the sand trays. Usually, we bring the chosen media with us to the table or easel. This activity has me thinking that perhaps wherever we are in the room we can experiment with it. So perhaps as we pause next to the easel markers, it's possible to invite a scribble on the easel, or a smudge of paint on the paint cabinet door list of paints to purchase. I am similarly reminded of my love for art stores where, following the marks of others, I can test pastels, pens, and pencils on the price tags. I have always found that soothing. Noah Hass-Cohen

Experience III: The Art Therapy Body Scan

The body scan is a mindfulness practice that can directly support relaxation and well-being. As such, it is invaluable to clients coping with health issues, eating disorders, disability, pain, and stress (Kabat-Zinn, 2005). It is integrated with the following art therapy experiential.

To begin the activity, each person prepares a sheet of paper that is as long as that individual's height. The sheets are cut from rolls of colored paper and taped to the floor. Next to the paper, participants roll out a blanket or mat, which they either lie on, sit on, or cover themselves with. While the body scan is ideally done lying down, it can also be done in a sitting position. For those sitting, the body-length roll of paper is taped to the wall. Participants either lie on their back or sit upright with their heels touching the floor. The options provided are also suggestive of empathic support of any physical conditions that the participants may have and that may prohibit lying on the floor. To achieve progressive awareness and relaxation, we mentally visit each body part. The beginning of this script is included below (a full version is available in Kabat-Zinn, 2005).

> *If you feel comfortable, please close your eyes; otherwise try to have them as unfocused as possible, looking into the distance. Notice where your breath is most viable. You may feel the rise and fall of your abdomen and chest, or the swelling and contracting of your rib cage against the floor, or the passage of breath through your nostrils. Notice the inhale and exhale of your breath. Take your breath down to your left little toe. Feel your little toe, whatever sensation that is here. Then go to the next toe and the next toe, to all five toes, notice the sensations here. Allow yourself to feel any and all sensations in the toes, if any. If you do not feel anything, allow yourself that. Now notice the soles of your feet. Feel the creases of the skin, the pad and rear of the sole and all the sensations here, if any. Now move your attention to the top of the foot and up to your ankle. Breathe into this upper part of this left foot. Notice the sensations you may or may not have here. Now notice your left ankle: the front, back, sides of it; how it presses against the floor or not; the three dimensions of it. Notice the sensations you may or may not have here. . . .*

The script continues to guide the listener's attention through the rest of the leg to the hips, through the other foot and leg, up the lower, middle, and upper back, and through the abdomen, chest, and internal organs to the hands, arms, shoulders, neck, and head. Once the whole body has been scanned, the script prompts a few deeper breaths connecting head to toe, and then beginning to gently move the arms and legs.

After having a moment to stir, we invite the studio participants to roll onto their sheet of paper on the floor. Those who had been sitting will stand against the paper, which is taped to the wall. Then, using one hand, they draw across the opposite side of their body using a light-colored marker, roughly tracing their silhouette. Those lying down will usually need to sit up

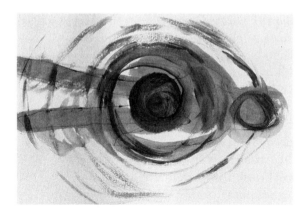

Figure 12.3 *My Body Scan.* At first, I was aware of following the prompts but after a while I realized that my concentration seemed to change quality and I was feeling a generalized all-encompassing relaxation. I had no idea how much time had passed and at the end I felt a deep warmth in the center of my body. Joanna Clyde Findlay

to trace around their legs and feet. We then invite each practitioner to map their mindfulness experience on the traced silhouette by representing their experience in color and shape with paints (Figure 12.3).

Sometimes the colorful mapping of the body moves across the silhouette from head to toe in the same order as the scan. Alternatively, as in Figure 12.3, the map will focus on one body part, like the belly, representing the most personally meaningful experience. Eliciting emotional expressions and revealing tension or discomfort, the body scan process can be a profound psychological experience. Images relating to loss of wholeness, broken hearts, inability to bear children, abortions, or mortality may surface. Having circulated the room to see each other's images, we may simply discuss the process of tracing the awareness, or discuss the images in detail depending on each person's level of comfort.

I found the body scan a remarkable experience. At first I could hardly believe we were taking so long just to notice our right foot and each toe. I was soon lulled by the repeated directions and noticed I was seeing each part prompted. I seemed to see it from the outside and feel it from the inside at the same time. I thought noticing sensations meant tension or pins and needles but often realized I was noticing images or memories. How my thighs feel fat, the burn from an accident I try to hide on my arm. Meanwhile, I felt myself relaxing, but not becoming sleepy. I realized that when a place did feel tense, the more I paid attention, the more, in fact, this feeling changed. I felt like I was get-

ting heavier and could fall through the floor yet I was feeling each part of my body. I had no idea how much time had passed. Lisa Kandaros

The discussion at the closing of the group revealed multiple applications of the body scan. Studio participants' reactions varied greatly; some realized this was the first time since childhood that they were able to pay close attention to their bodily sensations. For others, the activity accessed difficult memories, while for others, it was like a rediscovery of their living, breathing body. Remaining participants were able to access deep relaxation. Thus, imagery from focused attention reveals how an art therapy scan can contribute to self-esteem, body image, and pain work.

A key benefit of the art therapy based body scan is that by paying attention to our experience, our bodies and our thoughts as they are, we can learn to accept the experience without judgment and with kindness. This kind of kindness is associated with a reduction in pain (Kabat-Zinn, 2012). Aches, pains, and the limits of our body are encountered and pacified through focused awareness. Similarly, we let ourselves be aware of difficult personal experiences we cannot control, and instead of struggling against them, we see them for what they are, thereby reducing tension (Hayes et al., 2006). Therapists can integrate the body scan meditation into their self-care tools, develop their own scripts and the associated art making. According to Jon Kabat-Zinn (2012), for people with sleep and pain disorders, the body scan may bring on much-needed deep relaxation and rest.

Experience IV: A Mindful Mandala

A mandala activity can be used as a concentration mindfulness practice. The mandala, a circle, is drawn following a brief seated meditation. In Tibetan Buddhist traditions, intricate mandalas are made with colored sand. The mandala can represent the world, and its construction requires careful attention as it is created according to traditional specifications. Despite such care, this type of mandala making embodies the Buddhist principle of impermanence. After many days of work, the monks brush the exquisitely detailed sand paintings into a sand pile. The sand pile is collected into containers and, in a ceremonial ritual, is poured away into the sea or a river. In our studio, the mandala serves as a concentration and focusing device.

In preparation for the mandala pastel drawing, studio participants draw in pencil around a paper dinner plate or use a compass to draw a circle on a white sheet of paper. They also prepare a set of soft oil or water-soluble pastels offering a range of hues with at least 24 colors. Members are asked to find a

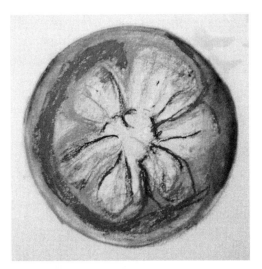

Figure 12.4 *Flowering Light.* Joanna Clyde Findlay

comfortable, supported sitting position, placing their feet on the floor, their hands on their laps, and closing their eyes if they are comfortable doing so. When a brief meditation period comes to a close, Joanna asks that they let their gaze fall upon their pastels. She then asks them to select a color that they are attracted to and begin to draw within the circle (Figure 12.4).

> *After the meditation, I had no clear idea of what I would draw. I just found I wanted golden warm colors around the outside of the circle moving towards a lighter center. When I began to draw towards the middle, I found myself tracing delicate light blue and green lines radiating outwards. As I worked, I became clearer about how the image needed to become a whole. I then added soft peach and yellow and when I sat back I realized petal shapes had emerged. This process helped me become more focused and balanced and I began to consider how this symbol related to my life.* Joanna Clyde Findlay

Another option for this practice is to use a preprinted mandala and color it in. Similar to the Tibetan mandala, which requires following a predetermined map, the preprinted details contribute significantly to the concentration that is required. In other words, the more detailed the mandala, the more concentration is needed. Because this is a learned practice, the preprinted mandalas that we offer vary in complexity. Likened to the use of tapes for meditation, preprinted mandalas can supply a useful structure to help focus our attention. Thus, the mandala activity can be very soothing and pleasurable as the intense concentration eases daily mind chatter.

> *I found this last practice the easiest. I had found the sitting medita-*
> *tion uncomfortable, because I felt I could not move and my back*
> *hurt, but I liked sitting at the table. I found drawing in the circle*
> *helped me. It gave me a focus and I found I started drawing from the*
> *center. Soon I realized that I was repeating a pattern of superposed*
> *stars. I felt steady and centered. I could have carried on, adding more*
> *and more. Although it was not perfectly symmetrical, I like the result*
> *and called it Now.* Patty Lewis

Mindful mandala making can support the therapist's self-development. Those who have prior experience with it might recognize the stabilizing effects of drawing in a circle. Jung (1963) suggested that making art within the unique shape of a circle generates self-integration and that mandala making can support the resolution of inner conflicts. For art therapists, this can become part of an ongoing journaling practice and reflective art making. Such informal mindfulness practices contribute to the kind of psychological flexibility, adaptability, empathy, and well-being that is vital for relation-based therapy (Siegel, 2010).

RELATIONAL NEUROSCIENCE: EVIDENCE FOR THE EFFECTIVENESS OF MINDFULNESS

Studies focusing on brain activity during mindfulness meditation practice have identified changes in the activation, density, and volume of specific brain structures. Mindfulness meditation practices stimulate significant cortical integration of sensory, visceral, emotional, and cognitive functions (Treadway & Lazar, 2009). A majority of research points to activation of higher-functioning brain regions, including the medial prefrontal cortex (mPFC), the dorsolateral prefrontal cortex (dlPFC), and the anterior cingulate cortex (ACC). This also noticeably includes the insular cortex in both hemispheres. These are the general regions most implicated during mindful meditation (Lazar et al., 2005; Treadway & Lazar, 2009). The dlPFC is involved in executive decision-making and attention while the ACC is associated with the synthesis of attention, motivation, and motor control. Mindfulness practices activate the left dlPFC (Treadway & Lazar, 2009) more than the right. Furthermore, structural changes in the thickening of the prefrontal cortex (PFC) occur over time in experienced practitioners (Lazar et al., 2005).

The insular cortex, folded deep inside the temporal and frontal lobes in each hemisphere, is also activated in meditation. It is associated with interoception, or the awareness of visceral "gut" feelings and the processing of transient bodily sensations (Treadway & Lazar, 2009). Functional imaging studies have implicated the insula in pain, anger, fear, disgust, happiness, and sadness. Acting like a switchboard, the insula receives information from sensory pathways via the thalamus and sends information to a number of other limbic-related structures, such as the amygdala (AMY), the ventral striatum, and the orbitofrontal cortex, as well as the motor cortices. In this way, the insula connects bodily sensations with emotions, thoughts, and decisions and shows structural transformations over time. Much like the PFC, the insula thickens in individuals who practice mindful meditation. A thicker insula cortex enables better coordination between these functions. This may in turn help reduce stress as it more efficiently resolves difficult emotional problems and internal bodily sensations (Hölzel et al., 2011; Lazar et al., 2005; Treadway & Lazar, 2009). However, many years of intensive practice are necessary to achieve increased density (Treadway & Lazar, 2009).

The processes triggered in mindful meditation seem to involve more left-sided activation of the PFC. It also involves a strengthening of the functional connectivity between the PFC and the amygdala (Siegel, 2012). It is suggested that this connection allows the left PFC to more effectively dampen the emotional responses in the amygdala alarm system.

Moreover, mindfulness training is thought to favor increased prefrontal regulation of limbic emotional responses, even among non expert practitioners. Accordingly, self-reports of mindfulness were correlated with more activity in the MPFC, as well as a down regulation of activity in the AMY during affect labeling tasks (Creswell, Way, Eisenberger, & Lieberman, 2007). Thus, top-down affect regulation functions and prefrontal region integrative functions support the growth of new synaptic connections and promote brain plasticity (Siegel, 2006). Increased gray matter concentration in brain regions involved in self-referential processing and perspective taking also suggests increased cognitive and psychological function (Hölzel et al., 2010).

In response to mindfulness practices, studies have pointed to the activation and structural neuroplasticity changes of other brain structures (Germer et al., 2005; Pace et al., 2009). These regions include those associated with learning and memory because meditators appear to also have significantly more gray matter density in the hippocampus (Hölzel et al., 2007, 2010; Treadway & Lazar, 2009). Previous studies demonstrated that gray matter modifications can result from learning abstract information motor skills (Draganski et al., 2004) and language skills (Mechelli et al., 2004). Structural changes occur in the limbic regions associated with the brain's emotional center. Furthermore, practitioners of the structured eight-week MBSR program have shown reductions in perceived stress, which was correlated with decreases in right basolateral AMY gray matter density (Hölzel et al., 2011). It now appears that actual brain changes can also be associated with changes in psychological measures, such as those that measure stress (Goldin, Ziv, Jazaieri, & Gross, 2013). In addition, it seems evident that the integrative effects of mindfulness practices reach beyond the PFC to extend more widely into lower, middle, and upper regions of the brain. That said, the precise means by which training-induced neuroanatomical plasticity occurs continues to be explored (Tang & Posner, 2012) but its benefits most likely result from practicing detachment from sources of wanting and suffering, along with selflessness (Dor-Ziderman, Berkovich-Ohana, Glicksohn, Goldstein, & Eason, 2008).

CREATE PRINCIPLES AND CLINICAL APPLICATIONS

Transformative Integrating is the primary focus of the studio art therapy activities in this chapter. Chapters 11 through 13 form the three cornerstones of Transformative Integrating. Mindful awareness gives rise to emotional spaciousness as it releases the individual from wanting things to be different than they are and provides opportunities for empathic affiliations. Empathizing becomes a foundation for insight and acceptance, which culminates in what is known as mindful compassion. In other words the CREATE principles of Creative Embodiment, Relational Resonating, and Adaptive Responding serve as doorways into mindful awareness. On the other hand, Transformative Integrating and Empathizing and Compassion arise as a consequence of the psychological and artistic space that mindful awareness opens up.

The art activities in this chapter include the collage collection process, media awareness and mindful walking, a body scan, and mandala drawing. By including mindfulness practices in conjunction with the art directives, we extend awareness to art therapy processes. Attentiveness to the present is linked to an in-the-moment existence, which can be bolstered by the studio work. Examples include increasing therapists' and clients' awareness of still versus active movements, interwoven with art making as well as minute-to-minute occurrences. Minute-to-minute occurrences include seeing, looking, listening, hearing, touching, smelling, and breathing. Client and therapist awareness is brought to the media qualities and to automatic versus intentional art making gestures. For example, the art therapy-based body scan encourages attention to mind-body relationships and the understanding of how bodily reactions inform our present psychological states. Focusing attention on touch, person-to-person right-to-left gestures, and bodily movements, the mindful collage selection stimulates awareness of the mind's constant labeling of pleasant or unpleasant experiences. The movement associated with mindful walking provides avenues for affect regulation and supports grounding.

In regard to Transformative Integrating, long-term mindfulness practices appear to structurally change the brain and promote psychobiological self-regulation and well-being. The synchronized client's and therapist's psycho-biological self-regulation promote bilateral and vertical resonance. This transformative integration synthesizes cognitive functions such as attention and insight with somatic experiences, tactile experiences, emoting, motivation, and motor control. We contend that sequencing mindfulness practices with mindful art therapy practices enhances the opportunity to experience integration. Examples again include the body scan art and the walking meditation with art marking. The two art therapy concentration practices, collage collection, and mandala making also enhance therapeutic mindful awareness and insight. Through these four examples, mindfulness is grounded in the here-and-now actions of tactile art making. One important contribution that this sequence may provide is the mitigation of dissociation. Clients with a history of chronic trauma or pain often report a tendency to dissociate or panic when they practice mindfulness meditation. Connecting meditation to tactile art making can circumvent this problem. Neurobiologically, dissociation is linked to an over-activated left hemisphere, specifically the PFC. Therefore, art making, which is associated with the parietal, temporal, limbic, and right-hemisphere functions, serves to synthesize and integrate psychological, emotional, and cognitive functions.

Empathizing and Compassion are embedded in how art therapists may want to approach the setup for the experientials and, most importantly, how the art making is discussed and interpreted. The collage affords the ability to empathically pay attention to the discarded collage images. Often symbolic of unwanted parts of the self, clients will crunch up and get rid of parts of the unwanted images. ATR-N practices advocate accepting these actions, yet looking into clients' discarded images, in order to gain insight into the clients' psychological functioning. Learning from mindfulness suggests that for some clients, empathically talking about these reactions and suggesting gently discarding those images may support self-acceptance and increase the capacity for empathizing. Softening reactions to self and others can decrease defensive positions and assist in shifting to kindness.

The art therapy walking meditation embodies the principle of Creative Embodiment. It recruits clients' walking in order to gain insight and increase intention. Walking meditation is about dwelling in a state of being while moving, as motion usually has a purpose. Standing in front of an easel, rising from one's chair to get needed media, and gesturing, cutting, modeling, and pounding clay are motions intended to express and relieve emotions as well as increase cognitions. Walking meditation serves to regulate anxiety and depression while increasing intentionality by purposefully slowing down. Furthermore, it teaches us that even when walking and paying attention to walking (i.e., not falling) we can be mindful of our surroundings, thus including art making as a walking meditation.

Relational Resonating witnesses a fluid, stable alignment with oneself and with another person, giving rise to self and relational compassion. Such mindful awareness entails a non-judgmental acceptance of others and supports secure attachment experiences. Propelled by the additional support of nonverbal communication, the experience of a mindful, attuned presence in the client-therapist relationship is a foundation for self-regulation via contingent communication. Perhaps the clearest illustration of the elevated empathy opportunity afforded by this principle is seen through the therapist's handling of unwanted images in the collage collection activity. Therapeutic embracing of discarded collage selections by the group exemplifies acceptance, flexibility, and respect.

Expressive art making with formal or informal mindfulness allows increased awareness of any emotions that arise, which are observed, acknowledged, and expressed. Furthermore, the Expressive Communicating principle supports clients' active integration of the recognition and identification of emotions as well as their manifestation. As clients select desirable images, they can tune inward, drawn in by the sounds and sensations involved. In this shift away from negative forces, they become mindful observers of the motions involved in each moment, including arm gestures, cutting and tearing sounds, and the chosen visuals. The sensation of sound is a powerful moment-to-moment container. In addition to bodily sensations, collage making paves the way for insight, and awakens emotions and thoughts. Mindfulness practices are about assisting clients to be in the moment, and to experience an increased sense of control, attention, acceptance, and tolerance for stress. In this respect, a shift away from negative thinking may occur for even the most traumatized client, bringing acceptance along with an adapted response.

Practicing the body scan may arouse previously unknown feelings of fear, loss, or pain. These emotions are usually more difficult to access as well as communicate. The body scan painting allows for the explicit expression and communication of these emotions while maintaining an inward felt sensation. Once mastered, clients learn that they can continue to do so as needed, reducing fear and anxiety. Art therapy directives have included asking clients where they experience emotions in their body and then asking them to place colors or images on a body outline or on a gingerbread type of silhouette (Riley, 2001). This is a cognitive-based directive as they think about where they experience bodily reactions. Adding the body scan practice to these exercises allows for the inclusion of actual somatic sensations, providing the opportunity to communicate how bodily reactions contribute to feelings and thoughts.

Mandala art making contributes to the understanding of the Adaptive Responding principle. Generated through centering, the round shape pulls the client's art making into the center, promoting a sense of control and concentration. With a goal of focused attention, these activities offer simple, accessible art making practices that can be soothing and pleasurable. For clients, centering practices, such as traditional mandala making or coloring, help focus on the present moment. When viewed through an adaptive response lens, this activity suggests the thin line between control and surrender via the practice of regulating this balance. The prevention of therapist burnout is an additional benefit gained by building a series of practices utilizing circle art.

CHAPTER 13

Empathizing and Compassion:
The Creative Arts

As I began sketching the plans for my altar, I became keenly immersed in my work and in the work of others. Sitting around the large table, I was moving back and forth between my work and others, noting, feeling, and becoming more and more aware of the meaning of what an altar is, an homage to our shared and personal experiences. For a moment, I was still, and then I saw the other people also sitting still in contemplation, looking inwards and summoning images. I realized I knew that process, too. I also recognized the feeling of leaning forwards to work closely, then moving back to see one's work. It felt like I was sensing other people and knowing them in an intimate way—I felt linked to everyone and their altar art as they worked in silence. In an obscure way, the more I become involved in my drawing, the more I found myself in silent communication; bonding together. Lisa Smith

EMPATHIZING IS A REFLECTION OF the ability to sense, recognize, understand, and respond to other people's emotions, thoughts, behaviors, belief systems, and experiences. Fueled by neurobiological mirroring and observation, empathy is the umbrella under which humans universally mentalize interpret, organize, and carry forward positive social interchanges and meaningful life experiences. In Greek, empathy means "to suffer with" (Walrond-Skinner, 1986). This emotional, developmental, cognitive, and social amalgam (Decety & Ickes, 2011) provides a pathway to compassionate insight for others' experiences. This chapter illustrates the Empathizing and Compassion principle of the CREATE model, which is informed by affective neuroscience, theory of mind, and attachment-based research.

Achieving a mindful and stable state that can help perceive what others intend supports the emergence of empathic resonance and compassionate responses (Gunuratana, 2002; Kabat-Zinn, 1994; Hanh, 2012). The phenomena of empathic association, mindfulness of mind states, and sensory awareness, as well as mentalization, are interconnected (Germer, 2009; Neff & Germer, 2013). For our purposes, we define empathy as including empathic concern and compassion. Growing from intersubjective experiences, empathy forms the foundation for the development of relational resonance and prosocial advances (Badenoch, 2008). These kinds of empathizing events, where one can experience the self and the other as compassionately connected, yet differentiated, help form and maintain therapeutic alliances and change. Intersubjectivity allows people to relate their experiences to those of others and is sustained by imitating, recognizing, perceiving, and anticipating actions. Innately, people tend to experience and express empathy and compassion toward those whom they feel attached to, mainly occurring when observing their loved ones experience pain (Singer, 2004; Watt, 2005). Although we do not experience their physical pain, we can sense it, evoking empathy and compassion. Empathic responses also occur when interpersonal communication is anticipated and imagined, Furthermore, like internal working models, empathic affiliations are an inborn states of mind that predispose people to intersubjective experiences and relational resonance (Duranti, 2010). Similar to hope and trust, empathizing is a unifying humanistic theoretical factor across clinical approaches.

In the therapist-client relationship, empathic relational resonance occurs as the brains and nervous systems of the therapist and the client mirror one another, vibrating and orchestrating together (Siegel, 2006, 2010). Such intersubjectivity involves automatic as well as active responsivity. This is achieved by mentally and emotionally placing oneself in another person's experiences (Husserl, 1989). It is a process of perspective taking that evolves and is supported developmentally across the life span (Hughes, 2004). As we describe throughout this chapter, similar processes most likely occur in the art therapy clinic. However, the art making and viewing of the art most likely add additional dimensions as they enhance empathic connectivity.

Interpersonal neurobiology holds that brain development changes concurrently with relationally induced variations in the experience of mother and baby (Ammaniti & Gallese, 2014). In other words, a human's nervous system is biologically wired for empathic interpersonal exchanges. Developmentally, mimicry, facial expressions, bodily communication, and emotional simulation begin at birth. These empathic social learning experiences are spontaneous and simultaneous. For example, as early as the third term, fetuses respond to familiar voices preferentially (Kisilevsky, Hains, Brown, Lee, Cowperthwaite et al., 2009), and in the neonatal room, babies will cry in response to other babies' cries. Such empathic responses can be emotionally contagious. It is from this base that intersubjective personal and social understanding develops (Stern, 2004).

The neurobiological bases of empathy are associated with the brain's emotional system function and with mirroring neurons and human mirroring systems interactions. While we touched upon the neurobiology of empathic relational resonances in earlier chapters, here we focus on mirroring. Mirror neurons (MN), which are found in monkeys and humans are located in the brain's frontal areas (Rizzolatti, Fadiga, Gallese, & Fogassi, 1996; Mukamel, Ekstrom, Kaplan, Iacoboni, & Fried, 2010). Human mirroring systems (MS) expand and involve several brain regions (Gallese, 2003; Rizzolatti & Craighero, 2004). Both function to contribute to people's felt knowledge of others. Specifically MN fire in recognition and anticipation of one's own and others' purposeful and successful movements involving the hands and mouth. When activated, the observer's reaction means, "I do what you do; I can do what you do; and I can recognize and anticipate what you will do." In other words, MN function is mostly about the recognition of purposeful doing.

More broadly dispersed across the nervous system, mirror neuron systems (MS) synchronize across people to support learning, communication, relational inferences, and interpersonal exchanges. For example, in the case of intersubjective pain, MS activate in response to interpersonal distress by arousing empathy (Singer, 2004; Watt, 2005). Also reactive to faces and other people, MS are involved in imitation and in reactions to positive and negative facial expressions (Iacoboni & Dapretto, 2006). When triggered, they stimulate an intersubjective response: "I can sense what you sense; I can feel what you feel; I experience what you experience; and I can plan for and anticipate what you will do." MS are involved in the observation and imitation of a broad spectrum of purposeful bodily movements. Linked with specific limbic structures, MS facilitate a social-emotional-based felt simulation of others' experiences as our own (Buccino et al., 2001; Fogassi et al., 2005; Gallese, 2004; Watkins, Strafella, & Paus, 2003). MS functions support the integration of bottom-up emotional expression and top-down executive regulation of emotions.

While affect regulation provides a cognitive dampening of overly exciting or disturbing emotions (Schore, 1994), empathizing allows acceptance of the disturbing emotion (Siegel, 2010). Together, this contrast generates insight and compassion toward oneself and others. In the interpersonal realm, the experience becomes "I experience, know, and accept you." Empathic resonance is nonverbal (Gallese, Eagle, & Migone, 2007). The clinical practice of empathizing requires holding, understanding, accepting, and respecting whatever it is that the client brings up or is representing. Such capacities are nonverbally embodied by gesture, smile, bodily posture, and intonation.

These are commonly used art therapy interactive strategies that support clients' ability to understand and share the feelings of another.

THREE CONDITIONS OF EMPATHY

Clinically speaking, empathic affiliations most likely require several dependent conditions (Decety & Jackson, 2004; Watt, 2005). First, a shared affective state occurs during an arousal-oriented situation or emotional experience (Jackson, Meltzoff, & Decety, 2005). This is often an automatic reaction (Husserl, 1970). Empathic responses are sensory, bodily, and emotional experiences that do not necessarily require an explicit or deliberate interpretive response (Gallese, 2003; Husserl, 1989). Facilitated by MN and MS, this response is an infectious feeling or immediate felt understanding of what the client that we care for knows and appreciates. Specific automatic art therapy processes can trigger empathy, such as handing media to a client or to each other in a group. Deliberate and specific art therapy directives, such as mother-child or other duo drawing, support intersubjectivity. The familiarity exists within ourselves to sense, experience, and work intuitively and sensitively with another. For art therapy, this is most likely because we sense what the client or artist made (Hass-Cohen, 2007). In essence, what we have learned from MN/MS research is that the brain generates a felt familiarity with what is anticipated and observed.

The second necessary condition of empathy is differentiation, or the "cognitive capacity to take the perspective of the other person while keeping self and other differentiated" (Jackson et al., 2005, p. 771). In part due to MN/MS function, the therapist might feel that he or she could have made what clients made, or feel their emotions. Yet the tangible artwork bears testimony to the client who created it or made each art mark or symbol. Keeping this delicate balance of self and togetherness flourishing is essential to therapeutic efficacy. The empathic close yet separate self and other represented in the art and art making can evoke emotional regulation and compassion, respectively. This differentiation is for the caregiver or the therapist to hold, understand, accept, and respect.

Maintaining prosocial intent is the third necessary condition. This is critical since there are individuals who can accurately sense others' affective states and take advantage of their vulnerabilities. In other words, empathy does not merely entail perceiving and understanding someone else's emotions; rather, it "must involve some motivation for the relief of the other's distress" (Jackson et al., 2005, p. 197). Mindfulness practices create space for empathic responses and, in the process, create a reciprocal supportive quality as empathic responses can also support mindfulness (Hanh, 2012). Empathy can also be directly supported by loving-kindness meditation (LKM) practices in which one sends well wishes to oneself, in general and when in distress, as well as toward others. It seems that this social practice reduces the stress response and ensuing inflammation in the body. Overall long-term practice of LKM can lead to shifts toward positive emotional and personal resources. Short-term LKM seems to more quickly support greater social connection with others (Fredrickson, Cohn, Coffey, Pek, & Finkel 2008; Hutcherson, Seppala, & Gross, 2008; Kok et al., 2013; Lutz, Brefczynski-Lewis, Johnstone, & Davidson, 2008). There are five traditional categories of loving-kindness: toward oneself, a friend or benefactor, a neutral person, a challenging person, and all sentient beings everywhere. The phrases include the sending of wishes for safety, happiness, physical and emotional well-being, acceptance, and freedom.

In art therapy, the nonjudgmental acceptance of process arts promotes a prosocial stance, and the universality of artistic expression can give rise to cross-cultural empathic affiliations. These pathways to self-acceptance are augmented by therapeutic art making, in which the therapist lends a third hand (Kramer, 1986). The therapist assists in organizing, accessing, and executing the client's intentions, providing ongoing prosocial support. Therapeutic goals are informed by empathetic and compassionate goals, including establishing self-states of well-being for self, relational states of wishing well for others and being supported by others, as well as investigating the possibility that compassionate traits can develop into states.

In the group and individual activities described in previous chapters, we came together to create, observe, react, and respond to the anticipated expressions of others. The art product and the art making are gateways to the intersubjective sharing of others' worldviews. In this chapter, the construction and presentation of an altar and the sharing of hand silhouettes are culminating group process events, contributing to a deeper mutual understanding: "I witness your art brimming full of symbols of your values, beliefs and experiences, and I know you beyond words. As I understand this experience in myself, I, too, can imagine or make my life's work. And as our hands join together, we support each other on our journey."

EMPATHIC ARTS: ALTARS AND MILAGROS

The experience of empathy and fostering intersubjective states can be held or transmitted by universal imagery, such as that of religious objects (Cosentino, 2006; Hass-Cohen, 2008b). The Altar experiential for this chapter originated from Noah's experiencing of religious and personal altars across her travels in the United States. Fueled by her appreciation for the desert, which reminds her of her country of origin, she discovered many outdoor altars that dot arid landscapes.

An example is the outdoor altar at the San José de Gracia Church in Las Trampas, New Mexico. It is dedicated to Santa Niño, Jesus Christ the Holy Child. In that part of the country, he is believed to wander the countryside at night spreading miracles, especially among the imprisoned, the poor, and the ill. Therefore, the personal objects placed on this outdoor altar often include shoes for the child Jesus, who supposedly wears them as he walks so much. Sometimes the shoes belong to sick children for whom the parents are seeking help. Regardless of one's religious affiliation, the image of a distressed parent placing little shoes on the altar is an empathic felt experience. Symbolizing both the ill children and their savior, the shoes also represent baby Jesus. Other symbolic objects include prayer rosaries, candles, and flowers (Figure 13.1).

Religious altars are designated spaces with fixed codes of use and decoration. From an ATR-N perspective, altars are spaces or representations with which we resonate empathically. These can be experiences in actual size or symbolism. Stunning examples await the visitor of *Multiple Visions: A Common Bond* at the Museum of International Folk Art in Santa Fe, New Mexico. In this exhibition, miniature figurines participate in communal celebrations of life and death from more than 100 nations. The community scenes are set on vibrant altar-like stages, inviting a detailed witnessing of day-to-day small town life. The museum visitors are welcomed to the small towns and can imagine themselves enjoying the open market, drinking in the sights, eating the foods, witnessing a wedding, celebrating a birth, or walking in a funeral procession. Remarkably, love, compassion, and joy radiate from facial features, gestures, and bodily positions. As visitors walk through the aisles, they

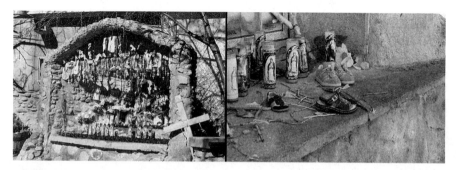

Figure 13.1 On Left, *Outdoor Altar in San José de Gracia, Las Trampas, New Mexico.* On right, one detail from same altar. This 18th-century church is one of the oldest surviving churches in New Mexico. Photo by Noah Hass-Cohen.

journey into an emotional and cultural world that is at the same time familiar and foreign. Perhaps the universality of the artifacts and scenes contribute to this felt sense and shared understanding. It is also likely that the rich and colorful snapshots may remind viewers of their own countries of origin. They are so vibrant that they remind the viewers of the scents associated with these senses. An example of artifacts that are similar to the ones found at the museum is the wedding altar in Figure 13.2, radiating a sense of community and supportive togetherness.

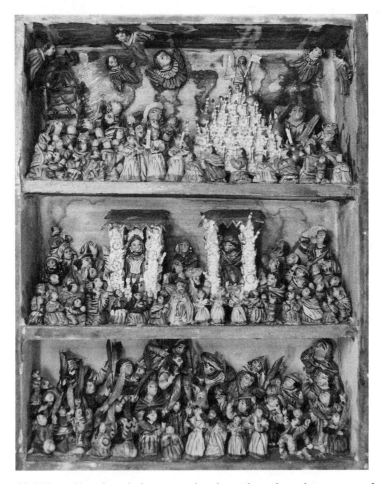

Figure 13.2 The wedding altar, which is contained in a box with two doors, depicts a group of people with objects that look like large leaves at the bottom, then the bride and groom in the middle, and finally at the top a representation of a wedding cake with candles. The representations have a religious nuance. Angels hover above the cake, which has an image of Jesus Christ on the top, and it looks like people are praying. From author's collection, Noah Hass-Cohen.

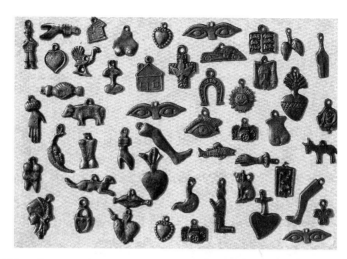

Figure 13.3 *Milagros are Religious Folk Charms that are Traditionally Used for Healing Purposes.* From author's collection, Noah Hass-Cohen.

Like the outdoor altar at San José de Gracia, altars are characterized by the presence of religious and compassionate offerings. The offering may be a precious or semi precious object. Milagros, which are miniature votive objects, are common altar offerings in South America. Typically small and symbolic, milagros represent the human body or images of people praying (Figure 13.3).

Frequently attached to altars and shrines, milagros are often purchased in churches, cathedrals, or from street vendors. In Spanish, the word milagro means "miracle" or "surprise." Also carried for protection and good luck, milagros are usually offered to a saint as a reminder of a petitioner's particular need, or in gratitude for a prayer answered. Furthermore, they assist in focusing attention on a specific ailment, based on the type of charm used. For instance, a milagro of a body part, such as a leg, might be used as part of a prayer for the improvement of a leg injury, or it might refer to a vow to travel to a holy place. Similarly, a heart might represent a variety of situations such as a heart condition, a romance, or sadness. Milagro symbolism may or may not be universal, but it is usually easy to identify with the forms, which frequently depict the human body. Depending on local customs, milagros come in a variety of shapes and dimensions and are created from many different materials. Ranging from flat to fully three-dimensional, they can be constructed from gold, silver, tin, lead, wood, bone, or wax. Although milagros are typically small, they can also be life size, which can boost empathic associations. The smaller the symbol, the more cognitive the associations, whereas the larger symbols resonate with implicit bodily imagery. In a church in Jericho, Noah found that most of the personal artifacts were wax-cast life-size limbs, suggesting pain, disease, or illness in a specific body part. The life-size images stimulate a surge of compassion for afflicted, sick, or healthy loved ones, as well as a wish for well-being. Realistically sized images also promote a sense of standing with a similar-minded group of people immersed in shared human experiences.

Following these experiences and information, we suggest to our creative milieu to create and decorate a life-sized hand that they will adorn with group and personal symbolism and to create a personal altar as homage to their experiences throughout the creative ATR-N arts group.

EXPERIENTIAL PRACTICES AND DIRECTIVES

Experience I: Hands Cutout

Inspired by the milagro art, we invite group members to focus their attention on their hands and think about any meaning hands hold for each of them, as well as for the group as a whole. We use this reflection, along with a hand tracing activity, to provide closure to a long-term group. The reflection invites culturally based interpersonal and personalized revelations. Our late colleague Shirley Riley (1999), who was a master at building relationships, introduced the Hands Cutout experiential to us. One hand is usually traced on regular smooth paper and is then cut out and pasted on a group mural. We are familiar with the Hands Cutout directive as we use it frequently for establishing solidarity and confidentiality, and enhancing therapeutic relationships (Galbraith et al., 2008). As empathic associations benefit from familiarity, we take pleasure in revisiting this staple intervention. However, we make two changes for purposes of consolidating the empathic associations built throughout the studio experiences.

First, placing both hands on a piece of textured paper, palms down, each person traces each hand with the other; the right hand traces the left and the left hand traces the right. Next, we say to everyone, "Draw on one hand a representation of what kind of closure you bring with you today. Include your sensations, emotions, feelings, and thoughts." On the other traced hand, they are requested to: "Do the same but for other group members: Include your hopes and regards for the group members, as well as your farewells. As you do so, decide how you will position your hands on the paper; next to each other, touching, or not touching." This is a conscious prosocial and empathy-oriented request. After the hand drawings are completed, each individual cuts out the hands from the paper and places them on a shared piece of paper, working either in pairs or in small groups (Figure 10.7).

Our hands are traced on textured paper (e.g., commercially available handmade paper). Alternatively, textured paper can also be made out of scraps found in the studio. Textures can be added through the process of rubbing the paper against various surfaces. Using textures engages the senses, especially touch, which intensifies the sensory experience. Sensory present moments have the potential to successfully compete with any negativity (Kerr, Sacchet, Lazar, Moore, & Jones, 2013). This is because attention is called to present experience, and not focused on past and future thoughts, which are often negative (Segal et al., 2012). Photographs of prehistoric hands, etched into rocks and stones, can also be used to stimulate sensory reactions. An example is a silhouette of a human right hand from the Chauvet Cave near the Ardèche River, France (http://rippleeffects.wordpress.com/2011/11/01/cave-of-forgotten-dreams-2010). Dated from the upper paleolithic period (c. 32,000 years old), the vivid handprint is surrounded by a deep blood-red. When looking at this ancient hand, its sensory qualities may stimulate an urge to stretch out one's own hand, mentally compare the two sizes and shapes, and reach out to the other across time. Group members often attest that they either sensed or felt their own fingers stretching out as they view these projected images. It is a symbolic empathic joining to an ancient man or woman across time. This simple gesture further promotes curious and open-minded wondering about the meaning of such Paleolithic creations. Closer in time are handprints of actors found on the Hollywood strip, which tourists come to visit, and for us, the handprints of our children who are long grown up (Figure 13.4).

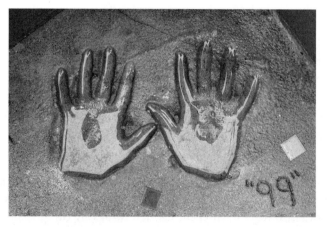

Figure 13.4 *Our Children's Handprints.* Imprinted in the concrete of our courtyard the prints remind me of other times and are daily reminders of love and the laughter of little ones. Noah Hass-Cohen.

Images of imprinted clay, on a wall, or in stone, and the texture and locale comes to symbolize "I sense as you sense," or become even a primitive altar where "You, me, and us" merge across time. In the same manner, group members also often reach out to touch each other's textured creations.

The second change from an ordinary way of implementing this directive is that we ask that the hands are placed in gestures of empathy toward the self and others. As each person is invited to make and decorate silhouettes of both hands, they may outline them together, separately, or engaged in some meaningful gesture. We work together, share materials, and accommodate each other as we stand around the tables. When everyone has finished, participants hold their hand silhouettes up against their chest and circulate around the social milieu, looking for other hand silhouettes with which they feel an empathic resonance. Individuals cluster together, sometimes attracted to each other's work by colors and vibe or the similarity of symbols, such as suns or hearts, or the position of the joined or cupped hands. Then in small groups or one at a time, people step up to a large sheet of butcher paper on the wall and glue their hand silhouettes onto the paper. A spontaneous rhythm takes over as the images of hands cover the wall, creating a tapestry of spread fingers. Some pairs of hands settle close to each other, others spread apart, and others touch. Consequently, this moment becomes a reflective opportunity to step back and consider the collective experience over the last months. The mural can be used to represent a culmination of a creative milieu's journey: From drawing of the initial hand silhouettes to a final celebration. Again, the difference between this and previous hand directives is that we more specifically ask for a recognizable hand gesture that holds the idea of empathy and that we use textured paper.

The therapist's steadying hand, the third hand (Kramer, 1986), is an implicit and explicit conveyor of empathy for which our participants have developed expertise. Our artists have been holding bits and ends of others' art pieces, and the creative space facilitators have helped hold, mend, and carry artwork. When such closeness was unwarranted or contraindicated, we engaged in other implicit ways of conveying our support. Examples include taping the paper to the table while one of our participants was working, providing soft towels to catch clay scraps, and wrapping up the art. The textured hand directive and these kinds of experiential simulations provide additional gateways to others' empathic resonance with emotional states.

As a follow-up, group members pair up for a therapist-client role-play and are asked to intentionally, empathically observe and mirror each other. They are asked to: "Draw a wish or an intention for yourself or for someone else." Role-play therapists are asked to pay attention to how their hands pick up the media and to the specific sounds of the first tentative scratches and the ensuing bold marks on the paper. Role-play therapists note body language on the part of the participant that suggests emotional communication. It is as if they are, together, being transported into the art and its language. Such direct and keen observation gives a felt emotional sense that we are involved in the activities of those we observe (Gallese, 2003). Accordingly, observation of art making is an embodied simulation that contributes to the art therapist's fuller knowledge of the client's inner art processes. For this reason, it is also important to give special attention to the tone of voice accompanying an art directive, as well as the manner in which the role-play therapist requests the artwork's title. Whether or not the client's art is touched, as well as the nature of facial and bodily expressions, conveys a sense of optimism that alleviates distress. Resulting embodied understanding conveyed through the therapist's actions and implicit emotions transfers to the client. The therapist is also asked to make imitative gestures that compassionately support the art maker. Mirrored grasping and creating of the client-artist and therapist transform mere observation. As such, the interpersonal impact of recognizing the mutuality of working together is brought to the forefront.

> *When reflecting upon how using the ATR-N model of empathy promotes MN/MS activations as a crucial element in our experience, I was struck by the manner in which we began our studio art experiences—by watching the Living Museum video. Right from the start, our groups begin to make their own art while seeing psychiatric patient artists making and talking about their art. That moment is often the first one in recognizing the other via their art making.*
> Joanna Clyde Findlay

Experience II: Art Therapy Altars

The Altar experiential is another transformative and integrative ATR-N activity. The guiding instructions are to: "Create an altar to honor and express your journey and that of others." Our discussion evolves around what altars are and what kind of interaction they invite as well as a consideration of the timing of such interactions; daily, weekly, or on anniversaries. Altars are personal and interpersonal spaces that hold meaningful spiritual and religious artifacts. Personally significant, home altars range from religious to nonreligious, as well as the ordinary or more unusual. Examples include a powder room table with perfumes and creams, a special family heirloom china cabinet, Buddhist individual, family, or business shrines, or a spiritual meditation space. People share pictures of actual altars kept at home, such as collections of meaningful objects, photographs, shells, mementos, and treasures from

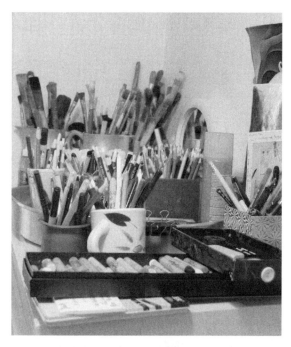

Figure 13.5 *My Personal Art Therapy Altar.* From back to front, a collection of paint brushes, colored pencils, markers, and pastels fill a table top. Noah Hass-Cohen

nature. These assemblies are places offering connections to memories, wishes, or prayers. Some, like Noah, regard the space devoted to their art media as a shrine (Figure 13.5).

Next, studio participants revisit their studio journey and are asked to recall the art, reflections, and shared activities. We may ask them to bring their portfolios to the studio. Whether at home or in the studio, we suggest that they recall using the varied media, remembering their movements in the room, and the group discussions, mindfully regathering their emotions, mentalizing thoughts and feelings, and reflecting in writing.

As they begin sketching ideas for their individual altar, the group members envision and share the symbols, colors, and forms that the idea of an altar suggests. Some will sort through their media boxes, finding fabric, colored paper, collage images, and special objects that they want to use. The discussion sets up a sense of togetherness and empathic anticipation as group members imagine what they and the others will be making at home to bring in the following week. In relation to other people's thoughts and feelings there is a sense of opaqueness, hopefully an absence of worry about performance, and genuine interpersonal interest.

Brought from home, the altars are shared during our last creative milieu meeting. The discussion centers on the interface of private and shared spaces where objects carry meaning in a relational context. Encouraged are reflection, sharing, and dialoging of felt senses and emotions, internal dialogues, and meta-cognitions, which are embodied in altar artifacts. As we witness and share the altars, we find that a process of empathic connectivity ensues. Openness to discovery and forgiveness are generated as we use each other as a predictable secure base (Bowlby, 1988).

We often focus our discussion around some core questions such as: What may the creator of the altar have been thinking? How may the creator see the world? What is she or he trying to convey to others? What feelings does looking at the altar arouse in you? How do you feel in your body when you experience the altar? In what ways do you feel connected to the creator of the altar? What would you like the creator of the altar to know about your experience? For example and remarkably, many in the group responded to the compassionate gift embedded in the symbolism of the brilliant glowing sun, shown in Figure 13.6.

Andrea's reflective golden orb was felt as constant, positive warmth, emanating light and confidence. The sun, which is neither rising nor setting, is fully present, perhaps representing unchanging empathy. Consequently, the altar is seen as bursting with color and texture, expressing richness and creativity. Participants responded that this felt like a celebratory space they could relate to as it expressed a shared journey.

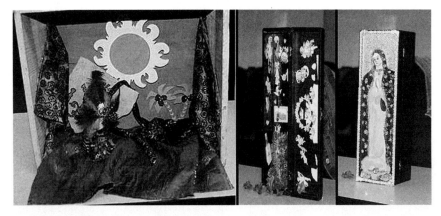

Figure 13.6 *Altar With a Sun.* Andrea Lewis (left). A reflective golden sun on a blue background shines over an exotic multicolored landscape. Textured red curtains frame the scene. The Guadalupe Virgin altar front (center) and back (right), Sylvia Garcia. A luminous yellow Virgin with an intricately decorated dark blue cloak is set on a textured shining golden surface. The rear of the Virgin's box appears like black lacquer with delicate mother-of-pearl decorations.

The second altar, the Guadaloupe Virgin, is enclosed in a box that can be opened, bringing to mind ancient icons and family heirlooms that have been packed away and carried across time. The Virgin Mary is perceived as supportive and loving, as she is in her shrines all across Latin America. A specific Catholic religious and cultural symbol, the Guadaloupe Virgin, in her delicate, intricate gold-decorated box, communicates honor and reverence. Her head, tilted in prayer communicates a kindly, loving, feminine presence. Observing this symbol, participants commented on a felt connection to all those who have sought such aid across time. The box opens and closes, suggesting a vulnerability that invokes softness and empathy. Coming up close to the image, one notices her inclined head, her praying hands that point upward, connecting body and face. Group members recount how the familiar posture invites hand-to-face, face-to-face, and body-to-body correspondence. It is as if at the same time that they are looking at the loving stance, they are experiencing it as well.

The Altar project incorporates shared social understanding, supports intersubjective resonance, and builds an anticipation of interpersonal connectivity. It expands upon the group's familiarity with each other and with therapeutic art making. These correspondences link across the mutual time spent creating together. Face-to-face and body-to-body observations, perceptions, and connections develop familiarity and empathy. Every week, the group has been creating art together, going home, processing their work, and coming back to create more art. Now, they are coming together to share their final creation and say goodbye; a collective goodbye that is also an homage to a collective experience. The ATR-N creative experience has evolved into an embodiment of the empathic shared experience embedded in the art making. Under the right conditions, each person knows what the others experience and feel through the familiarity of doingness.

RELATIONAL NEUROSCIENCE: MIRRORING

Mirroring functions form the neurobiological basis for the experiencing of empathic affiliations. In this section, we describe the neurobiology and function of MN and MS. The psychobiological representation of MN function is most easily revealed in the imitation of actions (Mukamel et al., 2010). In humans, MN are found in the ventral premotor cortex and the inferior parietal lobule (Keysers & Gazzola, 2010). The observer's neurons fire in response to action of another person and may prompt him or her to do what the other does or to have the impression that he or she can do so: "I do what you do; I can do what you do; and I can recognize and anticipate what you will do." Encompassing several neural pathways, and broader in their function, MS extend the understanding of others' physical actions to include the sensorial, emotional, and cognitive experiences. MN are found in MS motor areas and in occipital, temporal, insular, and parietal-visual areas (Rizzolatti & Craighero, 2004). The contagious ensuing MS experience is, "I can sense what you sense; I can feel what you feel; I can plan for what you will do; and I experience what you experience."

This crescendo of interpersonal mirroring leads to knowing the other and, under the right social conditions, contributes to acceptance: "I know and accept you." Knowing and understanding others' actions also has evolutionary and survival-based functions, and thus is not always linked to acceptance, empathy, and compassion. Personal affinity, caring, and MN/MS function provide a platform for empathic connectivity and empathic association will most likely arise when the observed person is familiar.

Mirror Neurons: "I Do What You Do, I Can Do What You Do and I Can Recognize and Anticipate What You Will Do."

A team of Italian researchers discovered mirroring cells when they were studying macaque monkeys' premotor brain cells (Rizzolatti et al., 1996). Such cells fire when macaques plan and carry out motor movements. The surprising finding was that they fired in response to hand-grasping actions performed by humans, even when the macaques were not performing the actions (Rizzolatti et al., 1996). Aptly named mirror neurons, these cells also fired in response to the recognition and anticipation of purposeful and successful actions (Iacoboni & Dapretto, 2006; Figure 13.7).

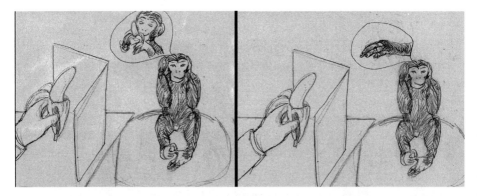

Figure 13.7 *Mirror Neurons in Action.* The cells fire in response when purposeful and/or successful actions are recognized and/or anticipated. On the left, a monkey observes a hand reaching for a banana, and his cells fire as if he is performing the same action. On the right, unable to see the banana ready to eat, the monkey can still anticipate holding the banana. Joanna Clyde Findlay

In the lab, macaque monkeys' MN fired in response to grasping, tearing, and holding familiar objects (Gallese, Gernsbacher, Heyes, & Iacoboni, 2011) and to observing and anticipating hand, mouth, and feet actions. Although with less intensity and frequency, the macaque monkeys' MN also responded to purposeful handling of tools, such as pliers (Ferrari, Rozzi, & Fogassi, 2005). The intensity of the firing response depended on how similar the tool-driven actions were to ones executed by the hand only. An overview of macaque monkey MN single-cell firing further suggests that when the self is engaged, when hands are used with specific grasping motions, and when the purpose of the motion is to eat, MN fire most strongly. These neurons also respond to social lip smacking and to the observation and anticipation of purposeful action, but not to scratching or miming (Iacoboni & Dapretto, 2006).

The neurobiology of the macaque monkey MS starts in the visual system. From there, neurons send information to the superior temporal sulcus (STS) and to an area in the parietal lobe (PF/7B), which in turn transmits information to the ventral premotor area (F5) that activates single-cell MN firing (Keysers & Gazzola, 2006). Thus, monkey imitation and learning rely on motor, temporal, and visual circuitry (Figure 13.8).

In humans, MN also activate in response to doing, seeing, and perceiving recognizable goal-oriented behaviors (Iacoboni & Dapretto, 2006). As in monkeys, imitation, observation, and anticipation of purposeful behaviors, as well as miming, begin early in life. Babies and infants quickly smile, open their mouths, and stick out their tongues in imitation of their caregivers.

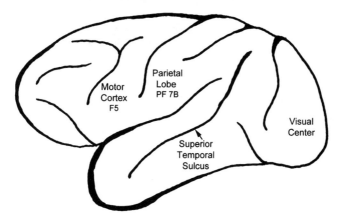

Figure 13.8 *Macaque MN in the Premotor Cortex of the Macaque Monkey.* Mirror neurons (F5) fire in response to actual or anticipated purposeful hand, foot, or mouth actions. MN receive information from parietal area PF/7B, the superior temporal sulcus (STS), and the visual center (Keysers & Gazzola, 2006; Perrett et al., 1984).

Mothers frequently mimic their infants' swallowing motions while feeding them. These interactive MN functions provide a gateway to understanding others' intentions as well as the ability to share common experiences.

Research on humans has shown evidence of MN in the executive area of the brain close to Broca's area that respond to observation. This suggests an evolutionary link to language development (Binkofski & Buccino, 2004; Buccino et al., 2001; Buccino, Binkofski, & Riggio, 2004). Language may have developed from imitation and gesture, using mouth/facial and hand/arm actions, as well as vocalizations (Rizzolatti & Arbib, 1998; Rizzolatti & Craighero, 2004). Perhaps this explains why the manipulation and purposeful grasping of art therapy media are experienced as nonverbal communicative language (Hass-Cohen, 2007). The activation of parallel observer and observed neuron regions facilitates direct self-other experiences of actions, perceived communication, auditory sounds, and intentionality. Because neurons that fire together tend to continue to fire together, MN functions are found in many human neural pathways (Keysers & Gazzola, 2010). Accordingly, research with either monkey or human participants shows that perceived auditory and visual speech, and a wide variety of other bodily actions such as communicative mouth movements, activate MN and MS in the doer of the actions and in the observer (Ferrari, Gallese, Rizzolatti, & Fogassi, 2003; Gallese et al., 2007; Watkins et al., 2003).

Mirror Neuron Systems: "I Can Sense What You Sense, I Can Feel What You Feel, I Can Plan for What You Will Do, and I Experience What You Experience."

In humans, MN/MS and other mirroring brain regions such as the insula fire in response to hand-to-hand, hand-to-face, face-to-face, and body-to-body actual, observed, perceived, and anticipated actions. Mirroring regions also fire in anticipation of communication with a person who is not yet in our visual field (Iacoboni & Dapretto, 2006).

The neurobiology of "I do as you do" and "I can do, understand, and anticipate what you do" is somewhat more complex for humans than for macaque monkeys. In order to infer from the self and from others' purposeful actions, information from the occipital and parietal regions is integrated with information from the temporal lobe. It is then forwarded to the MN found in the motor circuitry close to Broca's area (Buccino et al., 2001; Gallese, Keysers, & Rizzolatti, 2004; Iacoboni & Dapretto, 2006). MN are found in the premotor dorsal cortex, which can simultaneously represent multiple potential movement plans, and near Broca's language center. The presence of human MN near Broca's language center within the inferior frontal gyrus and the premotor ventral cortex correspond to monkey area F5. This location supports ideas that MN have a significant role for communication and language development. More recently, audiovisual MN were identified, supporting this hypothesis (Pineda, 2009). Broca's area responds to both self-produced and externally produced goal-directed movements, but not to visual body cues, and it encodes the motoric aspects of actions.

In parietal areas, the inferior parietal lobe, the intraparietal sulcus, and the superior parietal lobule fire in response to particular goal-oriented movements. The region just below the inferior parietal lobule responds to the use of tools (Naito & Ehrsson, 2006). In other words, motor-spatial information is integrated with visual and emotional inputs and forwarded to areas near the language production center, suggesting the integration of multiple sources of information into human observation, imitation, learning, and execution (Figure 13.9).

For example, it is likely that making art generates motor-spatial information that is integrated with visual and emotional inputs (Battaglia, Lisanby, & Freedberg, 2011). As it is verbalized and shared, the transformation provides the platform for integrative and empathic resonances. Learning and

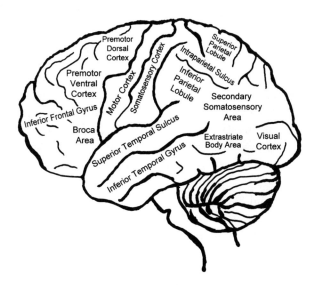

Figure 13.9 *Human Mirror Neuron and Mirror Systems.* Mirroring involves continuous matching between frontal inferences and temporal and parietal visual-motor-spatial processing, which causes MN frontal regions to fire. The frontal PFC areas are the premotor dorsal cortex, the inferior frontal gyrus, and the premotor ventral cortex, which are adjacent to Broca's language center. The temporal area associated with MN functions is the superior temporal sulcus. Parietal areas are the inferior parietal lobule, the intraparietal sulcus, and the superior parietal lobule. Visual processing includes the visual cortex, the secondary somatosensory cortex and the extrastriate body area.

execution are enhanced by imitation and observation, while empathy is enhanced by shared experiences.

Visual perception also involves empathic mirroring of bodily movements. More specifically, the right lateral occipital-temporal cortex has been shown to contain a neural system. Known as the extrastriate body area (EBA), it is specifically dedicated to the visual perception of the body, especially the human body (Downing, Jiang, Shuman, & Kanwisher, 2001). Neuroimaging demonstrates significant activation of MN and MS for body parts in motion as compared to static images of body parts (Buccino et al., 2001; Rizzolatti, Fogassi, & Gallese, 2001). The temporal area involved is the superior temporal sulcus, which responds to upper-limb movement observation. It receives information from the EBA. It is sensitive to inputs from brain regions that participate in the generation of movements and to self-produced movements, even in the absence of visual cues. Therefore, the EBA can differentiate self-produced movements from those produced by others. This is critical for processing the social significance of body-related visual signals in the superior temporal sulcus areas. Looking at moving targets also activates areas in visual processing pathways sensitive to implied movement (Blakemore & Decety, 2001; Kourtzi & Kanwisher, 2000).

Visual perception of static body parts also engages the EBA. The EBA shows a significantly stronger response when people are shown stationary pictures of human bodies and body parts than when they are shown inanimate objects or animal body parts (Downing et al., 2001). The ventral premotor cortex plays a critical role in understanding complete body postures (Urgesi, Moro, Candidi, & Aglioti, 2006). The parahippocampal area, found above the hippocampus, is another significant brain region for what has been called picture response theory (Epstein, Graham, & Downing, 2003; Epstein & Kanwisher, 1998). From an art therapy perspective, it is likely that collage images of bodies contribute to MN function and possibly to an increased sense of intersubjectivty as well as connection.

Neuroimaging further suggests that observing somebody being touched activates the same neural networks in one's own body. The same parts of the somatosensory cortex are activated whether someone is being touched or is watching someone else being touched (Keysers et al., 2004). The somatosensory cortex overlaps an area in the visual cortex that is activated when people view such actions. More specifically, the secondary somatosensory cortex posterior ventral area (S2-PV) also overlaps with the inferior parietal lobe where MNs can be found (Keysers et al., 2004).

Singer and colleagues (2004) discovered an activation of the secondary somatosensory cortex (S2) in an observer when his or her significant other's skin was punctured; the same neurons were activated in both people. More current neuroimaging studies show activation in the anterior insula and selected anterior medial cingulate cortex areas, which also activate in the processing of personal pain (Engen & Singer, 2013). One study showed that witnessing a romantic partner experience a shock activated the same brain regions in the beholder as the participant receiving the painful shock (Bernhardt & Singer, 2012).

Allodynia, or pain caused by a light touch, is thought to be a result of damage to regions of the parietal lobe (Bradshaw & Mattingly, 2001) where MN are located. Sometimes this term is also used for the pain one feels localized in a limb when seeing sudden injury to the same limb of another person. Similarly, viewing painful and traumatic images of bodily damage or mutilation causes neurons in the EBA to fire, creating a felt sense of immediate shock (Oya, Kawasaki, Howard, & Adolphs, 2002). Automatic and noncognitive activations of touch areas in the S2 and the cingulate cortex are very similar to activations seen in the premotor and posterior parietal cortex when we watch the actions of another person (Buccino et al., 2001). The mirroring activations of the same brain areas suggest that this embodied simulation enhances people's understanding of others' tactile experience (Gallese et al., 2007).

The activation and processing of MN/MS is reiterative. Frontal inferences about self and other continuously check for accuracy with ongoing visual, motor, and spatial stimulus processing. From a therapeutic perspective, mirroring and empathic affiliations are processes rather than products. In recognition of this reiterative process, we have purposefully named this chapter "Empathizing" instead of "Empathy." In line with the goals of therapy, the intention is to consistently engage in empathic endeavors. From an art therapy perspective, we wonder how sensory richness and targeted visual, spatial, and motor art-based activities promote such reiterative mirroring and empathy. Since revisiting and remaking multiple seen and felt images is required, the client re-experiences being seen and felt: "I, the therapist, see you, hear you; I sense you and understand you." This sentiment is continuously communicated and affirmed. Client and therapist can arrive at a felt sense that "I can do what the other does" through shared mechanisms. Witnessing, participating in, and anticipating kinetic action such as touching media, activating tools, and incorporating found images of people in movement are some of the processes involved.

The overview of human MN and MS function also suggests the strongest firing in response to purposeful and clear actions in meaningful contexts. In the following section, we review research, which suggested that MN and MS firing is driven more by the perception of goal-oriented actions and of interpersonal contexts than by the motor action itself. For example, when people deliberately or unconsciously mirror others, there is an increase in interpersonal empathic responses, liking, and interest (Chartrand & Bargh, 1999; Niedenthal, Mermillod, Maringer, & Hess, 2010). Thus, MN/MS functionally related brain areas present an embodiment of an ascending crescendo of "I and you" and "You and I" interpersonal metaphors. These include: "I do what you do; I can do what you do; I can recognize and anticipate what you will do; I can sense what you sense; I can feel what you feel; I can plan for what you will do; I experience what you experience; and I know and accept you."

Interpersonal Mirroring: "I Know and Accept You."

The interpersonal function of MN/MS is multifaceted. They are involved in imitation, perceived and anticipated communicative actions (Buccino et al., 2004), processing action-related sentences (Tettamanti et al., 2005), and interpersonal subjectivity (Gallese, 2010). Furthermore, interpersonal mind reading is a phenomenon whereby MN/MS functions enables social interdependence. "The interdependence between self and other that mirror neurons allow shapes the social interactions between people, where the concrete encounter between self and others becomes the shared existential meaning that connects them deeply" (Iacoboni & Dapretto, 2006, p. 265). A supporting interdependence example is how the distress of separation from loved ones activates parallel subcortical regions in both attached individuals (Watt, 2005). Thus, the mirroring of bodily movements and sensations, touching, facial expressions, and emotions sustains empathic interdependence.

Facial mirroring regions play an important role in understanding the correlations between particular emotions and facial expressions (Ekman, 2003). Neurons in the facial fusiform area (FFA) in the right hemisphere of the occipitotemporal cortex respond selectively to human faces. Signals are sent from the visual cortex to the FFA and to the prefrontal cortex, where contextual factors are processed, identified, and interpreted (Ekman, 2003; Kanwisher, 2000; Kanwisher, McDermott, & Chun, 1997; Tong et al., 2000). Moreover, connections between the mirroring and affect-processing brain regions suggest that even before an expression is interpreted, the recognition of facial expressions contributes to the intersubjective experience of empathy (Banissy, Garrido, Kusnir, Walsh, & Ward, 2011).

Babies' brains are also especially receptive to facial expressions, such as buccal muscle movements that involve the cheek, mouth, and tongue (Meltzoff & Moore, 1983). Developmentally, these automatic empathic responses primarily facilitate bonding and attachment, particularly as babies gaze at their caretakers' faces. This observation and contemplation begins to encode a lifetime repertoire for expressing and communicating compassion.

Facial expression interpretation is universal, thus providing the therapist with a shortcut to communicating, "I experience you and I know you." An exquisite form of self-regulation, the act of looking toward and looking away allows the person to self-soothe, much like a mother-baby interaction. Art therapy microskills involve a unique way of using face-to-face experiences. As clients shift their gaze away from the therapist, they focus on the art and have the opportunity to self-regulate in the therapist's presence. Then they can reenter the interpersonal relationship by bringing eye contact back to the interaction and talking about the art. Conversely, a therapist's ability to do this rhythmically and to actively engage in face-to-face communication is a critical clinical skill represented as a sequence: "I see you; I hear you; I feel you; I sense you." This mirroring function is also facilitated by functions of the FFA. This cortical region fires specifically and selectively in response to faces. For example, it sends signals to the amygdala upon the observation of fear-inducing faces. The amygdala then transmits input to the visual cortex and the prefrontal cortices for explicit memory processing (Hass-Cohen & Loya, 2008). Thus we recognize a fearful or sorrowful face and respond empathically to it before cognitive processing even takes place.

MN/MS are also involved in simulated embodiments of emotions. Neural networks activated during first-person, present experiences also activate in empathic experiences (Engen & Singer, 2013). Thus, when observing the emotional states of others, brain networks are activated as if the observer was experiencing these emotions firsthand. An analysis of 16 neuroimaging studies suggested that understanding another's actions evokes cognitive and emotional functions (Gallese et al., 2004). In such mirroring processes, the ACC is involved in the intersubjective simulation of emotion (Brune & Brune-Cohrs, 2006; Gallese et al., 2004; Watt, 2005). The MN/MS are connected to the limbic system via the insula and the amygdala. Moreover, the intersubjective experience of disgust, a visceral-emotional empathic response, is an example of brain structures joining in and acting as emotion-mirroring regions. In fact, the same regions are activated in those who observe others' facial expressions experiencing disgust, as in those actually experiencing the feeling. Neuroimaging reveals such activity in the left insula, the ACC, and the basal ganglia (Wicker et al., 2003). While the amygdala is the emotional center of the brain, the insula and the ACC are also significantly involved in emotional awareness (Bernhardt & Singer, 2012).

It may be possible for people to control their emotional empathic responses. When intentionally taking the perspective of another person, different neural areas were activated depending on relational closeness to the other (Engen & Singer, 2013). Empathy for a loved one showed increased activation in subcortical areas including the anterior insula, middle cingulate, and temporoparietal junction. In contrast, empathy for a stranger led to increased activation in cortical frontal regions (the superior frontal gyrus; Engen & Singer, 2013). This suggests that empathy for strangers is cognitively mediated. Similarly, the inferior frontal gyrus plays a further role in intentional empathy when one tries to identify with another person's affective state that is not consistent with what one is experiencing (Lamm, Meltzoff, & Decety, 2010).

Diminished cognitive empathy is associated with autism and antisocial psychopathy with diminished emotional empathy (Saxe, 2006). Lesions on the vmPFC have been found in individuals with low emotional empathy. Understanding the triadic relationship of the self, the other, and the situation is associated with dorsal medial prefrontal areas (dmPFC). Regions of the MPFC are activated in social cognition with the vmPFC, playing a role in emotional perspective taking such as empathy and sympathy, and the dmPFC in collaboration or the relationships between this triad (Saxe, 2006).

As discussed earlier in this chapter, empathic social responses are connected to the activation of MN/MS (Iacoboni & Dapretto, 2006; Keysers & Gazzola, 2006; Wicker et al., 2003). Regions of the prefrontal cortex, including subcortical limbic areas and other cortical regions, are also involved in social-emotional responses (Watt, 2005). Thus, activation of MN/MS is associated with affect regulation. Affect regulation is the capacity to manage one's emotions when faced with interpersonal-emotional occurrences (Schore, 1994). An expression of relational independence mostly involves cortical dampening of limbic-based emotions. When affect regulation is mediated by mirroring, it contributes to an acceptance of disturbing feelings. For example, empathy arises when the therapist mirrors the distressed person's body posture, tone, or facial expression. A comforting sensation, it is as if they share the same intersubjective space. The therapist becomes the compassionate companion who initiates interpersonal interactions that go beyond the self to include the other. Thus, it is an expression of differentiated interdependence. Notably, the use of art media lends additional opportunities for concrete and felt co-regulation, enhancing the art therapist's emotional ability to safely step into the client's picture. Moreover it is necessary to understand this companionship in a broader social context. Conceptualized as the neuroscience of second-person interactions, ideas that link motor and social functions are at the heart of a debate about MN/MS interpersonal functions (Schilbach et al., 2013). Putting together theory of mind, MN, and mentalizing functions brings together first-person experiences, third-person observations of others' behaviors, and second-person intersubjective worlds.

Findings from neuroimaging studies demonstrate that empathy and self-other perspectives do not involve a full neurological merger with the other (Decety & Lamm, 2006). For example, while watching a loved one experience pain, the same neural circuitry in the observer's brain is activated as in the brain of the person in pain. However, it does not involve the full pain circuitry. Researchers concluded, "only that part of the pain network associated with affective qualities, not sensory qualities, mediates empathy" (Singer et al., 2004, p. 1157). In other words, we feel for another person, but don't actually physically experience the pain. Such intersubjective, empathic reactions may be more fully explored within the context of art therapy. By nature, this framework relies on many aspects of meaningful visual, motor, and sensory processes that reflect MN firing. Once art therapists understand the neurological bases of empathy, they can better grasp the need to actively develop empathic relationships, the importance of therapist self-care, and the risks of secondary trauma for art therapists working with trauma images. Recognizing the empathic toll of witnessing and experiencing violence, abuse, and horror may convey to professionals the depth of their exposure and the necessity for the utmost self-care.

CREATE PRINCIPLES AND CLINICAL APPLICATIONS

The primary focus of the studio activities in this chapter is the CREATE principle of Empathizing and Compassion. However, while the chapter experientials include an ATR-N Altar and a group Hands Cutout mural directive, empathy as an embodied, active relational experience is present throughout this book and in all six CREATE principles. To this end, we have also included hypotheses about the application of the neuroscience of mirroring in this chapter's relational neuroscience section.

As illustrated above, the Creative Embodiment principle is closely linked to the experience of empathy. The function of MN suggests that imitation of purposeful action forms a fundamental neural basis for empathy. The movements, scratches, marks, and smudges inherent in clients' creation of an artwork elicit physical empathy and bodily involvement in the art therapist's response: "I can do what you do." Images of human parts or bodies in actual or implied action engage empathic resonance: "I do what you do." Hence, beginning a therapeutic relationship with a hand individually drawn, or ending group work with a Hands Cutout mural, gives therapists rapid access to an empathic connection. Seeing other group members make art supports the client's creative participation as MN fire in response to anticipated and implied movement. All the studio art making in this book mirrors this understanding. The response is, "I can anticipate what you will be doing." Art therapy gestures facilitate attachment as they echo early infant imitative dyadic learning through reciprocal movement. The mother-child sketches exemplify this understanding embodying a response such as, "I can feel what you might feel." Being together in the therapy room stimulates anticipation of purposeful action and nonverbal social interaction. This anticipation jump-starts an attachment process as client and therapist mirroring supports mutual understanding. Grasping and handling of the media, art tools, and the artwork embodies this process. At the beginning of therapy, clients' MN imitate the therapist's initial actions, such as picking up the crayon box, in anticipation of purposeful action (e.g., the client sees the therapist smudge pastel with fingers and then smudges too).

For the art therapist, MN/MS activation in response to the client reaching for the art media may initiate an exciting opportunity for empathic connectivity. MN/MS research invites art therapists to consider how purposeful use of hand gestures and tools may benefit clinical work. For example, it is likely that the intensity of therapist-client mirroring will depend on the client's familiarity with crayons or paintbrushes in comparison to hand-kneading clay, finger painting, or smearing media. It is also likely that the intensity of client MN firing will increase if the therapist's gestures are purposeful and goal oriented. Therefore, it is critical that art therapists explain the therapeutic goals of art making whenever possible. We hypothesize that under therapeutic conditions, it is likely that as the art therapist hands crayons, brushes, or even a tissue box to the client, his or her MN fire. The same is likely to be true for the therapist, whose MN fire in response to the client's handling and grasping of these objects. Consequently, MN firing is highly sensitive to actual or implied movement. As such, therapists must determine whether handing the tissue box or letting the client pick up tissues enhances empathy or, conversely, threatens safety.

Based upon this information, attending to the number of therapeutic exchanges in the clinical room is fascinating for expressive art therapists. Art therapy, sand tray, and play therapy each engage media grasping, often executed for the purposes of meaningful intentional activity. In anticipation of a therapist's hands purposefully offering soft oil pastels, a client may reach out to take them. Finally, we need to remember that therapists and clients have a mirroring reaction to content transmitted in art. It is therefore likely that empathic responses to simulated pain are foundational to countertransference reactions to the art, especially to complex PTSD art (King-West & Hass-Cohen, 2008). Clients' representation of psychological or physical pain in scratchy sharp lines and haunting PTSD images may arouse similar pain sensations within the therapist.

Most importantly, the discussion of MN/MS and the conceptualization of embodied reactions expand the principle of Creative Embodiment. It is proposed that survival-based movement, recognition of familiar actions, and implied movement form the bases for understanding universal icons, personal symbols, and social relationships. In this chapter, this is incarnated in our altar discussion and offerings. The altar of clients' lives need not be a formal altar. It is the collection of personal items, artifacts, and memories over the life span. The Altar directive merely provides a visual framework that allows for therapeutic exploration and social interaction. We expand more on these ideas in the epilogue.

Art therapy exchanges can foster interpersonal therapeutic empathic experiences key to the principle of Relational Resonating. The art therapist experiences a felt knowing of a client's state through witnessing the art making process and the art product during the dual drawing in Chapter 3. An intersubjective response, "I see you; I feel you," may arise since the dual drawing is a visual concretization of attuned verbal and nonverbal connections. Triggering MN functions, it may create trust and earned-secure attachment interactions. The inherently social nature of a shared art space, seeing others make art, and making art alongside others stimulates imitative change: "You, me, and us." Mutual client-therapist gestures may trigger automatic empathic reactions, which are the first condition for empathy. Examples include clients' hands reaching out to the tissue box, wiping tears from one's eyes, and facial expressions associated with upsetting emotions such as distress and depression. Even the holding of the head, the covering of the mouth, cheek, and face areas, or the anticipation of a client walking in the door may trigger a therapist's empathic response. It is also likely that the more attached the therapist is to his or her client, the more likely it is that he or she will be able to experience these empathic responses. Conversely, symptoms related to MN/MS dysfunction include isolation, lack of empathy, an inability to mentalize and assess another's intentions, and socialization difficulties (Ramachandran & Oberman, 2006). The experiential simulation supported by MN/MS functions can aid communication during crisis when language may be out of reach.

The second condition of empathy is differentiation. If emotional differentiation fails and the therapist cannot explicitly differentiate between his or her selfhood and that of the client, the therapist can become distressed and convey his or her distress personally. Such a contagious response can distract attention from the client's needs and may result in misattunement and may bypass the therapist's prosocial intent to alleviate suffering. This is in contrast to the therapist's ability to evoke secure attachment states as an example of empathic affiliation. We contend that art therapists are uniquely poised to remain empathically close yet separate from the other, as the client is clearly the author of the art product.

The opportunity for empathic connection extends outside the boundaries of the therapy room. Anticipating the felt sense of safety in entering the room is a foundation for relational connection. Clients journal at home and, in the process, anticipate sharing images with the therapist, hearing feedback, and continuing to draw. Making art at home or sharing previously made altars supports empathic bonds and provides access to private contemplative knowledge of another. Witnessing another's sacred place via a three-dimensional altar supports moments of shared episodic, implicit, and explicit memories: "I sense you; I see you; I hear you; I feel you; and I know you." When the therapist reaches to touch the client's page as the session ends and place it in the client's collage folder, the client knows the artwork will be safely stored inside. A feeling of being safely held and heard ensues.

The nonverbal color, sensory, and symbolic qualities of art therapy expression give a direct route to emotional communication that is critical to the affective responses of empathy that are key to the CREATE principle of Expressive Communicating. The therapist witnesses the creative process of the client, his or her movements, mark-making, and reactions, and thereby empathically understands the product through a felt sense of another's distress or happiness. The actual and expected impact of experiencing artwork can give rise to shared emotions, similar to those found in early childhood attuned dyads. Positive emotional states are amplified and negative ones modulated: "I sense you; I see you; I hear you; I feel you; and I know you." The excitation and vitality of expression in an empathic art therapy relationship establishes a feedback loop that supports further emotional investment and an increased expectation of reward in prosocial interpersonal exchanges: "I can sense you; I can see you; I can hear you; I can feel you; and I will know you." The repetitive experiences of attuned, empathic exchanges model the CREATE principle of Adaptive Responding: "I feel and can do what you do."

Imitation and anticipation of purposeful social interaction and verbal communication supports change. Repetitive experiences of attuned, empathic exchanges support improved coping within relationships, as in "I can do what you can do." This can jump-start the confidence to use materials where, for example, a client sees the therapist demonstrate how to handle clay and can imagine handling and expressing herself with clay as well. Similarly, it extends to a sense of potential, as seeing artwork on the studio walls arouses empathy. The client senses the possibility for change through witnessing its resiliency and hope through a response of "I can do what you do." For clients, seeing other clients' artwork on the walls assists in making the assumption, "If other clients made this art, so can I." Thus, the art products convey a culturally mediated understanding of self and other that promotes new possibilities. The role of perception in noncognitive observation suggests that nonpurposeful movements may arouse clients' anticipation of receiving empathic responses. This can include the mere presence of a therapist in the room and anticipation of what he or she will be offering. Empathy is aroused by the clients' art making as the therapist internally feels that he or she could have done what the client has done. Furthermore, when looking at the client's artwork, he or she can also experience what the client experiences. In this context, the art making, the art visuals, and their narratives provide a grand window of opportunity to understand one another deeply. Embedded in shared and empowering excitement, the art therapist and the client share the potential to join empathically as they watch each other's art making process, or engage in art making side by side.

The ATR-N art therapy directives of the last three chapters contribute to mindful awareness of automatic responses, thereby providing more space for empathic responses and supporting the principle of Transformative Integrating. Such neural integration of emotional sharing, meaning bottom-up information processing and linking subcortical awareness with cortical cognitions, contributes to increased awareness, acceptance, and interaction options. At the intersection of attuned attachment, the art therapist and client experience stable states of hope and well-being: "I sense you; I see you; I hear you; I feel you; and I know you."

CHAPTER 14

Reflections on the Love of Art Therapy: An Epilogue on Art, Art Therapy, and Neuroesthetics

Whenever I create, I base my creativity on instinct, on the process and the unfolding of form. It is rare that I have a distinct vision of the final product. Instead, I am free in the making of art and fully aware that along the way little sparks of imagination may invite me to try new forms or add new colors. I trust the process without ever knowing what the final product will be. (In those instances where I have an ounce of vision, the final product is usually more beautiful than the original image.) This is how I define my art. This is how I describe myself. Janine Stuppel

THE ART THERAPY RELATIONAL NEUROBIOLOGY (ATR-N) model, which is mapped by the CREATE principles, emerged from several intentions. One of these focused on understanding how the interpersonal neurobiology of emotion, cognition, and action are expressed in the dynamic interplay of brain and bodily systems during art therapy. The CREATE principles of Creative Embodiment, Relational Resonating, Expressive Communicating, Adaptive Responding, Transformative Integrating, and Empathizing and Compassion were envisioned as an integrative neuroscience-based model for the expressive art therapies (Hass-Cohen, 2008a). Writing this book has allowed us to articulate, develop, and show how to implement these principles. We have illustrated that an integrated, attuned, and regulated state of mind may emerge from novel sensory art making experiences in the therapist's presence. Achieving coherent mind states stabilizes the self and allows for a full empathic experience. As described in Chapter 13, a full empathic and compassionate response must include the motivation to relieve suffering. A fully engaged art therapist committed to this concept expands his or her efforts beyond a mere cognitive understanding of others' affective states. "In human empathy, however, the motivation to relieve suffering can be expressed through an enormously large N [number] of potential behaviors, running the gamut from direct physical rescue from life-threatening danger, to careful listening and reflecting upon the other person's emotional dynamics and history in psychotherapy, and many shades in between" (Watt, 2005, p. 196). Knowing and experiencing these values supports a nurturing relational base for client treatment as well as for therapist self-compassionate care.

Like empathy, self and other compassion emerges from mindfulness. When faced with whatever difficulties life brings with it, a self-compassion response is that of kindness rather than self-criticism. Like impermanence, imperfection is part of the shared human experience. Mindful turning inward and meditation practices assist in the ability to recognize, comprehend, accept, and act upon this understanding (Neff, 2009). Self and other compassion practices are complementary. For some it is easier to start with developing compassion for others. Compassion seems to involve three conditions: kindness, universality, and mindfulness (Neff, 2003). The same biases are often deeply rooted in art therapists' affiliations with those engaged in the arts and the art therapies. It seems that our love of art, art making, and artists can be explained as innately fueled by empathic and compassionate resonances. While love can emerge from compassion, we use the words compassion and love as very close constructs. In our ATR-N case, love means, warm, regulated, or prosocial feelings. In that vein, upholding compassionate interactions and kindness-based loving values are foundational art therapy tenets.

It is the coming together of our first and last principles, Creative Embodiment and Empathizing and Compassion that provides the framework for this conceptualization. Neurobiological activations in response to implied and actual movement, in particular that of mirror neurons and mirroring systems, evoke empathizing compassion, pleasure, and joy. Understanding these mirroring responses embodies and brings to life empathic reactions to art. As this intense writing project comes to its end, we suggest that this empathizing response facilitates and embodies the art therapist's love for art and art therapy. As such, this epilogue mostly focuses on art therapists' empathizing in response to the contemplation of works of art. In addition, it touches upon interactions with fellow art therapists and artists.

Empathizing skills are honed and revisited repeatedly in the art therapist's practice. Furthermore, empathizing, for the art therapist, arises in response to clients, works of art, art therapists and artists, and art making (Table14.1).

In Chapter 13, we discussed the first condition, meaning what arises in the art therapist in response to the client's art and art making. We also looked at what arises in the client in response to the art therapist's materials and the

Table 14.1 Four Conditions for Art Therapists
Empathizing and Joy

1. self of the client, their art, and art-making
2. contemplation of works of art
3. therapist's art-making
4. interactions with fellow art therapists and artists

handling of such materials. For both conditions, it is likely that the anticipation of a full experience of empathy arouses excitation and vitality. Knowing and experiencing that such compassionate experiences are possible is healing, for both the self of the therapist and the self of the client (Badenoch, 2008). These actual and anticipated experiences give rise to positive emotions. Furthermore, the recognition of the fact that such empathic experiences may be available contributes to art therapists' self-compassion, love, and appreciation of their day-to-day work. This is not intended to imply that art therapists must love their clients, love each other, or enjoy the same art. Yet we suggest that shared experiences contribute to mindful, empathic, and compassionate resonance, exciting us about art and art making. In fact, alongside love and joy, empathy and compassion are interactive mind states that are not limited by whom they are offered to, nor bound by specific situations or places. These empathic integrated and attuned states of mind are usually free from personal biases and have the potential to develop into a personal disposition for positivism and equanimity (Siegel, 2012).

Next, this epilogue focuses on art therapists' empathizing in response to the contemplation of works of art as well as touching upon their interactions with fellow art therapists and artists. This empathizing flourishes under "I, you, it" interactions. These kinds of interactions include at least one person, an intention to connect, and objects of mutual attention. Objects of attention range from the concrete, such as art media or symbolic art objects, to the abstract, such as the art therapy profession. An empathic reaction to the art emerges from conscious-cognitive and unconscious-automatic processing of the art object and forms the basis of a loving reaction to the art and to art therapy. The visual processing and sensory perception of salient art characteristics combine with the recognition of their universality. This integration promotes an empathic response. Additional awareness of how art therapy and art making can mitigate suffering reinforces this empathic reaction. Such complex empathic resonances provide a familiar context for social bonding with clients and fellow art therapists. Moreover, for art therapists, beholding art involves emotional and cognitive processing that contributes to an integrated and coherent state of mind, emerging as a satisfactory experience. It is most likely because art is a form of universal knowledge (Ramachandran & Hirstein, 1999). As such, it can be perceived as a constant and true way of knowing. In an impermanent world, such knowing can be very satisfying and pleasurable (Zeki, 1999). Pleasurable states are biologically motivating and arouse feelings of affection, joy, and love for the object or condition being contemplated, in this case art making and art therapy. Promoting equanimity, these mind states stimulate a love for the processes involved.

Neurobiologically, such states are likely activated through the interface of multiple neural pathways, which are discussed at great length in the earlier chapters. Many brain regions have been involved in empathizing and mirroring. The main ones include orbital and association cortices that process visual inputs (Zeki, 1999), the extrastriate body area (Downing et al., 2001), mirror neurons (Rizzolatti et al., 2001), motor areas (Battaglia et al., 2011; Urgesi et al., 2006), the sensory motor strip (Damasio, 2003), reward circuitry (Zeki), the medial prefrontal and anterior cingulate cortex (Gallese et al., 2004), orbitofrontal cortex (Frey & Petrides, 2002), and the insula (Wicker et al, 2003). The functions of these neural networks form the basis for empathic interpretation of the art characteristics and understanding of universal icons, personal symbols, social relationships, and the objective world (Figure 14.1).

Gallese (2003) provides support for how and why mirroring might be involved in empathic responses to inanimate art objects. He describes that as early as 1858, Lotze introduced empathy as a way people are able to put themselves into inanimate works of art. The ability to have a common, mirrored, and shared experience of action forms the basis of seeing the symbolic other as similar to the self and of the intersubjective experience of empathy. It

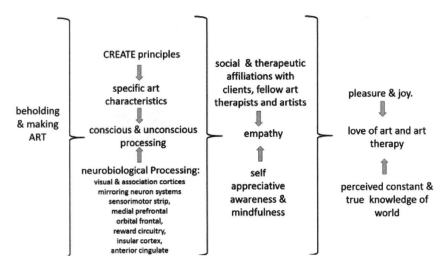

Figure 14.1 Toward the love of art therapy flow chart.

expands the understanding of the mirror neuron system's (MS) function to the following: "I recognize and remember someone else's action as one that I can do and one that I possibly may have experienced or could have experienced and yet am not experiencing right now." Thus, the experience of empathy requires bottom-up and top-down processing in the brain. Bottom-up processing sparks automatic identification with another's experience, while top-down information processing supports emotional self-regulation (Jackson et al., 2005). Additional top-down processing provides for executive prefrontal decisions that generate therapeutic beneficial actions, alleviating suffering (Decety & Lamm, 2006). Moreover, art making engages executive decision-making regions.

CONTEMPLATION OF WORKS OF ART

Conceptually, the sensory and action-based context of CREATE provides a foundation for its functional advantages. Similar ideas were reported in an account of a healing arts exhibit (Hass-Cohen, 2007). At the time, information about MS and mirroring functions, considered central to empathizing functions, inspired a description of art therapists' experiences. Taking advantage of this opportunity, Noah described how, when she actively looked at the *Mater Dolorosa* (Mother of Sorrow) she experienced a felt sense of mirroring (Hass-Cohen, 2007; Figure 14.2).

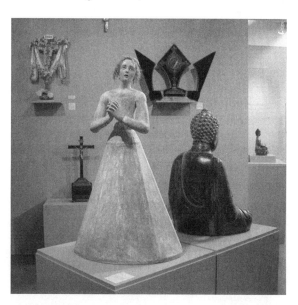

Figure 14.2 *Mater Dolorosa*, Mexico, wood, cloth, and paint. A young woman in a pale blue dress with her fingers interlaced and loosened hair looks upward. Collection of Sarah and John de Heras, courtesy of CAFAM.

Underneath my woolen wrap I found myself holding my hands together and looking up towards the face. The dynamic faded color made it seems as if her arms were moving while at the same time the chipped wooden texture of her skirt brought to mind her creator and raised questions about his motivation, pain, and passion for the arts. I also wanted to touch her whilst going around and around the circular hem of her dress. Her little smaller-than-life size was endearing, and her humanistic appearance in her faded blue chipped wood dress and her stance reminded me of a client. In that instance it was as if I was reaching out to both of them. Contemplating the sculpture, fellow art therapists shared that the embodied figure was bringing to life our learning of mirror neurons. Sharing the joy of a new understanding, we took out pads to create a rendition of the figure or an expressive reaction. Thus, in one situation, I now realized an experience of all four art therapy–based empathy conditions. During that day I encountered other images of Mary or the Madonna that mirrored my implicit memories of wringing my hands as my infant daughter went through ear surgery, of holding my own babies, and of remembered prayers. I also experienced calm as together the images held both sorrow and love and compassion. Regardless of the swirl of coalescing ideas and the emotional contradictions with my Jewish affiliation, being held compassionately took precedence. I have gone back to this image many times over the last few years and even now, as I am recalling the experience, I am finding new meaning and, as I write these words, I find myself saying, "I love this image." Noah Hass-Cohen

The *Mater Dolorosa,* her hands clasped together as if in a praying gesture, the frazzled hair, and uneven sheen all reflect her anguish and distress, which seemed to find a felt resonance in Noah's body. She recalls the *Mater Dolorosa*'s facial expression as the most alluring, her eyes looking up into the sky, simultaneously asking for the alleviation of the pain of her crucified son, as well as that of the world.

There are specific art-based characteristics that support empathic processing. Sensory and emotional experience infuse the beholder's visual processing due to the brain's unique attunement to any actual or implied physical motion within the image, even when the human figure is missing (Freedberg, 2007; Hass-Cohen & Loya, 2008). Foremost is any inclusion of actual recognizable movement. In this case, MS activation most likely supports our felt imitation of the muscular contraction and movement. "The tie-in to mirroring functions and to affect regulation suggests that empathy arises as a direct

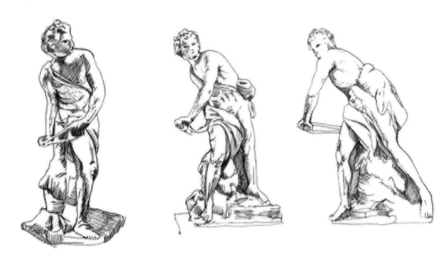

Figure 14.3 *David*, by 17th-century artist Gian Lorenzo Bernini. Illustration, Joanna Clyde Findlay

result of these kinds of observations" (Gallese & Di Dio, 2012). The picture of David by the 17th-century artist Gian Lorenzo Bernini, provides a striking example of these principles (Figure 14.3).

The aptly shown imminent and implied movement convinces us that as David will soon be firing his sling against Goliath. Several factors affect the strength of our reaction to actual or implied movement. The fit between the bodily form and the suggested movement, and the suggestion of a transition from one state to another, is part of it. Together with active viewing on the part of the beholder, these elements affect the ability to project one's own body image onto the work of art and establish a relationship with it (Gallese & Di Dio, 2012). The beholder's bodily involvement and sensory awareness are part of the active viewing of art, which is necessary in order to experience felt emotion. Studies involving observers looking at images that generated strong reactions revealed noteworthy connections. The somatosensory cortex organized itself in the same explicit activity pattern that would result if the observer's body were actually in the state simulated by the reaction to the image (Damasio, 2003), and evoked cortical excitation in brain motor areas (Battaglia et al., 2011). These findings might account for the empathic sensory responses experienced by people looking at intense pictures or paintings, such as a crucifixion scene or the image of a grieving mother. Additional specific examples stem from a picture of gripping hands, increasing corticospinal excitability as contrasted with an image of resting hands, or hands implying completed motions (Urgesi et al., 2006). Still images that imply motion also activate the motor and visual areas (Proverbio, Riva, & Zani, 2009; Urgesi et al., 2006).

Empathy for another person or vicariously experiencing another's affective state also depends on various personal trait factors. People who have problems with identifying and experiencing emotions will find it harder to empathize and be compassionate (Bernhardt & Singer, 2012). The same seems true for those with an insecure attachment style (Mikulincer, Gillath, & Shaver, 2002; Mikulincer & Shaver, 2001). In contrast, those with a strong and acute intuitive understanding of the image may experience a shock response to violent images of bodily harm. This may even be stronger than a response to seeing similar situations in reality, or imagining what they must have been like (Freedberg, 2007). At times, past events may become disturbing to an individual as a result of beholding such images. An example of this is the work of German artist Käthe Kollwitz, a survivor of two world wars. Her work depicted the horrors of both epochs. Her drawing style, which is almost sculptural, conveys a direct and painful impression of the twisting and tortured suffering bodies of mothers, fathers, children, and a nation.

Imagined touch by self, others, animals, or objects may also be empathically shared and felt before any cognitive understanding occurs. The multiple nails piercing Frieda Kahlo's skin in *Cracked Spine* (1994), while a rough metal armature holds her body up, is one such example. Another iconic work is Michelangelo's *The Creation of Adam"* from the Sistine Chapel ceiling, portraying the moment of creation, as God's finger is just about to touch Adam's, bequeathing life to him. In *The Scream* by Edvard Munch (1893), we recognize the gesture of holding the face with two hands, perhaps an attempt to hold in the pain. Similarly, a film example is a thrilling scene of a venomous arachnid spider giving Spiderman his powers. In another compelling example in a film called *For Colored Girls* (2010), we see the horrifying release of touch as the father of two infants that he had been dangling out the window lets go, his hands now open (Hass-Cohen & Chandler-Ziegler, 2013). Imagined touch, whether traumatic or positive, can cause tingling, prickling, or shivering sensations, common in shared empathic reactions (Freedberg, 2007). This reaction might be especially true for art therapists who are trained in fine arts and exposed to images of pain and suffering. It is also possible that even when the depicted body is still, we know that it has the capacity for movement. In addition, regardless of the body's state, the suggestion of body movement signifies a memory of when it was alive and moving. An example is the countless images of the dead Christ, a deceased body that generates an empathic hope for resurrection (Freedberg, 2009b). For Noah, reminders of her teenage clients' outline drawing of the bodies of children slain in the streets by gang members have a similar effect. She recalls hoping that they will come alive again in the haunting imagery. This last example helps clarify that not all distressed responses are empathically or compassionately based. In compassionate responses, the observer's distress is for those that are afflicted by the difficult experience and not centered in the observer's self-hood. Protecting oneself from viewing difficult murder scenes in *For Colored Girls* is quite often a needed response, as it reduces retraumatization. However, such an automatic empathic and self-protective response should not be confused with compassion.

Thus embodied empathizing literally signifies bringing bodily motion to life. Empathic attention is engaged as the MS fires in response to a recognized state of human affairs. This is partially because the activation of the MS also allows for both a general abstract representation of the actions of others and a coding of the intention for the action (Iacoboni & Dapretto, 2006). One's preconceptions about others' feeling states influence the quality of empathy given, similar to emotional regulation processes (Engen & Singer, 2012). Context, as well as relationship to another, also impacts the observer's empathic response. Consequently, imagery that references the human condition, even if abstractly, seems to have a stronger appeal to our compassion. In that manner, compassion is strongly and directly simulated by empathic engagement with facial expressions. We recognize a sorrowful face and respond empathically to it before cognitive processing even takes place (Elkins, 1999). Furthermore, the implicit recognition of faces or body positions may be triggered by the kind of work that the beholder does, or what life role he plays (Duranti, 2010; Freedberg, 2009b). The movement of represented facial expressions, especially those that involve gaze, and the mouth and cheek area, play a critical role in this reaction. People feel a compassionate imitative desire when they see buccal movements, which are movements of the cheek, jaw, and mouth (Freedberg, 2009a). Freedberg uses art examples to explain the variety of these movements. They can initiate anywhere from observing goal-oriented functions, such as grasping or ingesting food, to beholding singers or trumpeting angels blowing air with full cheeks into their instruments. In fact, the observation of buccal movement most likely enhances parallel areas in the brain (Ferrari et al., 2003); the observer's MS fires upon seeing an action, even if their relevant muscles do not move. The open shrieking mouth in Munch's *The Scream* appears to directly evoke both the grimace and the horror of such distress.

The empathic nature of the relationship that is automatically established between artworks and beholders capitalizes on mirroring, somatosensory, and cognitive and emotion-related components (Gallese & Di Dio, 2012). Automatic emotional response to artworks, as well as aesthetic judgment, are involved in these dynamic experiences. Such an evaluation requires the contribution of explicit cognitive appraisal, holistic grouping of the individual's values, knowledge, personal taste, interest in the artwork, prior knowledge, familiarity, and prosocial intent. These processing levels of aesthetic experience are tightly bound, yet not interchangeable. When the experience is enhanced by empathy, it is more likely to be accepted as positive, rewarding, and beautiful. As discussed, the beholder's experience of artworks consists of activating embodied simulation of actions, emotions, and corporeal sensations, which are universal mechanisms (Freedberg & Gallese, 2007).

As illustrated in Noah's reflection on the *Mater Dolorosa*, embodied sensorial intersubjectivity is mediated by universal, cultural, and personal narratives. Our empathic bodily responses provide sensory answers to the universal search for meaningful communication of human expression. An embodied simulation-driven observer response activates through triggering art characteristics and visible marks of the artist's creative gestures. Combined with a personal or culturally driven narrative, this integration of "how" and "what" of the art contributes to full empathy (Gallese & Di Dio, 2012). Examples in the previous chapters include the altars, milagros, *Mater Dolorosa*, and *David*. Simulated embodiment through size and weight of the art can add a powerful three-dimensional invitation to experience the art, suggesting that we move around it or be in it. We imagine our own limbs with the body-sized milagros. In the case of *David*, we are compelled to move around his muscular body in order to fully understand the moment when he will hurl the sling. It is the integration of the biblical story, where the smaller human fights the mighty giant, with the vivid depiction of action that gives rise to a compassionate response. Not limited to a biblical context, the universal phenomenon of the small fighting the mighty does not need to be associated with victory in order to inspire prosocial empathizing. In fact, it can represent a personal experience as well, as in Noah's case. *David*'s chiseled face bears a surprisingly strong resemblance to her teenage boyfriend, who was killed by friendly fire during his Israeli military service; she has carried his and the Bernini image with her throughout her adult life.

Thus the trigger of MS firing in response to art objects, particularly those with implied motion or body parts, is also enhanced by dynamic multisensory qualities of the art: "Multisensory, kinesthetic imagery was far more effective for healing than the flat, strictly visual two-dimensional variety" (Naparstek, 1994, p. 43). Art is a particularly rich field for locating multisensory, kinesthetic imagery, and is a wonderful means for stimulating a diversity of empathic resonances (Hass-Cohen, 2007).

THE LOVE AND JOY OF ART AND ART-MAKING

Regardless of whether one is looking at an art object or a client's or colleague's art, or if one is engaged in the struggles involved in creating, an overarching sense of acceptance, love, and joy arises. These mind states are not just a singular positive emotion or positive experience. Even when we are moved to cry with others and, in fact, cannot help resolve clients' tragedies nor ease their suffering right now, these accepting states can remain stable for therapists. Again, we are not implying that we appreciate and love all works of art equally, but that we have a permanent appreciation for the arts and therapeutic art products.

Positive aesthetic experiences have been associated with activating reward-related brain circuitry (Kawabata & Zeki, 2004). Such joy arises from several factors. One involves a feeling of pleasure from the consistent ability to make sense of the image. It is likely that looking at and experiencing the concrete and unchanging properties of objects provides a sense of consistency and pleasure (Zeki, 1999). This may contribute to a sense of security in finding dependable knowledge about the impermanent reality of the world. Perceptually, active looking gives way to the beholder's and the artist's brain process. At this point, superfluous visual information is eliminated in an effort to epitomize an indisputable, permanent, and tangible character of the art object and our life experience. As a side note, this process may be similar to long-term effects of concentration meditation (Brefczynski-Lewis, Lutz, Schaefer, Levinson, & Davidson, 2007). It is likely that the sitting Tibetan meditator or the sand mandala-making monks hold in their minds all the details of the art. Going back to our discourse, the observer is positioned in the same physical role as the creator, contributing to a strong identification and to marveling at the work. Identification with the artist also leads to an embodied feeling of his or her presence, ultimately connecting people across generations.

In the aforementioned *Mater Dolorosa*, the beholder's attention very quickly focuses on the gripping hands and upward pointing face, grouping them together as having the most salient meaning. Element assembly is a perceptual process that allows the brain to derive pleasure from extracting a figure from the background and ascertaining what is important. The resolution of visual ambiguity, together with the experience of safety, results in a cathartic "Aha" internal exhalation, accompanying our perceptual experience of the world. In the case of the *Mater Dolorosa*, the universality of the conscious or unconscious art enhances this experience. It is as if the beholder's experience moves from subjectivity to objectivity. Universality is furthered by the use of canonical art techniques (Di Dio, Macaluso, & Rizzolatti, 2007) and by the universal understanding of what is beautiful (Ramachandran & Hirstein, 1999). Moreover, Ramachandran's theory emphasizes that representations of human biological characteristics, such as pronounced hips and breasts, which are symbols of procreation, contribute to such rules. When we visit a museum or an art gallery, we do not simply perceive images, but rather contemplate objects whose presence in that specific physical space is justified and determined by their status as artworks (Gallese & Di Dio, 2012). Most certainly contributing to universality, this concept is also cognitively mediated because of several peculiar qualities. Our aesthetic experience is influenced by our museum culture, by the environment in which we were educated, by the aesthetic canons informing our time, and by our level of expertise and familiarity with the artworks we contemplate.

Artists learning from masters' works of art, report a similar reaction as works of art inspire them. When visiting an exhibit of Gustav Klimt drawings, for instance, our colleague, artist Robin Vance, went up close to the images of women and made drawing motions with her hand as if experiencing his hand and their posture and emotional state at the same time. We learn through sympathetic imitation and observation of another's known actions, which leads to identification with the artists and a desire to touch their art. In addition, someone else's actions are recognized as ones that we can do. As described previously, MS function in imitating actions, contributing to our understanding of visceral-emotional meanings from executed and perceived expressions (Gallese, 2003). Both representational and abstract art support the emergence of empathic response, yet it is original art that most strongly stirs these empathic responses (Vartanian & Goel, 2009). We connect with human experience across time and culture via experiencing art. As all client art making is original, this last finding suggests that this is a strength of our field; the original art of therapists and clients contributes to empathic resonance.

For the art therapist-artist, there is yet another layer of empathic connectivity: the recognition "I can make what you, client, or you, artist, make." The anonymous folk artist's hands, paintbrushes, and tools left residual marks on the wooden *Mater Dolorosa*, which can stimulate a longing to pick up a brush and renew the blue hue of her dress. It is as if the observer has a corporeal sense of the artist's movement behind his or her mark making (Freedberg, 2009b). Perhaps this is why many museum visitors want to touch the art. In this context, although Noah knew that she did not create the art, she still longed to be able to touch *Mater Dolorosa* or create something like her. Therein, perhaps, lies the longing of student artists to copy the master artists: not only to be like them, but also to be one with them. These movements involve recruitment of the very same neural structures that would normally be involved in the actual execution of the observed action; neurons in the premotor cortex and inferior parietal lobe fire, just as they would if we were actually engaged in the observed activity (Freedberg & Gallese, 2007). Connecting empathically with the movements, within the images of the artwork as well as with the movements inherent in artwork creation, gives new neurological depth to the common experience of physical empathy and bodily involvement when viewing art. As discussed earlier, compassion can be thought of as an emotional resonance; a recognition that "I have been there"; a self-projection into the past; and a cognitive response that takes the perspective of the other person while remaining differentiated (Jackson et al., 2005). In this context, the art therapist may long to support the image made by the client. This relates to Noah's desire to add a blue, soothing background to the white-on-black silhouettes of the gunned-down gang members. In other instances, we may notice and feel the absence of the human form as we seek it, wondering where it is. The art therapist's movement from observation to action is another route to empathy.

Art therapists' art making supports the development of compassion toward the self. It is in the struggle and joy of the art therapist making his or her own art that we can empathize with a client's process and experience of self-empathy. There is universality in the process of art making that lasts from gestation to completion. For empathic training purposes, it is easiest to start with learning self-compassion. The immediacy of the art process as well as sharing it with others may also support the development of emotional and prosocial empathy. Process art is easy to alter. It is possible to then pause and physically step back from the image or form and feel it, hearing the story it tells, and tell it to another, followed by altering, reworking, and continuing. There may be a need to add color or texture for emotion and meaning, or a need to go over and efface lines to alleviate any painful intensity, or accentuate positivity and growth (Figure 14.4).

Compassion training integrates self-regulation and self-compassion as well as compassion for others (Neff & Germer, 2013). This sequence, developing empathy for self and others, which gives rise to appreciative joy or love of art making, is central to the principle of Transformative Integrating.

For art therapists, there are immediate shared experiences which are based on a presupposed reality of shared encounters with art and art making. When art therapists have interactions and conversations with peers and colleagues, it's like being with soul mates. These biases are often deeply rooted in our affiliation with those engaged in the arts and art therapies. We want to underscore that engagement in art therapies provides not only an opportunity for empathic responses, but also an opportunity to affirm empathy's existence. It provides an opportunity to experience what it means to connect and to be understood. Perhaps one of art therapy's biggest professional assets is the opportunity to repeatedly concretize compassionate exchanges that can directly contribute to the buildup of shared collegial experiences. Without talking, art therapists have an understanding of what it means to make art,

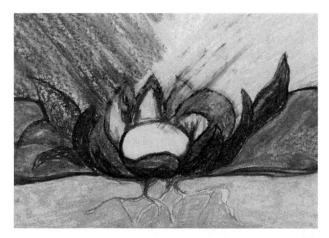

Figure 14.4 *Access to the Whole Source of Well-Being and Self-Kindness.* I found my mind went to plant-like forms, as often I find nature a source for calm and replenishment. I envisioned myself like a precious egg nestled in a lotus-like flower. The egg glows in the light of safety and nurture, held by strong leaves. It receives the warmth of the yellow sun and the blue energy of water and air. The plant's roots dig deep into a rich golden soil, receiving nourishment and strength. Talking with my friend prompted me to shower it with sunshine. We can recognize themes in our own art such as nature or cultural symbols and feel connected to universal experience and to our clients. Compassion for ourselves through the art-making process and symbols extends outward to our clients and our colleagues. Joanna Clyde Findlay

support the art making of clients, and understand the complexities of art that often cannot be verbalized. The arousal of compassion via the observation of art visuals is culturally mediated by process-based expressive art, while the shared social understanding is provided by the sense of intersubjectivity evoked (Figure 14.5).

The ideas discussed in this epilogue are supported by some empirical evidence. Following empathic compassionate training, increased brain activity

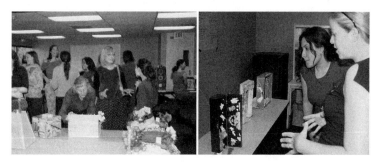

Figure 14.5 *Rich, Sensory Art, in a Relational Context.* This art evokes I-you inferences of motion and I-you experiential simulations of emotion. Zainab Pirbhai, MA, and Margaret McSwain, MA, resonate with the altars. Notice the resonance in body language.

was shown in regions associated with love and affiliation: the medial orbito-frontal cortex, the putamen (a shared motor system-limbic region), middle insula, and reward circuitry, specifically the ventral tegmental area and substantia nigra (Klimecki, Leiberg, Lamm, & Singer, 2012). As art therapists, we have seen and experienced how clients and fellow art therapists experience artwork and art making as a mirroring experience. Table 14.2 provides a summary of art characteristics, as we have discussed, that contribute to empathizing, empathy-based art therapy, and to the love of art and art therapy:

We should not assume that mirroring is the only condition that therapists and clients, especially those with disturbing histories, need in order to be self-compassionate and empathic. Rather, mirroring is a starting point. Under the guidance of the therapist, mirroring can support the development of self-compassion and empathy throughout treatment. This implicit self-compassion training must become an explicit set of therapeutic tools, which then guide toward the development of a compassionate self. Participating in studio art experiences, such as the ones discussed in this book, supports the development of self-compassion and learning how to extend compassion to clients and colleagues.

Table 14.2 Art Based Characteristics that Contribute to Empathizing and Compassionate Responses

- human images of simulated purposeful and/or implied hand, mouth, facial, and body movements
- naturalistic representation of identifiable body positions that we recognize (e.g., bending, lifting, and twisting)
- images of being touched by self or others
- recognizable universal human situations such as the potential for life and movement in a still body representation
- recognizable facial expressions in art, especially in the areas of eyes, mouths, and cheeks
- striking absence of the human form, which causes us to look for it, wondering where it is
- images of universal and cultural experiences
- timeless existence of art objects, which provides a comforting sense of constancy
- concrete characteristics of the artwork, size, weight, and medium, which supports the development of salient meaning in the beholder's mind
- the size and weight of the sculpture, which engages the beholder to move around it, be in it, and touch it
- explicit and implicit art-making marks such as carved wooden notches and the thick paste of paint, which embody how the artist's movements created the artwork
- process art, which focuses on basic emotions: "I identify with your response"
- art content that relates to the expression of suffering or its easing

For many years, we have been privileged to sense how selves enter into self-other relationships through art therapy expressions. It is likely that the experience of actual and anticipated feelings of empathy, which arouse excitation and vitality, evoke prosocial positive emotions. Knowing that such empathic compassionate experiences may be possible is truly healing for the client. It is what makes art therapists love their work. Finally, we have claimed that it is not only the aesthetics but also the experience of empathy toward art that excites and propels people toward art exhibits. Empathy, the embodied image, and the artist evoke the love of art.

Glossary: Relational Neuroscience Key Terms

accidental touch. Unnecessary touching that occurs while accomplishing a task.

acetylcholine (ACh). An excitatory neurotransmitter that supports memory and learning functions. In the central nervous system and the peripheral nervous system motor circuits, it stimulates arousal and attention circuits.

adrenal gland. Endocrine glands above the kidneys responsible for releasing the stress hormones cortisol, epinephrine, and noradrenaline.

adrenaline. See **epinephrine**.

adrenal medulla. At the heart of the adrenal gland, the adrenal medulla secretes epinephrine (adrenaline), norepinephrine (noradrenaline), and a small amount of dopamine in reaction to stress.

adrenocorticotropic hormone (ACTH). During the endocrine system's stress response, the pituitary gland secretes ACTH, stimulating the adrenal glands above the kidneys to secrete cortisol into the bloodstream.

affect. A person's subjective experience of basic emotions.

affect regulation. Higher brain regions dampen mid- and lower-neuropathway reactions. Relational attunement, mindfulness, and self-compassion practices contribute to integration of emotive and cognitive brain centers, as in the case of long-term meditators.

afferent. An afferent nerve transmits sensory information from sense organs toward a processing center in the central nervous system. Afferent refers to the direction of movement inward.

allodynia. A condition in which pain is experienced due to a stimulus that does not usually provoke pain.

allostasis. The process of attaining stability, or homeostasis, through behavioral or physiological change.

Alzheimer's disease. The most widespread form of dementia, which has no cure, and causes progressive degeneration and eventually leads to death. Mindfulness practices may delay aging and degenerative processes.

ambivalent attachment. Adult insecure attachment style in which a person wants relationships but due to anxiety finds relationships challenging.

amygdala. Situated in the limbic system, the amygdala consists of two almond-shaped structures that set off the sympathetic nervous system's stress response. Amygdala reactions play a role in implicit processing of emotion (especially fear) and memory. Also, central nucleus of the amygdala (CEN); dorsal lateral amygdala (D-LA).

anterior. At the front of a designated biological structure.

anterior cingulate cortex (ACC). Located in the cerebral cortex, the ACC mediates affect and mind-body conflicts such as anxiety, connecting the limbic brain with cortical regulation. The ACC helps notice cognitive and emotional processing errors and enables visuospatial and memory processing, reward-based learning, and social awareness. See **cingulate cortex.**

arousal. The stimulation of neural networks or structures and their corresponding functions.

association areas and/or pathways. Circuits in the occipital, parietal, temporal, and frontal regions of the cortex that carry multimodal sensory or motor information to other cortical areas in order to support complex integration functions.

attachment. The predisposition of infant mammals and humans to call on their mothers to establish a safe, secure base of exploration. Patterns of attachment formed establish a model for intimate relationships throughout life.

attachment system. Set of behaviors that allow a person to attain and retain closeness to a differentiated other, in the context of fear, exploration, caregiving, and peer affiliation.

attunement. A term from developmental or attachment theory that points to a person's emotional capacity to identify with another's state of being. Attunement occurs before actual interaction with the other person as well as throughout any subsequent interactions.

auditory cortex. Areas in the temporal lobe that process auditory information from the hearing organs.

autobiographical coherency. A style of narrative about the self that is integrated and accurate.

autobiographical memory. A category of episodic memory that links a sense of one's self to one's past, present, and future.

autobiographical memory functions. The self-function, comprising internal processes of conceptualizing and managing the self; the directive function, guiding present actions and plans for the future; and the social function, which is used to connect and communicate with others.

basal ganglia. Located in the central brain region, these are subcortical structures that provide feedback to the cortex and modify voluntary motor movements. The basal ganglia interface with emotional-motor areas that support flexible emotional function.

basic emotions. These are six emotions: anger, disgust, fear, happiness, sadness, and surprise. They are universally recognized across cultures.

bed nucleus of the stria terminalis (BNST). A site within the hypothalamic-pituitary-adrenal axis. Acute stress and threat monitoring influence its activity.

bottom-up processing. Learning that is based on processing of low-order sensory or emotional features. This is a step-by-step process that leads to higher-order perceptions. See **top-down processing**.

brain stem. Connects the spinal cord with subcortical brain regions. It directs basic involuntary body functions like heart rate and breathing. The brain stem and thalamus co-regulate sensory information coming from the body as well as motor information going out to the body.

Broca's area. An area associated with language processing, speech production, and comprehension in the left frontal lobe.

buccal muscle movements. Movements in the cheeks, which are paired on both sides of the face.

catecholamines. A category of neurotransmitters that includes dopamine, norepinephrine (noradrenaline), and epinephrine (adrenaline).

caudate. A structure within the basal ganglia in the limbic system related to multimodal information processing and inhibition.

central nervous system (CNS). The brain and spinal cord.

central sulcus. A noticeable landmark of the brain, dividing the parietal lobe from the frontal lobe and the primary motor cortex from the primary somatosensory cortex, also called the central fissure.

cerebellum. A brain lobe involved in complex motor movements and procedural learning that evaluates visuospatial signals corresponding to self and/or others' movements. It is situated at the back of the brain beneath the visual cortex, adjacent to and behind the brain stem.

cingulate cortex. A structure in the neocortex located above the corpus callosum that is divided into anterior (front) and posterior (back) sections. Its role is to integrate a multitude of sensory, memory, and executive functions. See **anterior cingulate cortex**.

cingulate gyrus. Included in the limbic system, this structure receives input from the thalamus and the neocortex and is implicated in emotion formation and processing, learning, and memory.

circuitry. Neural pathways that link and enable communication between various structures or regions in the brain and/or the body.

cognitions. Mental processes that incorporate calculating, reasoning, problem solving, and decision making.

complex trauma. A psychological injury due to prolonged exposure to social and/or interpersonal trauma, which culminates in the lack or loss of control, helplessness, and deformations of identity and sense of self.

conditioned stimulus response (CSR). A previously neutral stimulus that ultimately comes to induce a conditioned response.

consolidation. The means by which internalized representations and short-term memories become fixed with preexisting long-term memories.

controlling touch. Touch that attempts to direct behavior, aim for compliance, or request mental or perceptual attention.

co-regulation. Affect regulation that occurs in a relationship.

corpus callosum (CC). A wide band of nerves between the right and left hemispheres that connects and facilitates communication.

cortex. The outer layer of any organ or structure. It often refers to the cerebral or neocortex ("new" cortex), which is the most recently evolved and most human brain structure. See **neocortex.**

cortical. Concerning the cerebral cortex.

corticotropin releasing hormone (CRH). A hormone released by the hypothalamus. CRH sets off the endocrine system's HPA stress response. It excites the pituitary to release adrenocorticotropin (ACTH) into the bloodstream. See **ACTH, stress response.**

cortisol. An endocrine stress hormone discharged from the adrenal gland that aids in stopping the HPA stress response. It moves through the vascular system to the pituitary and hypothalamus, where it stimulates reduced ACTH and CRH secretions. Cortisol increases glucose metabolism, generating additional energy and changes in immune responses. See **ACTH, stress response**.

critical (sensitive) periods. Vulnerable periods of development when biological structures and functions are sensitive to experiential and environmental influences. Such effects can permanently define and change structure and functioning in the brain. See **experience-dependent maturation**.

default mode network (DMN). A brain region that is activated when individuals turn attention inward. Associated with creativity and reflective and divergent thinking.

dementias. A broad category of brain diseases that cause long-term loss of the ability to think and reason clearly that are acute enough to affect a person's day-to-day functioning.

dendritic connectivity. Electrical stimulation from branched projections of the neuron via synapses linking neurons, at various points throughout the dendritic tree.

diencephalon. Transmits sensory information between brain regions and directs many autonomic functions of the peripheral nervous system. It is one of the two divisions of the forebrain including the thalamus, hypothalamus, posterior portion of the pituitary gland, and the pineal gland.

dismissive attachment style. An adult insecure attachment style in which a person seems to avoid attachment and is overly independent and invulnerable to feelings associated with being closely attached to others.

disorganized attachment. An attachment style that shows a lack of clear attachment behavior. In young children, actions and responses to caregivers are often a mix of behaviors including simultaneous approach-avoidance or freezing, which enables a degree of proximity in the face of a frightening or unfathomable caregiver. In adults, it is expressed in obliviousness to relational issues.

dissociation. A large variety of experiences, ranging from mild detachment from immediate surroundings to more severe detachment from physical and emotional experience.

dopamine (DA). A central nervous system neurotransmitter or neuromodulator that is connected to experiences of reward, pleasure, and salience. DA is important in motor functions, motivation, learning, and memory.

dorsal. A descriptor that indicates the upper or top region of a referenced biological structure.

dorsal lateral amygdala (D-LA). Top part of the amygdala that is responsive to a stressor.

dorsal medial prefrontal cortex (dmPFC). Upper front part of the prefrontal cortex involved in planning complex cognitive behavior, personality expression, decision making, and regulating social behavior.

dorsal stream (where-how or parietal stream). Circuitry in the parietal lobe that rapidly integrates vision with action. Enabling rapid reaction to the environment, it is sensitive to motion and implied motion. This visual stream changes its functions to accommodate peripheral information in people with visual impairments.

dorsolateral prefrontal cortex (DLPC). A region in the frontal lobe that coordinates working and contextual memory, focuses attentional processes, directs spatial information, and guides and inhibits behavior based upon left-hemisphere reasoning. It also manages cognitive conflicts, sets goals, makes plans, perseveres, monitors, and self-regulates.

dysregulation. The disruption or stoppage of necessary functions. Dysregulation results in reduced ability to maintain or reestablish homeostatic functioning.

entorhinal area. An area of the brain located in the medial temporal lobe that operates as a hub in an extensive network for memory and navigation.

epinephrine (E) / adrenaline. A neurotransmitter released by sympathetic nerves and the adrenal gland's medulla. Epinephrine mobilizes fight-or-flight responses by accelerating body responses that facilitate emergency functioning while decelerating nonemergency functions. See **short-term stress response, long-term stress response,** and **noradrenaline.**

episodic memory. Long-term mental maps of an individual's experience of past events that are embedded in specific time and context: what, when, how, and where. These memories can be explicit and conscious or implicit and unconscious. See **implicit/nondeclarative memory** and **explicit/declarative memory.**

executive decision making. Associated with verbal and integrated functions such as art making.

experience-dependent maturation. The impact of genes and the environment on developing areas of the brain during critical periods,. Structure, volume, density, and function can be boosted or reduced by environmental impacts only during these times. See **critical periods.**

explicit/declarative memory. Conscious, intentional recall of formerly learned information from past experiences and/or facts for deliberate exposition and task performance.

extrastriate body area (EBA). A lower region of the visual cortex engaged in the visual perception of the human body and body parts.

facial fusiform area (FFA). An area of the human visual system that is implicated specifically in facial recognition.

fear response. A reaction to a threat perceived unconsciously or consciously in the amygdala that triggers a fight, flight, or freeze response.

feedback. A readjustment in a system's response due to supplementary input once the system's response has started (learning or allostatic responses). For example, the pressure needed to work clay will vary due to the resistance felt based upon feedback during the process.

fight-or-flight response. A rapid sympathetic nervous system reaction to threats or stressors. The body is prepared for defense or escape by norepinephrine and epinephrine release.

freeze response. A swift sympathetic nervous and/or polyvagal system reaction to perceived threats or stressors. This actual shutdown of bodily systems, in particular breathing, if persistent, can lead to death.

frontal lobe. The brain's chief executive area in charge of incorporating and integrating perceptual, volitional, cognitive, motor, and emotional processes. The frontal lobe helps plan, coordinate, control, and execute behavior.

fusiform face area (FFA). A region in the temporal cortex near the occipital lobe implicated in color, word, number, and especially face processing (fusiform gyrus). The FFA senses face configurations and similarities. The ventral area is particularly sensitive to familiarity.

glucocorticoids. Discharged by the adrenal gland's cortex in response to serious injury or stressors, these are corticosteroids implicated in fat metabolism, and regulation of blood pressure and inflammation. See **cortisol.**

gray matter. Made up of unmyelinated neurons that surround myelinated neuropathways in the brain and spinal cord. See **myelination.**

gray matter density. Increased connections between unmyelinated neurons that contribute to a heavier and less vulnerable brain. Supports aging and stress-related functioning. Recorded postmortem for people engaged in mental activities, such as higher education.

gustatory areas. Two substructures in the insular lobe and the frontal lobe in charge of the perception of taste.

gyrus/gyri. Ridge(s) on the cerebral cortex generally surrounded by one or more sulci (depressions or furrows). See **sulcus.**

haptic processing. The process of recognition of objects through touch. This involves a mix of somatosensory perception of patterns on the skin's surface (e.g., edges, curvature, and texture) and proprioception of hand position.

hemispheric integration. The balancing of right and left hemispheric functions.

high-road indirect pathway. The slower, more detailed processing of potentially threatening sensory stimuli through the thalamus to cortical areas compared to more immediate low-road responses. See **low-road response.**

hippocampus. Seahorse-shaped limbic structure in the central brain region that is sensitive to stress. It is implicated in spatial navigation, learning, and initiating and consolidating explicit memory processes.

homunculus. The out-of-scale model of a human drawn or sculpted to reflect the relative space human body parts occupy in the somatosensory cortex (sensory homunculus) and the motor cortex (motor homunculus) with such areas as lips and hands emphasized. Displays intramodal neuroplasticity. That is, areas dedicated to feeling amputated limbs are functionally taken over for other human body parts.

hormones. Chemicals produced by glands in the endocrine system to communicate messages through fluid-based systems in the body.

hypothalamic-pituitary-adrenal (HPA) axis. A circuit of endocrine glands that release stress hormones. The HPA axis moderates the nervous, immune, and endocrine management of bodily needs during chronic or recurrent stress. See **hypothalamus, pituitary gland, adrenal gland, CRH, ACTH, and cortisol.**

hypothalamus (HY). A structure in the lower brain that connects nervous system and endocrine functioning, particularly autonomic functions. It strongly influences body functioning during developmental and stress states.

immune system. A protective bodily system that distinguishes organism cells from foreign cells and debris. Innate immune responses provide general defense against invaders. Adaptive immune responses offer specific immune responses to invaders.

implicit emotions. Emotions that are out of conscious awareness.

implicit/nondeclarative memory. Automatic, nondeclarative, or procedural memory, such as used during tasks not requiring conscious recall, like walking or talking. Implicit memories are free of time or place-of-origin markers.

impulse control. The capacity to resist a temptation, urge, or impulse.

inferior parietal lobes. Lower parts of the parietal lobes.

inhibit. The stopping or blocking of activation or functioning in neurons or brain structures.

insecure attachment. An organized or consistent category of attachment. For child attachment styles, this includes resistant-ambivalent anxious and avoidant types; the bond between an adult and infant that is without trust or consistency. The adult or caregiver may fail to respond to the infant's needs. For adults, corresponds to preoccupied and dismissive styles.

instrumental touch. Type of touch that accomplishes a task in itself.

insula or insular cortex. A structure that is responsible for processing interoceptive stimuli and tracking the self and other's ongoing body states. It helps moderate extreme emotions, awareness, and expressions of bodily conditions like pain. Insula function is implicated in theory of mind and empathic functioning.

internal working model (IWM). An internal representation of the outside world and one's own possible actions structured around the accessibility and responsiveness of a caregiver.

interoception. Perception of sensations in one's internal organs.

intraparietal sulcus. This region is implicated in perceptual-motor coordination (e.g., directing eye movements and reaching) and visual attention, and located horizontally on the parietal lobe.

kindling. A neuronal response to a stimulus that augments over time, affecting memory and associated with trauma. Traumatic kindling is suggested to be due to amygdala and hippocampal conditioning. It contributes to flashbacks and passive coping.

kinesthetic. Pertaining to the sensation of bodily position, weight, muscle tension, and movement.

lateral geniculate nucleus (LGN). Region in the thalamus.

lateralization. When either hemisphere specializes in a brain function. For example, most language tasks are lateralized to the left hemisphere.

left hemisphere. The side of the brain dominant in cognitive and language functions, sequential processing, explicit awareness, and conscious functions.

left inferior frontal gyrus. The left lower region of the frontal lobe, commonly known as Broca's area, that is extremely important for language production and verb comprehension.

limbic system. A theoretical, rather than anatomical, term that groups central brain structures that regulate, evaluate, and integrate emotions and sensations into motivational states, survival responses, and memories.

locus coeruleus (LC). A brain stem structure in the reward system, linked to anxiety and fear reactions, that secretes norepinephrine and serotonin.

longitudinal fissure. A cleft down the central surface of the brain that anatomically separates the right cerebral hemisphere from the left. It delineates the boundary between the right and left hemispheres.

long-term (chronic) stress response. A slow, more sustainable endocrine response to threats and stressors. This reaction modifies body functioning so that ongoing stress or survival challenges can be managed. See **hypothalamic-pituitary-adrenal axis.**

long-term memory. A type of memory that retains needed information across time, whereas short-term memory holds less information for a shorter time, up to 20–30 seconds, unless the information is rehearsed.

low-road response (direct path). Potentially threatening sensory stimuli are directed through the thalamus directly to the amygdala, which stimulates the sympathetic nervous system's fight-or-flight reaction. See **high-road response.**

mammalian brain. The second of the three triune brain parts, also known as the limbic system. Humans share this brain with older mammals like dogs, cats, and horses.

medial frontal lobes. Forward sections of the frontal lobes nearest to the midline that separates the hemispheres.

medial prefrontal cortex (MPFC). The forward section of the prefrontal cortex. The core activity of this brain region is considered to be coordination of thoughts and actions according to internal goals.

medial sections of the default mode network. The middle part of a functional neuronal network associated with introspective thought, including activities like rumination, daydreaming, or retrieving memories. This network includes the medial prefrontal cortex and the posterior cingulate cortex, as well as the ventral precuneus and parts of the parietal cortex.

medial temporal lobe. The internal surface of each temporal lobe, which includes the hippocampal area, entorhinal cortex, and amygdala. These conduct multifunctional processing and serve memory functions.

medulla. A structure's central portion, like the adrenal medulla of the adrenal cortex, or the medulla (oblongata) in the brain stem. Autonomic life functions (breathing and blood pressure) and sensory and motor signals are transmitted to higher brain centers via the medulla. The adrenal medullar cortex is associated with the short-term stress response.

mentalization. A coherent, cognitive, and secure emotional foundation for mentalizing and understanding intentions is needed to accurately attribute thoughts, desires, and objectives to others, and to predict or explain their actions.

mentalizing. The capacity to understand the mental state of oneself and others.

mesocortical circuit. A pathway facilitated by dopamine activity that connects the ventral tegmentum to the cerebral cortex, in particular the frontal lobes. It is one of the four principal dopamine pathways in the brain.

mesolimbic dopaminergic projections. Neurons that project to numerous areas of the brain from the mesocorticolimbic dopamine system, widely implicated in the drug and natural reward circuitry of the brain.

metacognition. Knowing how and when to use certain stratagems for learning or problem solving, or thinking about thinking.

midline neuropathways. Associated with the default mode network.

mirror neurons. Triggered when a purposeful task is performed, observed being performed, or viewed as a person's intent. Nonpurposeful actions do not stimulate them.

mirror neuron system. Mechanism of mirror neurons proposed to be central mimicry, imitation, simulation, and perhaps empathy. Situated in the parietal cortex, frontal premotor cortex, and the superior temporal sulcus. The specific region activated depends on what is being observed.

motivation. Internal and external factors that stimulate desire and energy for the pursuit, direction, persistence, and intensity of achieving a goal.

motor strip (primary motor cortex). Forms a thin band along the center of the frontal lobe and contains distinct areas for most body parts. There is a large and direct pathway to the lower motor neurons of the brain stem and spinal cord. Cortical neurons connect from those areas to a specific body part, such as a hand, and direct its action.

motor system. Part of the central nervous system that is involved with movement.

myelination. A thin white layer that develops over neuronal axons as they mature as an outgrowth of glial cells. Myelin enables faster, more efficient communication and distinguishes white matter from gray matter (unmyelinated neurons).

neocortex. The top layer of the cerebral hemispheres. It is involved in higher functions such as sensory perception, precise motor control, spatial reasoning, abstract and rational thought, and, in humans, language.

nervous system. Includes the brain, spinal cord, sensory organs, and all of the nerves that connect these organs with the rest of the body and communicate among its parts.

neurogenesis. The growth of new neurons, either during prenatal development or, in adults, in the hippocampus, a brain structure highly involved in learning as well as explicit and spatial memory.

neuromodulator. A messenger released from a neuron in the central nervous system. It may not be released at synaptic sites, like neurotransmitters. It often acts through second messengers and can produce long-lasting effects.

neuron. The basic building block of the nervous system. It receives information through specialized receptor sites and transmits information to other neurons and cells using electrical impulses and chemical messengers. A typical neuron possesses a cell body (soma), dendrites, and an axon.

neuropeptides. Signaling molecules in the brain that operate as either neurotransmitters or hormones. They can cross the blood-brain barrier and link brain and bodily functions.

neuroplasticity or plasticity. The brain's ability to reorganize itself by forming new neural connections throughout life, observed via an increase, decrease, or change in synaptic connections. It can strengthen, renew, or repair neural networks.

neurotransmitter. A chemical messenger that carries, boosts, and modulates signals between neurons and other cells in the body. It transmits information across a synapse between neurons to communicate.

noradrenaline. See **norepinephrine.**

norepinephrine (NE). A stress hormone central in the maintenance of alertness, drive, and motivation. Noradrenaline is released from the adrenal medulla during the SAM axis from the brain stem's locus coeruleus. Integral to the fight-or-flight response, it directly increases heart rate, triggering the release of glucose from energy stores and increasing blood flow to skeletal muscles. See **short-term stress response, long-term stress response,** and **adrenaline.**

nucleus accumbens. An area at the bottom of the forebrain crucial in pleasure circuitry, including laughter, reward, and reinforcement learning.

occipital face association area (OFA). A facial expression processing area in the visual cortex. The OFA reacts to isolated, inverted, or upright facial parts in images.

occipital lobe. Also called the visual cortex, it is one of the four main lobes or regions of the cerebral cortex. This region receives visual input from the retina, processes it into what we see, and forwards it to other cortical structures for further integration.

olfactory lobes. Creating the sense of smell, they incorporate the forebrain's olfactory bulb, tract, and cortex. Smell stimuli bypass the thalamus and connect directly to the amygdala, thereby rapidly influencing emotional processing.

orbital frontal cortex (OFC). Located toward the bottom rather than the top of prefrontal regions, this region enables individuals to adapt their behavior in response to unexpected rewards or adversities integrating and moderating emotional processes, along with holding and processing of autobiographical memory. The right OFC helps control affective decision-making.

oxytocin (OXY). A chemical messenger in the brain controlling key aspects of the reproductive system, including childbirth, breast-feeding, stress reduction, and aspects of human affiliative and bonding behavior. OXY is secreted in the hypothalamus and released into the blood by the pituitary.

parasympathetic nervous system. A branch of the nervous system responsible for triggering the relaxation response and a sense of well-being.

parietal lobes or cortex. The parietal lobe is one of the four lobes of the neocortex. Located at the back of the head directly under the skull, it assists in the processing of visual images and other forms of sensory, kinesthetic, and proprioceptive input. The parietal lobes enable cohesive complex awareness of one's body-self within the environment.

peripheral nervous system (PNS). Made up of the nerves and ganglia outside of the brain and spinal cord, the PNS includes the autonomic and somatic nervous systems and enables mind-body functions via the central nervous system.

pituitary gland. Connected to the hypothalamus, it is known as the body's master gland, controlling the activity of most other hormone-secreting glands. Hypothalamic releasing factors excite pituitary hormones to circulate and alter the body's glandular functioning. See **ACTH, oxytocin, HPA axis,** and **stress response.**

polyvagal theory. The theory proposes a biological basis or social nervous system based upon phylogenic stage-based activation of the vagus nerve. Social engagement relates to body immobilization, motivation, and social communication. The vagus nerve permits self-soothing, calming, and sympathetic adrenal inhibition.

pons. Area in the brain stem.

positive feedback. An initial change that will bring about additional change in the same direction.

postcentral gyrus. See **somatosensory cortex.**

posterior. A direction descriptor indicating a region toward the back of a designated biological structure.

posterior cingulate cortex. The back of the cingulate cortex region. It activates during emotion and memory retrieval, particularly during autobiographical memory retrieval. See **cingulate cortex.**

precuneus. A structure identified in the default mode network implicated in visual association processing.

prefrontal cortex (PFC). Located in the front of the brain behind the forehead, the PFC is critical in directing executive functions, problem solving, and anticipating impactful events. It helps regulate perceptions, maintain attention, and mediate affect and behavior.

premotor area. Associated with the planning of motor actions; sends information to the motor strip.

preoccupied attachment. An organized insecure adult attachment style. People with this style are anxiously focused on intimacy, approval, and responsiveness from their partners.

proprioception. The sense of knowing where our limbs are in space and the effort needed for movement without having to look.

protoconversation. An adult-infant interaction, made up of words, sounds, and gestures, that attempts to convey meaning before the onset of language in the child.

putamen. A paired round structure situated at the base of the forebrain and one of the nuclei that make up the basal ganglia. Together with the caudate nucleus, it may be referred to as the corpus striatum. The main function of the putamen is to regulate movements and influence various types of learning. It employs dopamine to perform its functions.

pyramidal motor neuronal system. Vertically connects the motor system.

raphe nucleus. Located in the brain stem, these nuclei function to release serotonin in the brain. It is implicated in motivation, affect processing, and slow-wave sleep.

recall. Ability of memory to retrieve events or information from the past, with or without cues.

recognition. The capacity to recognize previously encountered information, external experiences, or other internal representations.

reconsolidation. An updating consolidation that modifies retrieved memory with current information. Perceptions in the present may combine with these internal representations from the past and alter memories each time they are recalled.

regulation. The capacity to constrain or control processes that would otherwise disorganize or interfere with well-being and healthy functioning.

rehearsal. Refers to mental, visual, phonological, and emotional techniques for helping us remember information in order to revive, maintain, or elaborate upon memory or understanding.

relaxation response. A parasympathetic nervous system branch response that changes the physical and emotional reaction to stress.

reptilian lower brain. The third part of the triune brain, which directs temperature control, fight-or-flight fear responses, and defending territory, similar to the brains of reptiles.

reticular activating system (RAS). Consists of several neuronal circuits connecting the brain stem to the cortex, involved in regulating basic functions such as sleep.

retrosplenial cortex (RSC). An important part of a network of brain regions that reinforce a range of cognitive functions, including episodic memory, navigation, imagination, and planning for the future.

reward system. A circuit wherein the cerebral cortex signals the ventral tegmental area of the brain to release the chemical dopamine into the amygdala, the prefrontal cortex, and the nucleus accumbens. This effect regulates and controls behavior by inducing pleasurable results.

right hemisphere (RH). The side of the brain implicated in holistic, nonverbal, and emotional processing; preconscious and visual spatial awareness; feelings and intuitions; and the impact of immediate stress and reactions on the body.

salience. The state or quality by which a stimulus stands out relative to nearby stimuli. Saliency directs attention and learning.

secondary somatosensory area (S2). A second region adjacent to the primary somatosensory cortex (S1). It receives processing instructions from S1.

secure attachment. An organized category of attachment. Young children with secure attachment are visibly upset when their caregivers leave, happy when they return, and seek comfort from caregivers when frightened. In adults, recognized in coherent collaborative discourse and tendency to have trusting, long-term relationships.

selective serotonin reuptake inhibitor (SSRI). Pharmaceutical that allows serotonin, which is a pleasurable neurotransmitter, to stay in the bodily system longer (between the synapses). Widely used as an antidepressant. Approved for post-trauma treatment. See **raphe nucleus.**

semantic memory. Lasting memory for information unrelated to specific episodic events and/or autobiographical memories.

sensorimotor strip. A combined structure of the primary motor cortex and the primary somatosensory cortex.

sensory system. Nervous system structures consisting of neural pathways that receive stimuli from the internal and external environment and conduct this information to parts of the brain such as the thalamus or parietal area for processing. See **afferent neurons.**

serotonin (5-HT). Serotonin is a neurotransmitter found in the digestive tract, the central nervous system, blood platelets, and the pineal gland that generally has a calming effect and produces a sense of well-being. Low levels are linked to depressive and obsessive-compulsive disorders.

short-term (acute) stress response. Rapid fight, flight, or freeze reactions to threats and/or stressors that galvanize the body for instant action. It also shuts down unnecessary bodily functions. See **SAM axis.**

social evaluation. The brain's evolution to continuously be alert and respond to social and relational cues, triggers, and situations.

somatosensory cortex or area (somatosensory strip, SSA). Brain region that acts like a map representing the body for sensory input. It is behind the central sulcus in the parietal lobe.

spinal cord. The principal pathway for information connecting the brain and peripheral nervous system. It is part of the central nervous system protected within the backbone, or vertebral column.

stress response. A stress response is a biological and psychological response experienced on encountering a threat. The goal is to enable survival and a return to normal functioning. See **HPA axis, SAM axis, and amygdala.**

subcortical. Brain regions underneath the cerebral cortex that modify and generate involuntary or automatic functions outside of awareness. Their role reveals adaptations from earlier periods of evolutionary development.

substantia nigra. A brain structure located in the mesencephalon (midbrain) that controls voluntary movement, regulates mood, and produces dopamine.

superior colliculus (SC). A visual reflex center in the midbrain that plays a role in helping orient the head and eyes to all types of sensory stimuli. It localizes attention to quick, peripheral movements, and features of the spatial environment independently of the thalamus.

superior parietal lobule. A region critical for sensorimotor integration and spatial orientation that maintains an internal representation of the body's state. It is located at the upper rear of the parietal lobes.

superior temporal sulcus (STS). A long trench in the temporal lobe that is critical to social competence or theory of mind. It is a junction where visual, somatosensory, and auditory inputs come together. The STS distinguishes salient stimuli and supports facial processing, emotional learning, and deciphering the beliefs and perspectives of other people. The right STS area identifies motion.

sympathetic adrenal medulla (SAM) axis. The SAM response immediately readies the body to cope with survival threats or stressors. The sympathetic nervous system triggers the medulla of the adrenal glands to release adrenaline and noradrenaline.

sympathetic nervous system. One of the major parts of the autonomic nervous system, along with the parasympathetic nervous system. Its overall action is to activate the body's nervous system fight-or-flight response. Nonetheless, it continuously works to maintain homeostasis.

synapse. A small gap separating neurons or a neuron and a muscle or a gland. Neurotransmitters carry nerve impulses across synapses to transfer information and enable continued activation of postsynaptic neurons.

synaptic pruning. Neurological regulatory processes by which extra neurons and synaptic connections are eliminated, bringing changes in neural structure and more efficient synaptic configurations.

temporal-amygdala-orbitofrontal network. A network that among its several functions connects the texture and color of objects with emotions, novelty, and sense of self.

temporal association cortex. Involved in complex perceptual functions and recognition of faces and objects beyond the simple detection of sensory stimuli. In humans the association areas are by far the most developed part of the cerebral cortex.

temporal lobes. Located in the cerebral cortex near the ear, they treat inputs involved in memory and complex visual, auditory, linguistic, emotional, and motivational functions. These functions are key to comprehending language, evaluating interpersonal interactions, deriving meaning, and nonverbal response-oriented activities. The right temporal lobe is linked to nonverbal response-oriented activities in particular.

temporoparietal junction (TPJ). A region where the temporal and parietal lobes meet that integrates information both from the external environment and from within the body. The TPJ helps to distinguish and understand others' beliefs as well as predict their behavior (theory of mind).

thalamus. A pair of egg-shaped structures just above the brain stem between the cerebral cortex and the limbic system. It acts as a sensory gateway and communicates nearly all sensory and motor information between the body/brain stem and cortical/subcortical areas.

theory of mind. The ability to ascribe mental states, desires, intents, and beliefs to other people and the use of these states to explain and predict the actions of those other persons.

top-down processing. Cognitive-driven information processing that regulates subcortical sensory or affect-based, limbic processes. See **bottom-up processing.**

vagus/vagal nerve. The longest cranial nerve, critical to the parasympathetic nervous system, which extends from the brain stem to the abdomen, via various organs including the heart, esophagus, and lungs. Excessive stimulation of the vagus nerve is responsible for slowing the heart rate and causing the freeze response.

vascular system. The blood distribution network made up of arteries, veins, and capillaries.

ventral. A descriptor signifying the lower surface of a biologically designated structure.

ventral medial prefrontal cortex (vMPFC). An area in the prefrontal cortex concerned with the processing of risk and fear reactions, and decision making. It is located in the frontal lobe at the bottom of the cerebral hemispheres.

ventral stream (what or temporal stream). A pathway carrying visual information from the visual cortex to the temporal lobe for object and form vision. This pathway combines shape, color, and significance with object recognition and meaning. It is the connection between the temporal lobe and the limbic system that allows emotion, recognition, and memory to affect the meaning given to visual attributes.

ventral striatum. An area of the striatum that interfaces with motor and limbic structures, considered a reward center.

ventral tegmental area. A group of neurons that are the origin of the dopaminergic cell bodies of the dopamine system or natural reward circuitry of the brain. It is located close to the midline on the floor of the midbrain.

vertical integration. A process by which vertical neural networks integrate, such as the motor system.

visual cortex. Area of neocortex responsible for decoding, encoding, and distribution of visual stimuli. The visual cortex is located in the occipital lobe. See **occipital lobe.**

visual dominance. About 70% of the population process information visually (in comparison to other senses such as touch).

visual system. Central nervous system structures involved in visual perception. Includes two pathways that help integrate visual information in the temporal and frontal lobes. See **dorsal stream, ventral stream.**

Wernicke's area. Located on the left side of the brain in the temporal lobe, it is implicated in the comprehension of language and syntax.

white brain matter. White tissue seen in the brain and spinal cord composed of nerve fibers and the myelin sheath on neurons' axons. See **myelination.**

working memory. The active part of our memory system that temporarily holds and processes information for current tasks.

References

Adler, J. M. (2013). Clients' and therapists' stories about psychotherapy. *Journal of Personality, 81*(6), 595–605.

Adolphs, R. (2004). Emotional vision. *Nature Neuroscience, 7*(11), 1167–1168.

Ainsworth, M. S., Blehar, M. C., & Waters, E. (1978). *Patterns of attachment: A psychological study of the strange situation.* Oxford, U.K.: Lawrence Erlbaum.

Akshomooff, N. A., & Courchesne, E. (1992). A new role for the cerebellum in cognitive operations. *Behavioral Neuroscience, 106*(5), 731–738.

Alexopoulos, G. S. (2005). Depression in the elderly. *Lancet, 365*, 1961–1970.

Allen, G., & Courchesne, E. (2003). Differential effects of developmental cerebellar abnormality on cognitive and motor functions in the cerebellum: An fMRI study of autism. *American Journal of Psychiatry, 160*, 262–273.

Allen, G., Fonagy, P., & Bateman, A. (2008). *Mentalizing in clinical practice.* Washington, DC: American Psychiatric Publishing.

Allen, J. G. (2001). *Traumatic relationships and serious mental disorders.* New York, NY: Wiley.

Allen, J. G. (2005). *Coping with trauma: Hope through understanding* (2nd ed.). Washington, DC: American Psychiatric Publishing.

Allen, J. G. (2006). Mentalizing in practice. In J. G. Allen & P. Fonagy (Eds.), *The handbook of mentalization based treatment* (pp. 3–30). Chichester, U.K.: Wiley.

Allen, J. G. (2012). *Restoring mentalizing in attachment relationships: Treating trauma with plain old therapy.* Washington, DC: American Psychiatric Publishing.

Allen, J. J., Urry, H. L., Hitt, S. K., & Coan, J. A. (2004). The stability of resting frontal electroencephalographic asymmetry in depression. *Psychophysiology, 41*, 269–280.

Allen, J. S., Bruss, J., & Damasio, H. (2005). The aging brain: The cognitive reserve hypothesis and hominid evolution. *American Journal of Human Biology, 17*(6), 673–689.

Allen, P. B. (1995). *Art is a way of knowing: A guide to self-knowledge and spiritual fulfillment through creativity.* Boston, MA: Shambhala.

Allison, K. C., & Friedman, L. S. (2004). Soothing a sensitive gut. *Newsweek, 144*(13), 71.

Alyusheva, A. R., & Nourkova, V. V. (2012). Identity formation and autobiographical memory: Two interrelated concepts of development. *World Academy of Science, Engineering and Technology, 6*, 263–266.

Ammaniti, M., & Gallese, V. (2014). *The birth of intersubjectivity: Psychodynamics, neurobiology, and the self.* New York, NY: Norton.

Ammaniti, M., Gallese, V., & Altman, J. (1969). Autoradiographic and histological studies of postnatal neurogenesis. IV. Cell proliferation and migration in the anterior forebrain, with special reference to persisting neurogenesis in the olfactory bulb. *Journal of Comparative Neurology, 137*(4), 433–457.

American Psychiatric Association. (1994). *Diagnostic and statistical manual of mental disorders* (4th ed.). Arlington, VA: American Psychiatric Publishing.

Amodio, D. M., & Frith, C. D. (2006). Meeting of minds: The medial frontal cortex and social cognition. *Nature Reviews Neuroscience, 7*(4), 268–277.

Andreasen, N. (2011). A journey into chaos: Creativity and the unconscious. *Mens Sana Monographs, 9*(1), 42–53.

Andreasen, N. C. (2005). *The creating brain: The neuroscience of genius*. New York, NY: Dana Press.

APA Presidential Task Force on Evidence-Based Practice. (2006). Evidence-based practice in psychology. *American Psychology, 61*, 271–285.

Appleton, V. (2001). Avenues of hope: Art therapy and the resolution of trauma. *Art Therapy: Journal of the American Art Therapy Association, 18*(1), 6–13.

Ardiel, E. A., & Rankin, C. H. (2010). Importance of touch in development. *Pediatric Child Health, 15*(3), 153–156.

Asen, E., & Fonagy, P. (2012). Mentalization based therapeutic interventions for families. *Journal of Family Therapy, 34*(4), 347–370.

Asplund, C. L., Todd, J. J., Snyder, A. P., & Marois, R. (2010). A central role for the lateral prefrontal cortex in goal-directed and stimulus-driven attention. *Nature Neuroscience, 33*(4), 507–510.

Atchley, R. A., Keeney, M., & Burgess, C. (1999). Cerebral hemispheric mechanisms linking ambiguous word meaning retrieval and creativity. *Brain Cognition, 40,* 479–499.

Bach-y-Rita, P. (1972). *Brain mechanisms in sensory substitution*. New York, NY: Academic Press.

Backos, A. K., & Pagon, B. E. (1999). Finding a voice: Art therapy with female adolescent sexual abuse survivors. *Art Therapy: Journal of the American Art Therapy Association, 16*(3), 126–132.

Badre, D., & D'Esposito, M. (2009). Is the rostro-caudal axis of the frontal lobe hierarchical? *Nature Reviews Neuroscience, 10,* 659–669.

Badre, D., Hoffman, J., Cooney, J. W., & D'Esposito, M. (2009). Hierarchical cognitive control deficits following damage to the human frontal lobe. *Nature Neuroscience, 12*(4), 515–522.

Badenoch, B. (2008). *Being a brain-wise therapist: A practical guide to interpersonal neurobiology*. New York, NY: Norton.

Baer, R. A. (2003). Mindfulness training as a clinical intervention: A conceptual and empirical review. *Clinical Psychology, 10*(2), 125–143.

Baer, R. A. (Ed.). (2006). *Mindfulness-based treatment approaches: Clinician's guide to evidence base and applications*. San Diego, CA: Elsevier.

Baeken, C., Marinazzo, D., Van Schuerbeek, P., Wu, G. R., De Mey, J., Luypaert, R., & De Raedt, R. (2014). Left and right amygdala-mediofrontal cortical functional connectivity is differentially modulated by harm avoidance. *PLoS ONE, 9*(4), e95740.

Baird, B., Smallwood, J., Mrazek, M. D., Kam, J. W. Y., Franklin, M. S., & Schooler, J. W. (2012). Inspired by distraction: Mind wandering facilitates creative incubation. *Psychological Science, 23*(10), 1117–1122.

Baizer, J. S. (2014). Unique features of the human brainstem and cerebellum. *Frontiers of Human Neuroscience, 8,* 202.

Baker, C. I., Dilks, D. D., Peli, E., & Kanwisher, N. (2008). Reorganization of visual processing in macular degeneration: Replication and clues about the role of foveal loss. *Vision Research, 48*(18), 1910–1919.

Bakermans-Kranenburg, M. J., & van IJzendoorn, M. H. (2007). Research review: Genetic vulnerability or differential susceptibility in child development: The case of attachment. *Journal of Child Psychology and Psychiatry, 48*(12), 1160–1173.

Ball, B. (1998). *I, you and the art: The interactive space in art therapy with children* (Doctoral dissertation, New York University, New York, NY).

Baranowsky, A. B., Gentry, J., & Schultz, D. (2010). *Trauma practice: Tools for stabilization and recovery* (2nd exp. and rev. ed.). Cambridge, MA: Hogrefe.

Barlow, D. H. (2002). *Anxiety and its disorders: The nature and treatment of anxiety and panic* (2nd ed.). New York, NY: Guilford.

Barnes, L. L., de Leon, C. F., Wilson, R. S., Bienias, J. L., & Evans, D. A. (2004). Social resources and cognitive decline in a population of older African Americans and whites. *Neurology, 63*(12), 2322–2326.

Barnes, S. J. (1989). *The Rothko Chapel: An act of faith*. Houston, TX: Rothko Chapel.

Barnhofer, T., Crane, C., Hargus, E., Amarasinghe, M., Winder, R., & Williams, J. M. G. (2009). Mindfulness-based cognitive therapy as a treatment for chronic depression: A preliminary study. *Behaviour Research and Therapy, 47*, 366–373.

Baron-Cohen, S., Leslie, A. M., & Frith, U. (1985). Does the autistic child have a "theory of mind"? *Cognition, 21*(1), 37–46.

Barry, R. A., Kochanska, G., & Philibert, R. A. (2008). G × E interaction in the organization of attachment: Mothers' responsiveness as a moderator of children's genotypes. *Journal of Child Psychology and Psychiatry, 49*(12), 1313–1320.

Bat Or, M. (2010). Clay sculpting of mother and child figures encourages mentalization. *The Arts in Psychotherapy, 37*, 319–327.

Bateman, A., & Fonagy, P. (2011). *Handbook of mentalizing in mental health practice*. Washington, DC: American Psychiatric Publishing.

Bateson, G. (1972). *Steps to an ecology of mind: Collected essays in anthropology, psychiatry, evolution, and epistemology*. Chicago, IL: University of Chicago Press.

Bath, H. I. (2008). Calming together: The pathway to self-control. *Reclaiming Children and Youth, 16*(4), 44–46.

Battaglia, F., Lisanby, S. H., & Freedberg, D. (2011). Corticomotor facilitation during observation and imagination of a work of art. *Frontiers in Human Neuroscience, 5*, 1–6.

Bechara, A., Tranel, D., & Damasio, H. (2000). Characterization of the decision-making deficit of patients with ventromedial prefrontal cortex lesions. *Brain, 123*(11), 2189–2202.

Beck, A. T., Rush, A. J., Shaw, B. F., & Emery, G. (1979). *Cognitive therapy of depression*. New York, NY: Guilford.

Beckes, L., & Coan, J. A. (2011). Social baseline theory: The role of social proximity in emotion and economy of action. *Social and Personality Psychology Compass, 5*, 976–988.

Bekinschtein, P., Oomen, C. A., Saksida, L. M., & Bussey, T. J. (2011). Effects of environmental enrichment and voluntary exercise on neurogenesis, learning and memory, and pattern separation: BDNF as a critical variable? *Seminars in Cell and Developmental Biology, 22*(5), 536–542.

Belkofer, C., & Konopka, L. (2008). Conducting art therapy research using quantitative EEG measures. *Art Therapy: Journal of the American Art Therapy Association, 28*(4), 56–63.

Belkofer, C. M., Van Hecke, A. V., & Konopka, L. M. (2014). Effects of drawing on alpha activity: A quantitative EEG study with implications for art therapy. *Art Therapy: Journal of the American Art Therapy Association, 31*(2), 61–68.

Bell, V. (2001). *The executive system and its disorders*. Retrieved from http://www.neuro.spc
.org/vaughan/ExecutiveFunctionLecture.pdf

Benes, F. M., Turtle, M., Khan, Y., & Farol, P. (1994). Myelination of a key relay zone in the
hippocampal formation occurs in the human brain during childhood, adolescence, and
adulthood. *Archives of General Psychiatry, 51*(6), 477.

Benish, S. G., Imel, Z. E., & Wampold, B. E. (2008). The relative efficacy of bona fide psychotherapies for treating posttraumatic stress disorder: A meta-analysis of direct comparisons. *Clinical Psychology Review, 28,* 746–758.

Bernhardt, B. C., & Singer, T. (2012). The neural basis of empathy. *Annual Review of Neuroscience, 35,* 1–23.

Berntsen, D., Willert, M., & Rubin, D. C. (2003). Splintered memories or vivid landmarks?
Qualities and organization of traumatic memories with and without PTSD. *Applied Cognitive Psychology, 17*(6), 675–693.

Berry, D. S., & Hansen, J. S. (1996). Positive affect, negative affect and social interaction.
Journal of Personality and Social Psychology, 71, 796–809.

Beutler, L. E. (2009). Making science matter in clinical practice: Redefining psychotherapy.
Clinical Psychology Science Practice, 6, 301–317.

Binkofski, F., & Buccino, G. (2004). Motor functions of the Broca's region. *Brain and Language, 89,* 362–369.

Bird, A., & Reese, E. (2006). Emotional reminiscing and the development of an autobiographical self. *Developmental Psychology, 42*(4), 613.

Bishop, C. M. (1995). *Neural networks for pattern recognition*. Oxford, U.K.: Clarendon.

Blagov, P. S., & Singer, J. A. (2004). Four dimensions of self-defining memories (specificity,
meaning, content, and affect) and their relationships to self-restraint, distress, and repres-
sive defensiveness. *Journal of Personality, 72*(3), 481–511.

Blakemore, S. J. (2008). The social brain in adolescence. *Nature Reviews Neuroscience, 9*(4),
267–276.

Blakemore, S. J. (2012). Development of the social brain in adolescence. *Journal of the Royal
Society of Medicine, 105*(3), 111–116.

Blakemore, S., & Decety, J. (2001). From the perception of action to the understanding of
intention. *Nature Reviews Neuroscience, 2*(8), 561–567.

Blakemore, S. J., & Choudhury, S. (2006). Development of the adolescent brain: Implications for executive function and social cognition. *Journal of Child Psychology and Psychiatry,
47*(3–4), 296–312.

Blakemore, S. J., den Ouden, H., Choudhury, S., & Frith, U. (2007). Adolescent development of the neural circuitry for thinking about intentions. *Social Cognitive and Affective
Neuroscience, 2*(2), 130–139.

Bluck, S. (2003). Autobiographical memory: Exploring its functions in everyday life. *Memory,
11*(2), 113–123.

Bluck, S., & Alea, N. (2005). The self-reported uses of autobiographical memory. *Social Cognition, 23*(1), 91–117.

Bluck, S., & Alea, N. (2011). Crafting the TALE: Construction of a measure to assess the
functions of autobiographical remembering. *Memory, 19*(5), 470–486.

Bluck, S., Alea, N., Habermas, T., & Rubin, D. C. (2005). A tale of three functions: The self-
reported uses of autobiographical memory. *Social Cognition, 23*(1), 91–117.

Bluck, S., & Habermas, T. (2000). The life story schema. *Motivation and Emotion, 24*(2),
121–147.

Bohart, A. C., & Tallman, K. (1999). *How clients make therapy work: The process of active self-
healing*. Washington, DC: American Psychological Association.

Bohn, A., & Berntsen, D. (2008). Life story development in childhood: The development of life story abilities and the acquisition of cultural life scripts from late middle childhood to adolescence. *Developmental Psychology, 44*(4), 1135.

Bostan, A. C., Dum, R. P., & Strick, P. L. (2010). The basal ganglia communicate with the cerebellum. *Proceedings of the National Academy of Sciences, 107*(18), 8452–8456.

Bowen, S., Witkiewitz, K., Clifasefi, S. L., Grow, G., Chawla, N., Hsu, S. H., Carroll, H. A., Harrop, E., Collins, S. E., Lustyk, M. K., & Larimer, M. E. (2014). Relative efficacy of mindfulness-based relapse prevention, standard relapse prevention, and treatment as usual for substance use disorders: A randomized clinical trial. *JAMA Psychiatry, 71*(5), 547–556.

Bowlby, J. (1988). *A secure base: Parent-child attachment and healthy human development.* New York, NY: Basic Books.

Bowlby, J. (1999). *Attachment: Attachment and loss* (Vol. 1, 2nd ed.). New York, NY: Basic Books.

Bradford, G. K. (2012). On the question of sanity: Buddhist and existential perspectives. *Journal of Transpersonal Psychology, 44*(2), 224–239.

Bradley, M. M., & Lang, P. J. (1999). *Affective norms for English words (ANEW): Stimuli instruction, and affective ratings* (Tech. Rep. C-1). Gainesville, FL: University of Florida, Center for Research in Psychophysiology.

Bradshaw, J. L., & Mattingley, J. B. (2001). Allodynia: A sensory analogue of motor mirror neurons in a hyperaesthetic patient reporting instantaneous discomfort to another's perceived sudden minor injury? *Journal of Neurology, Neurosurgery & Psychiatry, 70*(1), 135–136.

Brady, K. T., Dansky, B. S., Back, S. E., Foa, E. B., & Carroll, K. M. (2001). Exposure therapy in the treatment of PTSD among cocaine-dependent individuals: Preliminary findings. *Journal of Substance Abuse Treatment, 21*(1), 47–54.

Brefczynski-Lewis, J. A., Lutz, A., Schaefer, H. S., Levinson, D. B., & Davidson, R. J. (2007). Neural correlates of attentional expertise in long-term meditation practitioners. *Proceedings of the National Academy of Sciences, 104*(27), 11483–11488.

Bremner, J. D. (2002). *Understanding trauma-related disorders from a mind-body perspective: Does stress damage the brain?* New York, NY: Norton.

Bremner, J. D. (2003). Long-term effects of childhood abuse on brain and neurobiology. *Child and Adolescent Psychiatric Clinics of North America, 12*(2), 271–292.

Bremner, J. D. (2006). The relationship between cognitive and brain changes in posttraumatic stress disorder. *Annals of the New York Academy of Sciences, 1071,* 80–86.

Bressler, S. L., & Menon, V. (2010). Large-scale brain networks in cognition: Emerging methods and principles. *Trends in Cognitive Sciences, 14,* 277–290.

Brett, E. A., & Ostroff, R. (1985). Imagery and posttraumatic stress disorder: An overview. *American Journal of Psychiatry, 142*(4), 417–424.

Brewer, J. A., Mallik, S., Babuscio, T. A., Nich, C., Johnson, H. E., Deleone, C. M., Minnix-Cotton, C. A., Byrne, S. A., Kober, H., Weinstein, A. J., Carroll, K. M., & Rounsaville, B. J. (2011). Mindfulness training for smoking cessation: Results from a randomized controlled trial. *Drug and Alcohol Dependence, 1*(1–2), 72–80.

Brewin, C. R., Andrews, B., & Valentine, J. D. (2000). Meta-analysis of risk factors for posttraumatic stress disorder in trauma-exposed adults. *Journal of Consulting and Clinical Psychology, 68*(5), 748–766.

Brewin, C. R., Gregory, J. D., Lipton, M., & Burgess, N. (2010). Intrusive images in psychological disorders: Characteristics, neural mechanisms, and treatment implications. *Psychological Review, 117*(1), 210–232.

Bridgham, T., & Hass-Cohen, N. (2008). Art therapy and acquired immune deficiency syndrome (AIDS): A relational neuroscience case conceptualization. In N. Hass-Cohen & R. Carr (Eds.), *Art therapy and clinical neuroscience* (pp. 270–281). London, U.K.: Jessica Kingsley.

Briere, J. (2013). Mindfulness, insight, and trauma therapy. In C. K. Germer, R. D. Siegel, & P. R. Fulton (Eds.), *Mindfulness and psychotherapy* (2nd ed., pp. 208–224). New York, NY: Guilford.

Briere, J., & Scott, C. (2012). *Principles of trauma therapy: A guide to symptoms, evaluation, and treatment* (2nd ed.). Thousand Oaks, CA: Sage.

Bringhurst, D. L., Watson, C. W., Miller, S. D., & Duncan, B. L. (2006). The reliability and validity of the Outcome Rating Scale: A replication study of a brief clinical measure. *Journal of Brief Therapy, 5*(1), 23–30.

Brown, C. (2008). Very toxic—handle with care: Some aspects of the maternal function in art therapy. *International Journal of Art Therapy: Inscape, 13*(1), 13–24.

Brown, E. E., Robertson, G. S., & Fibiger, H. C. (1992). Evidence for conditional neuronal activation following exposure to a cocaine-paired environment: Role of forebrain limbic structures. *Neuroscience, 12*(10), 4112–4121.

Bruce, S., & Muhammad, Z. (2009). The development of object permanence in children with intellectual disability, physical disability, autism, and blindness. *International Journal of Disability, Development & Education, 56*(3), 229–246.

Brück, C., Kreifelts, B., & Wildgruber, D. (2011). Emotional voices in context: A neurobiological model of multimodal affective information processing. *Physics of Life Reviews, 8*(4), 383–403.

Brune, M., Brune-Cohrs, U. (2006). Theory of mind: Evolution, ontogeny, brain mechanisms and psychopathology. *Neuroscience and Biobehavioral Reviews, 30,* 437–455.

Buccino, G., Binkofski, F., Fink, G. R., Fadiga, L., Fogassi, L., Gallese, V., Seitz, R. J., Zilles, K., Rizzolatti, G., & Freund, H. J. (2001). Action observation activates premotor and parietal areas in a somatotopic manner: An fMRI study. *European Journal of Neuroscience, 13,* 400–404.

Buccino, G., Lui, F., Canessa, N., Patteri, I., Lagravinese, G., Benuzzi, F., Porro, C., & Rizzolatti, G. (2004). Neural circuits involved in the recognition of actions performed by nonconspecifics: an fMRI study. *Journal of Cognitive Neuroscience, 16*(1), 114–126.

Buckner, R. L., Andrews, J. R., & Schacter, D. L. (2008). The brain's default network: Anatomy, function, and relevance to disease. *Annals of New York Academy of Science, 1124,* 1–38.

Bunge, S. A., & Zelazo, P. D. (2006). A brain-based account of the development of rule use in childhood. *Current Directions in Psychological Science, 15*(3), 118–121. doi:10.1111/j .0963-7214.2006.00419.

Burgess, N., Maguire, E. A., & O'Keefe, J. (2002). The human hippocampus and spatial and episodic memory. *Neuron, 35*(4), 625–641.

Burkitt, E., & Newell, T. (2005). Effects of human figure type on children's use of colour to depict sadness and happiness. *International Journal of Art Therapy: Inscape, 10*(1), 15–22.

Burns, R. C., & Kaufman, S. H. (1970). *Kinetic family drawings (K-F-D): An introduction to understanding children through kinetic drawings.* London, U.K.: Brunner/Mazel.

Burrus, C. (2013). Developmental trajectories of abuse: An hypothesis for the effects of early childhood maltreatment on dorsolateral prefrontal cortical development. *Medical Hypotheses, 81*(5), 826–829.

Buschkuehl, M., Jaeggi, S. M., Hutchison, S., Perrig-Chiello, P., Däpp, C., Müller, M., et al. (2008). Impact of working memory training on memory performance in old-old adults. *Psychological Aging, 23*(4), 743–753.

Bush, G., Luu, P., & Posner, M. (2000). Cognitive and emotional influences in anterior cingulate cortex. *Trends in Cognitive Sciences, 4*(6), 215–222.

Cane, F. (1983). *The artist in each of us.* Craftsbury Common, VT: Art Therapy.

Cannon, W. (1942). Voodoo death. *American Anthropologist, 44,* 169–181.

Carlson, N. R. (2013). *Foundations of behavioral neuroscience* (9th ed.). New York, NY: Pearson Education.

Carlsson, G., Uvebrant, P., Hugdahl, K., Arvidsson, J., Wiklund, L. M., & von Wendt, L. (1994). Verbal and non-verbal function of children with right- versus left-hemiplegic cerebral palsy of pre- and perinatal origin. *Developmental Medicine and Child Neurology, 36,* 503–512. doi:10.1111/j.1469-8749.1994.tb11880

Carmody, J., Baer, R. A., Lykins, E. L. B., & Olendzki, N. (2009). An empirical study of the mechanisms of mindfulness in a mindfulness-based stress reduction program. *Journal of Clinical Psychology, 65*(6), 613–626.

Carr, R. (2008a). Neurotransmitters, neuromodulators and hormones: Putting it all together. In N. Hass-Cohen & R. Carr (Eds.), *Art therapy and clinical neuroscience* (pp. 76–91). London, U.K.: Jessica Kingsley.

Carr, R. (2008b). Sensory processes and responses. In N. Hass-Cohen & R. Carr (Eds.), *Art therapy and clinical neuroscience* (pp. 43–61). London, U.K.: Jessica Kingsley.

Carter, R. (2010). *Mapping the mind* (2nd ed.). Los Angeles, CA: University of California Press.

Carter, R., Aldridge, S., Page, M., & Parker, S. (2009). *The human brain: An illustrated guide to its structure, function and disorders.* London, U.K.: Dorling Kindersley.

Carver, C. S., & Harmon-Jones, E. (2009). Anger is an approach-related affect: Evidence and implications. *Psychological Bulletin, 135*(2), 183–204.

Cassidy, J., & Shaver, P. R. (2010). *Handbook of attachment: Theory, research, and clinical applications* (2nd ed.). New York, NY: Guilford.

Catani, M., Dell'Acqua, F., & de Schotten, M. (2013). A revised limbic system model for memory, emotion and behaviour. *Neuroscience and Biobehavioral Reviews, 37*(8), 1724–1737. doi:10.1016/j.neubiorev.2013.07.001

Cavada, C., Company, T., Tejedor, J., Cruz-Rizzolo, R. J., & Reinoso-Suarez, F. (2000). The anatomical connections of the macaque monkey orbitofrontal cortex. *Cerebral Cortex, 10*(3), 220–242.

Cavanna, A. E., & Trimble, M. R. (2006). The precuneus: A review of its functional anatomy and behavioural correlates. *Brain, 129,* 564–583. doi:10.1093/brain/awl004

Chakravarthy, V. S., Joseph, D., & Bapi, R. S. (2010). What do the basal ganglia do? A modeling perspective. *Biological Cybernetics, 103*(3), 237–253.

Champagne, F., & Meaney, M. J. (2001). Like mother, like daughter: Evidence for non-genomic transmission of parental behavior and stress responsivity. *Progress in Brain Research, 133,* 287–302.

Chandler, M. J., Lalonde, C. E., Sokol, B. W., & Hallett, D. (2003). Personal persistence, identity development, and suicide: A study of Native and Non-native North American adolescents. *Monographs of the Society for Research in Child Development, 68*(2), 2–73.

Chang, F., Mullin, E., Trantham, S., & Surrey, J. (2013). Mindfulness and person centered expressive arts therapies. In L. Rappaport (Ed.), *Mindfulness and the arts therapies: Theory and practice.* London, U.K.: Jessica Kingsley.

Chapman, L. (2014). *Neurobiologically informed trauma therapy with children and adolescents: Understanding mechanisms of change.* New York, NY: Norton.

Chapman, L., Morabito, D., Ladakakos, C., Schreier, H., & Knudson, M. (2001). The effectiveness of art therapy interventions in reducing posttraumatic stress disorder (PTSD) symptoms in pediatric trauma patients. *Art Therapy: Journal of the American Art Therapy Association, 18*(2), 100–104.

Chartrand, T. L., & Bargh, J. A. (1999). The chameleon effect: The perception-behavior link and social interaction. *Journal of Personality and Social Psychology, 76,* 893–910.

Chávez-Eakle, R. A., Graff-Guerrero, A., García-Reyna, J. C., Vaugier, V., & Cruz-Fuentes. C. (2007). Cerebral blood flow associated with creative performance: A comparative study. *Neuroimaging, 38*(3):519–528.

Chilton, G. (2014). *An arts based study of the dynamics of expressing positive emotions within the intersubjective art making process* (Doctoral dissertation, Drexel University, Philadelphia, PA).

Chiron, C., Jambaque, I., Nabbout, R., Lounes, R., Syrota1, A., & Dulac, O. (1997). The right brain hemisphere is dominant in human infants. *Brain, 120*(6), 1057–1065.

Choi, S., & Goo, K. (2012). Holding environment: The effects of group art therapy on mother–child attachment. *Arts in Psychotherapy, 39*(1), 19–24.

Christian, D. (2008). The cortex: Regulation of sensory and emotional experience. In N. Hass-Cohen & R. Carr (Eds.), *Art therapy and clinical neuroscience* (pp. 62–74). London, U.K.: Jessica Kingsley.

Chused, J. F. (2007). Non-verbal communication in psychoanalysis: Commentary on Harrison and Tronick. *Journal of the American Psychoanalytic Association, 55,* 875–882.

Cicione, R. M., Fontaine, L. A., & Williams, C. N. (2002). Trauma relief unlimited: An outcome study of a new treatment method. *Trauma and Loss: Research Interventions, 2*(2), 25–32.

Cirlot, J. E. (1990). *Dictionary of symbols* (2nd ed.). Oxon, U.K.: Routledge.

Clarkin, J. F., & Levy, K. N. (2004). The influence of client variables on psychotherapy. In M. J. Lambert (Ed.), *Bergin and Garfield's handbook of psychotherapy and behavior change* (5th ed., pp. 194–226). New York, NY: Wiley.

Clyde Findlay, J. (2008). Immunity at risk and art therapy. In N. Hass-Cohen & R. Carr (Eds.), *Art therapy and clinical neuroscience* (pp. 207–220). London, U.K.: Jessica Kingsley.

Clyde Findlay, J., Lathan, M. E., & Hass-Cohen, N. (2008). Circles of attachment: Art therapy albums. In N. Hass-Cohen & R. Carr (Eds.), *Art therapy and clinical neuroscience* (pp. 191–205). London, U.K.: Jessica Kingsley.

Coan, J. A. (2010). Adult attachment and the brain. *Journal of Social and Personal Relationships, 27,* 210–217.

Coan, J. A., Schaefer, H. S., & Davidson, R. J. (2006). Lending a hand: Social regulation of the neural response to threat. *Psychological Science, 17,* 1032–1039.

Coates, S. (2006). Preface. In J. G. Allen & P. Fonagy (Eds.), *The handbook of mentalization-based treatment* (pp. xvi–xvii). Chichester, U.K.: Wiley.

Coffman, K. A., Dum, R. P., & Strick, P. L. (2011). Cerebellar vermis is a target of projections from the motor areas in the cerebral cortex. *Proceedings of the National Academy of Sciences, 108*(38), 16068–16073.

Cohen, B., & Cox, C. (1995). *Telling without talking: Art as a window into the world of multiple personality.* New York, NY: Norton.

Cohen, J. A., Mannarino, A. P., & Deblinger, E. (Eds.). (2006). *Treating trauma and traumatic grief in children and adolescents.* New York, NY: Guilford.

Cohen Kadosh, K., Johnson, M. H., Dick, F., Cohen Kadosh, R., & Blakemore, S. J. (2013). Effects of age, task performance, and structural brain development on face processing. *Cerebral Cortex, 23*(7), 1630–1642.

Cohen, M., Granger, S., & Fuller-Thomson, E. (2013). The association between bereavement and biomarkers of inflammation. *Behavior Medicine*. [Epub ahead of print]

Cole, P. M., Teti, L. O., & Zahn-Waxler, C. (2003). Mutual emotion regulation and the stability of conduct problems between preschool and early school age. *Development and Psychopathology, 15*(1), 1–18.

Collignon, O., Dormal, G., Albouy, G., Vandewalle, G., Voss, P., Phillips, C., & Lepore, F. (2013). Impact of blindness onset on the functional organization and the connectivity of the occipital cortex. *Brain, 136*(Pt 9), 2769–2783.

Connors, M. E. (2011). Attachment theory: A "secure base" for psychotherapy integration. *Journal of Psychotherapy Integration, 21*(3), 348–362.

Conway, M. A. (2009). Episodic memories. *Neuropsychologia, 47*(11), 2305–2313.

Conway, M. A., & Pleydell-Pearce, C. W. (2000). The construction of autobiographical memories in the self-memory system. *Psychological Review, 107*(2), 261.

Conway, M. A., Singer, J. A., & Tagini, A. (2004). The self and autobiographical memory: Correspondence and coherence. *Social Cognition, 22*(5), 491–529.

Cook, A., Blaustein, M., Spinazzola, J., & van der Kolk, B. (Eds.). (2003). *Complex trauma in children and adolescents: White paper*. National Child Traumatic Stress Network. Retrieved from http://www.nctsnet.org/nctsn_assets/pdfs/edu_materials/ComplexTrauma_All.pdf

Corrigan, J. D., Selassie, A. W., & Orman, J. A. L. (2010). The epidemiology of traumatic brain injury. *Journal of Head Trauma Rehabilitation, 25*(2), 72–80.

Cosentino, H. (2006). *Healing a cultural exploration: View point, social anthropology*. Los Angeles, CA: Craft and Folk Art Museum Publishers.

Costafreda, S. G., Brammer, M. J., David, A. S., & Fu, C. H. (2008). Predictors of amygdala activation during the processing of emotional stimuli: A meta-analysis of 385 PET and fMRI studies. *Brain Research Reviews, 58*(1), 57–70.

Courtois, C. C., & Ford, B. (Eds.). (2009). *Treating complex traumatic stress disorders*. New York, NY: Guilford.

Cozolino, L. (2010). *The neuroscience of psychotherapy: Healing the social brain* (2nd ed.). New York, NY: Norton.

Cozolino, L. (2013). *The social neuroscience of education: Optimizing attachment and learning in the classroom*. New York, NY: Norton.

Craig, A. D. (2003). Interoception: The sense of the physiological condition of the body. *Current Opinion in Neurobiology, 13*, 500–505.

Crenshaw, D., & Mordock, J. (2005). *A handbook of play therapy with aggressive children*. Lanham, MD: Aronson.

Creswell, J. D., Way, B. M., Eisenberger, N. I., & Lieberman, M. D. (2007). Neural correlates of dispositional mindfulness during affect labeling. *Psychosomatic Medicine, 69*(6), 560–565.

Crone, E. A. (2009). Executive functions in adolescence: Inferences from brain and behavior. *Developmental Science, 12*(6), 825–831.

Cyders, M. A., Burris, J. L., & Carlson, C. R. (2011). Disaggregating the relationship between posttraumatic stress disorder symptom clusters and chronic orofacial pain: Implications for the prediction of health outcomes with PTSD symptom clusters. *Annals of Behavioral Medicine, 41*(1), 1–12. doi:10.1007/s12160-010-9221-5

Dadds, M. R., Bovbjerg, D. H., Redd, W. H., & Cutmore, T. R. (1997). Imagery in human classical conditioning. *Psychological Bulletin, 122*(1), 89–103.

Damasio, A. (2005). *Descartes' error: Emotion, reasoning, and the human brain*. New York, NY: Penguin.

Damasio, A. R. (2003). *Looking for Spinoza: Joy, sorrow and the feeling brain.* Orlando, FL: Heartcourt.

Daniels, J. K., McFarlane, A. C., Bluhm, R. L., Moores, K. A., Clark, C. R., Shaw, M. E., Williamson, P. C., Densmore, M., & Lanius, R. A. (2010). Switching between executive and default mode networks in posttraumatic stress disorder: Alterations in functional connectivity. *Journal of Psychiatry and Neuroscience, 35*(4), 258–266.

D'Argembeau, A., Lardi, C., & Van der Linden, M. (2012). Self-defining future projections: Exploring the identity function of thinking about the future. *Memory, 20*(2), 110–120.

David, P. (1999). *The power of touch: The basis for survival, health, intimacy, and emotional well-being.* Carlsbad, CA: Hay House.

Davidson, R. J. (2004). Well-being and affective style: Neural substrates and biobehavioural correlates. *Philosophical Transactions of the Royal Society B: Biological Sciences, 359*(1449), 1395–1411.

Davidson, R. J., & Begley, S. (2012). *The emotional life of your brain: How its unique patterns affect the way you think, feel, and live, and how you can change them.* New York, NY: Hudson Street.

Davidson, R. J., & McEwen, B. S. (2012). Social influences on neuroplasticity: Stress and interventions to promote well-being. *Nature Neuroscience, 15*(5), 689–695.

Deater-Deckard, K., & Petrill, S. A. (2004). Parent-child dyadic mutuality and child behavior problems: An investigation of gene-environment processes. *Journal of Child Psychology and Psychiatry, 45*(6), 1171–1179.

De Bellis, M. D., Keshavan, M. S., & Shifflett, H. (2002). Brain structures in pediatric maltreatment-related posttraumatic stress disorder: A sociodemographically matched study. *Biological Psychiatry, 52,* 1066–1078.

DeBoard, M. S., Kilian, S. C., Naramor, T. L., & Brown, W. S. (2003). Normal development of bimanual coordination: Visuomotor and interhemispheric contributions. *Developmental Neuropsychology, 23*(3), 399–421.

Decety, J., & Ickes, W. (2011). *The social neuroscience of empathy.* Cambridge, MA: The MIT Press.

Decety, J., & Jackson, P. L. (2004). The functional architecture of human empathy. *Behavioral and Cognitive Neuroscience Reviews, 3*(2), 71–100.

Decety, J., & Lamm, C. (2006). Human empathy through the lens of social neuroscience. *Scientific World Journal, 6,* 1146–1163.

Decety, J., & Michalska, K. (2010). Neurodevelopmental changes in the circuits underlying empathy and sympathy from childhood to adulthood. *Developmental Science 13*(1), 886–899. doi:10.1111/j.1467-7687.2009.00940.x

de Kloet, E. R. (2012). Stress and the hippocampus. In T. Bartsch (Ed.), *The clinical neurobiology of the hippocampus: An integrative view* (p. 77). Oxford, U.K.: Oxford University Press.

de Kloet, E. R., Joels, M., & Holsboer, F. (2005). Stress and the brain: From adaptation to disease. *Nature Reviews Neuroscience, 6*(6), 463–475.

Demaree, H. A., Everhart, D. E., Youngstrom, E. A., & Harrison, D. W. (2005). Brain lateralization of emotional processing: Historical roots and a future incorporating "dominance." *Behavioral and Cognitive Neuroscience Reviews, 4*(1), 3–20.

Demiray, B., & Bluck, S. (2011). The relation of the conceptual self to recent and distant autobiographical memories. *Memory, 19*(8), 975–992.

Deoni, S. C. L., Mercure, E., Blasi, A., Gasston, D., Thomson, A., Johnson, M., Williams, S. C., & Murphy, D. G. M. (2011). Mapping infant brain myelination with magnetic resonance imaging. *Journal of Neuroscience, 31*(2), 784–791.

Diamond, G., Siqueland, L., & Diamond, G. M. (2003). Attachment-based family therapy for depressed adolescents: Programmatic treatment development. *Clinical Child and Family Psychology Review, 6*(2), 107–127.

Diamond, L. M. (2001). Contributions of psychophysiology to research on adult attachment: Review and recommendations. *Personality and Social Psychology Review, 5*, 276–295.

Diamond, M. C., Krech, D., & Rosenzweig, M. R. (1964). The effects of an enriched environment on the histology of the rat cerebral cortex. *Journal of Comparative Neurology, 123*(1), 111–119.

Di Dio, C., Macaluso, E., & Rizzolatti, G. (2007). The golden beauty: Brain response to classical and renaissance sculptures. *PLoS ONE, 2*(11), e1201. doi:10.1371/journal.pone .0001201

Doidge, N. (2007). *The brain that changes itself: Stories of personal triumph from the frontiers of brain science.* New York, NY: Penguin.

Dor-Ziderman, Y., Berkovich-Ohana, A., Glicksohn, J., Goldstein, A., & Eason, C. (2008). Mindfulness-induced selflessness: A MEG neurophenomenological study. *Frontiers of Human Neuroscience, 24*(7), 582.

Downing, P. E., Jiang, Y., Shuman, M., & Kanwisher, N. (2001). A cortical area selective for visual processing of the human body. *Science, 293*(5539), 2470–2473.

Draganski, B., Gaser, C., Busch, V., Schuierer, G., Bogdahn, U., & May, A. (2004). Changes in grey matter induced by training. *Nature, 427*, 311–312.

Draganski, B., Gaser, C., Kempermann, G., Kuhn, H. G., Winkler, J., Buchel, C., & May, A. (2006). Temporal and spatial dynamics of brain structure changes during extensive learning. *Journal of Neuroscience, 26*(23), 6314–6317.

Drago, V., Crucian, G. P., Foster, P. S., Cheong, J., Finney, G. R., Pisani, F., & Heilman, K. M. (2006). Lewy body dementia and creativity: Case report. *Neuropsychologia, 44*, 3011–3015.

Drury, S. S., & Giedd, J. (2009). Inside the adolescent brain. *Journal of the American Academy of Child and Adolescent Psychiatry, 48*(7), 677–678.

Duerden, E. G., Arsalidou, M., Lee, M., & Taylor, M. J. (2013). Lateralization of affective processing in the insula. *Neuroimage, 78*, 159–175.

Duranti, A. D. (2010). Husserl, intersubjectivity and anthropology. *Anthropological Theory, 10*(1), 1–20.

Eason, C. (2008). *Fabulous creatures, mythical monsters, and animal power symbols: A handbook.* Westport, CT: Greenwood.

Ebisch, S. J., Ferri, F., & Gallese, V. (2014). Touching moments: Desire modulates the neural anticipation of active romantic caress. *Frontiers in Behavioral Neuroscience, 8*, 60.

Ehlers, A., & Clark, D. M. (2000). A cognitive model of posttraumatic stress disorder. *Behavior Research and Therapy, 38*, 319–345.

Eisenberger, N. I., Taylor, S. E., Gable, S. L., Hilmert, C. J., & Lieberman, M. D. (2007). Neural pathways link social support to attenuated neuroendocrine stress responses. *NeuroImage, 35*, 1601–1612.

Ekman, P. (1992). An argument for basic emotions. *Cognition and Emotion, 6*, 169–200.

Ekman, P. (1999). Basic emotions. In T. Dalgleish & M. J. Power (Eds.), *Handbook of cognition and emotion*, (pp. 45–60). New York, NY: Wiley.

Ekman, P. (2003). *Emotions revealed: Recognizing faces and feelings to improve communication and emotional life.* New York, NY: Times Books.

Eliot, L. (1999). *What's going on in there? How the brain and mind develop in the first five years of life.* New York, NY: Bantam.

Elkins, J. (1999). *Pictures of the body: Pain and metamorphosis.* Stanford, CA: Stanford University Press.

Elkis-Abuhoff, D. L., Goldblatt, R. B., Gaydos, M., & Corrato, S. (2008). The effects of clay manipulation on somatic dysfunction and emotional distress in Parkinson's patients. *Art Therapy, 25*(2), 122–128.

Elliot, A. (1999). Approach and avoidance motivation and achievement goals. *Educational Psychologist, 34*(3), 169–189.

Elston, G. N. (2003). Cortex, cognition and the cell: New insights into the pyramidal neuron and prefrontal function. *Cerebral Cortex, 13*(11), 1124–1138. Retrieved from http://cercor.oxfordjournals.org/cgi/pmidlookup?view=long&pmid=14576205

Elwert, F., & Christakis, N. A. (2008). The effect of widowhood on mortality by the causes of death of both spouses. *American Journal of Public Health, 98*(11), 2092–2098.

Engen, H., & Singer, T. (2013). Empathy circuits. *Current Opinion in Neurobiology, 23*(2), 275–282.

Epstein, R., Graham, K. S., & Downing, P. E. (2003). Viewpoint-specific scene representations in human parahippocampal cortex. *Neuron, 37*(5), 865–876.

Epstein, R., & Kanwisher, N. (1998). A cortical representation of the local visual environment. *Nature, 392*(6676), 598–601.

Erikson, E. H. (1959). *Identity and the life cycle.* New York, NY: International Universities Press.

Eriksson, P. S., Perfilieva, E., Björk-Eriksson, T., Alborn, A. M., Nordborg, C., Peterson, D. A., & Gage, F. H. (1998). Neurogenesis in the adult human hippocampus. *Nature Medicine, 4*(11), 1313–1317.

Erricker, C. (2011). *Buddhism made simple.* London, U.K.: Hodder Education.

Esch, T., & Stefano, G. B. (2005). The neurobiology of love. *Neuroendocrinology Letters, 3*(26), 175–192.

Euston, D. R., Gruber, A. J., & McNaughton, B. L. (2012). The role of medial prefrontal cortex in memory and decision making. *Neuron, 76*(6), 1057–1070.

Exner, J. E. (1980). But it's only an inkblot. *Journal of Personality Assessment, 44,* 563–576.

Farb, N., Segal, Z. V., & Anderson, A. K. (2013). Mindfulness meditation training alters cortical representations of interoceptive attention. *Social Cognitive and Affective Neuroscience, 8*(1), 15–26.

Ferrari, P. F., Gallese, V., Rizzolatti, G., & Fogassi, L. (2003). Mirror neurons responding to the observation of ingestive and communicative mouth actions in the monkey ventral premotor cortex. *European Journal of Neuroscience, 17*(8), 1703–1714.

Ferrari, P. F., Rozzi, S., & Fogassi, L. J. (2005). Mirror neurons responding to observation of actions made with tools in monkey ventral premotor cortex. *Journal of Cognitive Neuroscience, 17*(2), 212–226.

Field, T. (Ed.). (2004). *Touch and massage in early child development.* Calverton, NY: Johnson and Johnson Pediatric Institute.

Fish, B. (2012). Art Response art: The art of the art therapist. *Art Therapy: Journal of the American Art Therapy Association, 29*(3), 138–143.

Fivush, R. (2007). Maternal reminiscing style and children's developing understanding of self and emotion. *Clinical Social Work, 35,* 37–46.

Fivush, R. (2011). The development of autobiographical memory. *Annual Reviews of Psychology, 62,* 559–582.

Fivush, R., Habermas, T., Waters, T. E., & Zaman, W. (2011). The making of autobiographical memory: Intersections of culture, narratives and identity. *International Journal of Psychology, 46*(5), 321–345.

Fivush, R., Haden, C. A., & Reese, E. (2006). Elaborating on elaborations: Maternal reminiscing style and children's socio-emotional outcome. *Child Development, 77*, 1568–1588.

Fjorback, L. O., Arendt, M., Ornbol, E., Fink, P., & Walach, H. (2011). Mindfulness-based stress reduction and mindfulness-based cognitive therapy—a systematic review of randomized controlled trials. *Acta Psychiatrica Scandinavica, 124*(2), 102–119.

Foa, E. B., Keane, T. M., Friedman, M. J., & Cohen, J. A. (Eds.). (2009). *Effective treatments for PTSD: Practice guidelines from the International Society for Traumatic Stress Studies* (2nd ed.). New York, NY: Guilford.

Fogassi, L., Ferrari, P. F., Gesierich, B., Rozzo, S., Chersi, F., & Rizzolatti, G. (2005). Parietal lobe: From action organization to intention understanding. *Science, 308*(5722), 662–667.

Fogel, A., & Garvey, A. (2007). Alive communication. *Infant Behavior and Development, 30*, 251–257.

Foley, E., Baillie, A., Huxter, M., Price, M., & Sinclair, E. (2010). Mindfulness-based cognitive therapy for individuals whose lives have been affected by cancer: A randomized controlled trial. *Journal of Counseling and Clinical Psychology, 78*(1), 72–79.

Follmer, G., Sun, S., Bunnell, S. L., & Lindboe, K. (2013). Making sense of traumatic memories: Memory qualities and psychological symptoms in emerging adults with and without abuse histories. *Memory, 21*(1), 125–142.

Fonagy, P., & Bateman, A. (2004). *Psychotherapy for borderline personality disorder: Mentalization-based treatment.* Oxford, U.K.: Oxford University Press.

Fonagy, P., Gergely, G., Jurist, E., & Target, M. (Eds.). (2005). *Affect regulation, mentalization, and the development of self.* London, U.K.: H. Karnac.

Fonagy, P., & Target, M. (1997). Attachment and reflective function: Their role in self organization. *Development and Psychopathology, 9*, 679–700.

Fonagy, P., & Target, M. (1998). Mentalization and the changing aims of child psychoanalysis. *Psychoanalytic Dialogues, 8*(1), 87–114.

Ford, J. D. (2009). Neurobiological and developmental research: Clinical implications. In C. Courtois & J. Ford (Eds.), *Treating complex traumatic stress disorders: An evidence-based guide* (pp. 31–58). New York, NY: Guilford.

Ford, J. D., Racusin, R., Ellis, C. G., Daviss, W. B., Reiser, J., Fleischer, A., & Thomas, J. (2000). Child maltreatment, other trauma exposure, and posttraumatic symptomatology among children with oppositional defiant and attention deficit hyperactivity disorder. *Child Maltreatment, 5*(3), 205–217.

Fox, M. D., Corbetta, M., Snyder, A. Z., Vincent, J. L., & Raichle, M. E. (2006). Spontaneous neuronal activity distinguishes human dorsal and ventral attention systems. *Proceedings of the National Academy of Sciences, 103*, 10046–10051.

Fox, S. E., Levitt, P., & Nelson III, C. A. (2010). How the timing and quality of early experiences influence the development of brain architecture. *Child Development, 81*(1), 28–40.

Frank, J. D., & Frank, J. B. (1993). *Persuasion and healing: A comparative study of psychotherapy* (3rd ed.). Baltimore, MD: Johns Hopkins University Press.

Frank, J. D., & Frank, J. B. (2004). Therapeutic components shared by all psychotherapies. In A. Freeman, M. J. Mahoney, P. DeVito, & D. Martin (Eds.), *Cognition and psychotherapy* (2nd ed., pp. 45–78). New York, NY: Springer.

Franklin, M. (2010). Affect regulation, mirror neurons, and the 3rd hand: Formulating mindful empathic art interventions. *Art Therapy: The Journal of the American Art Therapy Association, 27*(4), 160–167.

Fredrickson, B. L. (2004). The broaden and build theory of positive emotions. *Philosophical Transactions of the Royal Society of London Biological Sciences, 359*, 1367–1377.

Fredrickson, B. L., Cohn, M. A., Coffey, K. A., Pek, J., & Finkel, S. M. (2008). Open hearts build lives: Positive emotions, induced through loving-kindness meditation, build consequential personal resources. *Journal of Personality and Social Psychology, 95,* 1045–1062.

Freedberg, D. (2007). Empathy, motion and emotion. In K. Herding & A. Krause Wahl (Eds.), *Wie sich Gefühle Ausdruck verschaffen: Emotionen in Nahsicht* (pp. 17–51). Berlin, Germany: Driesen.

Freedberg, D. (2009a). Choirs of praise: Some aspects of action understanding in fifteenth century painting and sculpture. In D. Levine & J. Freiberg (Eds.), *Medieval renaissance baroque: A cat's cradle for Marilyn Aronberg* (pp. 65–81). Lavin, NY: Italica Press.

Freedberg, D. (2009b). Movement, embodiment, emotion. In T. Dufrenne & A.-C. Taylor (Eds.), *Cannibalismes disciplinaires: Quand l'histoire de l'art et l'anthropologie se rencontrent* (pp. 37–61). Paris, France: INHA/Musée du quai Branly.

Freedberg, D., & Gallese, V. (2007). Motion, emotion, and empathy in esthetic experience. *Trends in Cognitive Sciences, 11*(5), 197–203.

Freton, M., Lemogne, C., Bergouignan, L., Delaveau, P., Lehéricy, S., & Fossati, P. (2013). The eye of the self: Precuneus volume and visual perspective during autobiographical memory retrieval. *Brain Structure and Function, 219*(3), 959–968.

Frey, S., & Petrides, M. (2002). Orbitofrontal cortex and memory formation. *Neuron, 36*(1), 171–176.

Friedman, M. J., Keane, T. M., & Resick, P. A. (2010). *Handbook of PTSD: Science and practice.* New York, NY: Guilford.

Frisch, M. J., Franko, D. L., & Herzog, D. B. (2006). Arts-based therapies in the treatment of eating disorders. *Eating Disorders, 14*(2), 131–142.

Frith, C. (2009). Role of facial expressions in social interactions. *Philosophical Transactions of the Royal Society B: Biological Sciences, 364*(1535), 3453–3458.

Frith, C. D., & Frith, U. (1999). Interacting minds—a biological basis. *Science, 286*(5445), 1692–1695.

Frith, C. D., & Frith, U. (2003). Development and neurophysiology of mentalizing. *Philosophical Transactions of the Royal Society B: Biological Sciences, 358*(1431), 459–473.

Frith, C. D., & Frith, U. (2006). The neural basis of mentalizing. *Neuron, 50*(4), 531–534.

Frith, U. (2001). Mind blindness and the brain in autism. *Neuron, 32*(6), 969–979.

Furth, G. M. (1988). *The secret world of drawings: Healing through art.* Boston, MA: Sigo.

Galbraith, A., Subrin, R., & Ross, D. (2008). Alzheimer's disease: Art creativity and the brain. In N. Hass-Cohen & R. Carr (Eds.), *Art therapy and clinical neuroscience* (pp. 254–269). London, U.K.: Jessica Kingsley.

Gallace, A., & Spence, C. (2010). Touch and the body: The role of the somatosensory cortex in tactile awareness. *Psyche, 16*(1), 30–67.

Gallegos, D. R. (2009). Learning in Alzheimer's disease is facilitated by social interaction and common ground. *Dissertation Abstracts International: Section B: The Sciences and Engineering, 69*(7-B).

Gallese, V. (2003). The roots of empathy: The shared manifold hypothesis and the neural basis of intersubjectivity. *Psychopathology, 36,* 171–180.

Gallese V. (2010). Embodied simulation and its role in intersubjectivity. In T. Fuchs, H. C. Sattel, & P. Henningsen (Eds.), *The embodied self, dimensions, coherence and disorder* (pp. 78–92). Stuttgart, Germany: Schattauer.

Gallese, V., & Di Dio, C. (2012). Neuroesthetics: The body in esthetic experience. In V. S. Ramachandran (Ed.), *The encyclopedia of human behavior* (pp. 687–693). New York, NY: Academic Press.

Gallese, V., Eagle, M. N., & Migone, P. (2007). Intentional attunement: Mirror neurons and the neural underpinnings of interpersonal relations. *Journal of the American Psychoanalytic Association, 55*(1), 131–176.

Gallese, V., Gernsbacher, A. M., Heyes, C., Hickok, G. & Iacoboni, M. (2011). Mirror neuron forum. *Perspectives on Psychological Science, 6*, 369– 407.

Gallese, V., Keysers, C., & Rizzolatti, G. (2004). A unifying view of the basis of social cognition. *Trends in Cognitive Sciences, 8*(9), 396–403.

Gantt, L. M., & Tinnin, L. W. (2007). Intensive trauma therapy of PTSD and dissociation: An outcome study. *Arts in Psychotherapy, 34*(1), 69–80.

Gantt, L. M., & Tinnin, L. W. (2009). Support for a neurobiological view of trauma with implications for art therapy. *Arts in Psychotherapy, 36*(3), 148–153.

Garrido, M. J., Kusnir, L., Duchaine, F., Walsh, B. V., & Ward, J. (2011). Superior facial expression, but not identity recognition, in mirror-touch synesthesia. *The Journal of Neuroscience, 31*(5), 1820–1824.

Gavron, T. (2013). Meeting on common ground: Assessing parent-child relationships through the joint painting procedure. *Art Therapy: Journal of the American Art Therapy Association, 30*(1), 12–19.

Gavron, T. (2014a). עבוד עדיל (אקספסילוטי) עבומ עדיל (אימפליסיוטי) עלבומ עדימ -הריצי תסובמב הכרדה. Graduate School of Creative Arts Publication, *4*(1), 406–400. In Hebrew

Gavron, T. (2014b). Personal communication, September 16, 2014.

Gazzaniga, M. S. (2002). The split brain revisited. *Scientific American Special Edition, 12*(1), 27–31.

George, C., Kaplan, N., & Main, M. (1996). *Adult attachment interview protocol.* Unpublished manuscript. University of California at Berkeley, CA.

Gerber, N. (2014). The essential components of doctoral-level education for art therapists. *Arts in Psychotherapy, 33*, 98–112.

Gerber, N., Templeton, E., Chilton, G., Cohen Liebman, M., Manders, E., & Shim, M. (2012). Art-based research as a pedagogical approach to studying intersubjectivity in the creative arts therapies. *Journal of Applied Arts and Health, 3*(1), 39–48.

Gerlach, K. D., Spreng, R. N., Gilmore, A. D., & Schacter, D. L. (2011). Solving future problems: Default network and executive activity associated with goal-directed mental simulations. *NeuroImage, 55*(2011), 1816–1824.

Germer, C. (2009). *The mindful path to self-compassion: Freeing yourself from destructive thoughts and emotions.* New York, NY: Guilford.

Germer, C. K., Siegel, R. D., & Fulton, P. R. (Eds.). (2005). *Mindfulness and psychotherapy.* New York, NY: Guilford.

Giedd, J. N. (2004). Structural magnetic resonance imaging of the adolescent brain. *Annals of New York Academy of Science, 1021,* 77–85.

Giedd, J. N., Blumenthal, J., Jeffries, N. O., Rajapakse, J. C., Vaituzis, A. C., Liu, H., et al. (1999). Development of the human corpus callosum during childhood and adolescence: A longitudinal MRI study. *Progress in Neuro-psychopharmacology and Biological Psychiatry, 23*(4), 571–588.

Gil, E. (2010). *Working with children to heal interpersonal trauma: The power of play.* New York, NY: Guilford Press.

Gilbert, S. J., Williamson, I. D. M., Dumontheil, I., Simons, J. S., Frith, C. D., & Burgess, P. W. (2007). Distinct regions of medial rostral prefrontal cortex supporting social and nonsocial functions. *Social Cognitive and Affective Neuroscience, 2*(3), 217–226.

Gillath, O., Giesbrechtb, B., & Shaver, P. R. (2009). Attachment, attention, and cognitive control: Attachment style and performance on general attention tasks. *Journal of Experimental Social Psychology, 45*(4), 647–654.

Gillespie, J. (1994). *The projective use of mother-and-child drawings: A manual for clinicians.* New York, NY: Brunner/Mazel.

Goldberg, E. (2001). *The executive brain: Frontal lobes and the civilized mind.* New York, NY: Oxford University Press.

Goldberg, E. (2005). *The wisdom paradox.* New York, NY: Gotham.

Goldberg, E. (2009). *The new executive brain: Frontal lobes in a complex world.* New York, NY: Oxford University Press.

Goldenberg, G. (2009). Apraxia and the parietal lobes. *Neuropsychologia, 47*(6), 1449–1459. doi:10.1016/j.neuropsychologia.2008.07.014. 18692079

Goldin, P., Ziv, M., Jazaieri, H., & Gross, J. J. (2013). MBSR vs. aerobic exercise in social anxiety: fMRI of emotion regulation of negative self-beliefs. *Social Cognitive and Affective Neuroscience, 8*, 65–72.

Golomb, C. (1992). *The child's creation of a pictorial world.* Berkeley, CA: University of California Press.

Gottman, J. M., & Driver, J. L. (2005). Dysfunctional marital conflict and everyday marital interaction. *Journal of Divorce and Remarriage, 43*(3–4), 63–77.

Grabenhorst, F., Rolls, E. T., Margot, C., da Silva, M. A. A. P., & Velazco, M. I. (2007). How pleasant and unpleasant stimuli combine in different brain regions: Odor mixtures. *Journal of Neuroscience, 27*, 13532–13540.

Grafman, J., & Litvan, I. (1999). Importance of deficits in executive functions. *Lancet, 354*, 1921–1923.

Graham, J. E., Christian, L. M., & Kiecolt-Glaser, J. K. (2006). Stress, age, and immune function: Toward a lifespan approach. *Journal of Behavioral Medicine, 29*(4), 389–400.

Granic, I., O'Hara, A., Pepler, D., & Lewis, M. D. (2007). A dynamic systems analysis of parent-child changes associated with successful "real-world" interventions for aggressive children. *Journal of Abnormal Child Psychology, 35*(5), 845–857.

Greenberg, L. (2011). *Emotion focused therapy.* Washington, DC: American Psychological Association.

Grey, A. (2012). *The sacred mirrors.* Retrieved from http://www.alexgrey.com.

Grice, H. P. (1975). Logic and conversation. In P. Cole & J. Morgan (Eds.), *Syntax and semantics* (Vol. 3, pp. 41–58). New York, NY: Academic Press.

Grice, H. P. (1991). *Studies in the way of words.* Cambridge, MA: Harvard University Press.

Gringage, B. D. (2003). Diagnosis and management of post-traumatic stress disorder. *American Family Physician, 68*(12), 2401–2409.

Gross, C. G. (2000). Neurogenesis in the adult brain: Death of a dogma. *Nature Reviews Neuroscience, 1*, 67–73.

Gross, J. J., & Barrett, L. F. (2011). Emotion generation and emotion regulation: One or two depends on your point of view. *Emotion Review, 3*(1), 8–16.

Gunuratana, B. H. (2002). *Mindfulness in plain English.* Somerville, MA: Wisdom Publications.

Gusnard, D. A., Akbudak, E., Shulman, G. L., & Raichle, M. E. (2001). Medial prefrontal cortex and self-referential mental activity: Relation to a default mode of brain function. *Proceedings of the National Academy of Science, 98*(7), 4259–4264.

Habermas, T. (2011). Autobiographical reasoning: Arguing and narrating from a biographical perspective. *New Directions for Child and Adolescent Development, 131*, 1–17.

Habermas, T., & Bluck, S. (2000). Getting a life: The emergence of the life story in adolescence. *Psychological Bulletin, 126*(5), 748.

Habermas, T., & de Silveira, C. (2011). The development of global coherence in life narratives across adolescence: Temporal, causal, and thematic aspects. *Developmental Psychology, 44*(3), 707–721.

Habermas, T., Ehlert-Lerche, S., & de Silveira, C. (2009). The development of the temporal macro-structure of life narratives across adolescence: Beginnings, linear narrative form, and endings. *Journal of Personality, 77*(2), 527–559.

Hagmann, P., Cammoun, L., Gigandet, X., Meuli, R., Honey, C. J., Wedeen, V. J., & Sporns, O. (2008). Mapping the structural core of human cerebral cortex. *PLOS Biology, 6*(7), e159.

Hall, M., & Irwin, M. (2001). Physiological indices of functioning in bereavement. In M. S. Stroebe, R. O. Hansson, W. Stroebe, & H. Schut (Eds.), *Handbook of bereavement research: Consequences, coping, and care* (pp. 473–492). Washington, DC: American Psychological Association.

Hamamé, C. M., Vidal, J. R., Ossandón, T., Jerbi, K., Dalal, S. S., Minotti, L., Bertrand, O., Kahane, P., & Lachaux, J. P. (2012). Reading the mind's eye: Online detection of visuospatial working memory and visual imagery in the inferior temporal lobe. *Neuroimage, 59*(1), 872–879.

Harel, J., Kaplan, H., Avimeir-Patt, R., & Ben-Aaron, M. (2006). The child's active role in mother-child, father-child psychotherapy: A psychodynamic approach to the treatment of relational disturbances. *Psychology and Psychotherapy: Theory, Research and Practice, 79*, 23–36.

Hanh, T. N. (1976). *The miracle of mindfulness: An introduction to the practice of meditation.* Boston, MA: Beacon.

Hanh, T. N. (2011). *The long road turns to joy: A guide to walking meditation* (rev. ed.). Berkeley, CA: Parallax.

Hanh, T. N. (2012). *The pocket Thich Nhat Hanh.* Boston, MA: Shambhala.

Harlow, H. (1958). The nature of love. *American Psychologist, 13*(12), 673–685.

Harlow, H. F., & Zimmerman, R. (1959). Affectional response in the infant monkey: Orphaned baby monkeys develop a strong and persistent attachment to inanimate surrogate mothers. *Science, 130*(3373), 421–432.

Harmon-Jones, E. (2007). Asymmetrical frontal cortical activity. In E. Harmon-Jones & P. Winkielman (Eds.), *Social neuroscience, integrating biological and psychological explanations of social behavior.* New York, NY: Guilford.

Harrist, A. W., & Waugh, R. M. (2002). Dyadic synchrony: Its structure and function in children's development. *Developmental Review, 22*(4), 555–592.

Hart, S. (2008). *Brain, attachment, personality: An introduction to neuroaffective development.* London, U.K.: Karnac.

Hass-Cohen, N. (1992). *Towards a theory of art therapy* (Unpublished master's thesis, Loyola Marymount University, Los Angeles, CA).

Hass-Cohen, N. (2003). Art therapy mind body approaches. *Progress, Family Systems Research, and Therapy, 12*, 24–38.

Hass-Cohen, N. (2006a). Art therapy and clinical neuroscience in action. *GAINS Quarterly, Premier Edition,* 10–12.

Hass-Cohen, N. (2006b). Markers of insecure attachment classifications in eight to nine year family drawings: Applications from research. *GAINS Autumn Quarterly,* 20–23.

Hass-Cohen, N. (2007). Cultural arts in action: Musings on empathy. *GAINS Summer Quarterly,* 41–48.

Hass-Cohen, N. (2008a). CREATE: Art Therapy Relational Neuroscience principles (ATR-N). In N. Hass-Cohen & R. Carr (Eds.), *Art therapy and clinical neuroscience* (pp. 283–309). London, U.K.: Jessica Kingsley.

Hass-Cohen, N. (2008b). Partnering of art therapy and clinical neuroscience. In N. Hass-Cohen & R. Carr (Eds.), *Art therapy and clinical neuroscience* (pp. 35–36). London, U.K.: Jessica Kingsley.

Hass-Cohen, N. (2008c). Who are we? Updating personal and collective memories. "My Complement, My Enemy, My Oppressor, My Love." An art therapist's view of Kara Walker's retrospective exhibit. *Global Association for Interpersonal Neurobiology Studies, GAINS Spring Quarterly*, 19–29.

Hass-Cohen, N. (2015). Review of the neuroscience of chronic trauma and adaptive resilient responding. In J. King, *Art therapy, trauma and neuroscience: Theoretical and practical perspectives*. London, New York: Routledge Publishers.

Hass-Cohen, N., & Carr, R. (Eds.). (2008). *Art therapy and clinical neuroscience*. London, U.K.: Jessica Kingsley.

Hass-Cohen, N., & Chandler-Ziegler, K. A. (2014). Vicarious trauma and resiliency focused supervision and expressive writing activity. In R. Bean, S. Davis, & M. P. Davey (Eds.), *Clinical supervision activities for increasing competence and self-awareness*. New York, NY: Wiley.

Hass-Cohen, N., & Clyde Findlay, J. (2009). Pain, attachment, and meaning making: Report on an Art Therapy Relational Neuroscience assessment protocol (a case study). *Arts in Psychotherapy, 36*(4), 175–184.

Hass-Cohen, N., Clyde Findlay, J., Carr, R., & Vanderlan, J. (2014). "CHECK, change and/or keep what you need": An Art Therapy Relational Neurobiological (ATR-N) trauma intervention. *Art Therapy, 31*(2), 69–78.

Hass-Cohen, N., & Kim, S. (2014). *Art mediated interpersonal touch and space: A phenomenological study with Korean female art therapy students*. Manuscript submitted for publication.

Hass-Cohen, N., & Loya, N. (2008). Visual system in action. In N. Hass-Cohen & R. Carr (Eds.), *Art therapy and clinical neuroscience* (pp. 92–110). London, U.K.: Jessica Kingsley.

Hass-Cohen, N., Veeman, T., Chandler-Ziegler, K. A., & Brimhall, A. (2014). A disaster experiential activity and reflection (DEAR): Developing international and national disaster competencies. In R. Bean, S. Davis, & M. P. Davey (Eds.), *Clinical supervision activities for increasing competence and self-awareness*. New York, NY: Wiley.

Hayes, S. C., Luoma, J., Bond, F., Masuda, A., & Lillis, J. (2006). Acceptance and commitment therapy: Model, processes, and outcomes. *Behaviour Research and Therapy, 44*(1), 1–25.

Hayes, S. C., Strosahl, K. D., & Wilson, K. G. (2012). *Acceptance and commitment therapy: The process and practice of mindful change* (2nd ed.). New York, NY: Guilford.

Hebb, D. O. (2002). *The organization of behavior: A neuropsychological theory*. Mahwah, NJ: Lawrence Erlbaum. (Original work published 1949.)

Heisler, L. K., Cowley, M. A., Kishi, T., Tecott, L. H., Fan, W., Low, M. J., Smart, J. L., Rubinstein, M., Tatro, J., Zigman, J. M., Cone, R. D., & Elmquist, J. K. (2003). Central serotonin and melanocortin pathways regulating energy homeostasis. *Annals of the New York Academy of Sciences, 994*(1), 169–174.

Henry, J. P., & Wang, S. (1999). Effects of early stress on adult affiliative behavior. *Psychoneuroendocrinology, 23*(8), 863–875.

Herculano-Houzel, S. (2010). Coordinated scaling of cortical and cerebellar numbers of neurons. *Frontiers in Neuroanatomy, 4*(12), 1–8.

Herman, J. L. (1992). Complex PTSD: A syndrome in survivors of repeated and prolonged stress. *Journal of Traumatic Stress, 5*(3), 377–391.

Herman, J. L. (1997). *Trauma and recovery: The aftermath of violence from domestic abuse to political terror* (2nd ed.). New York, NY: Basic Books.

Hertenstein, M. J., Holmes, R., McCullough, M., & Keltner, D. (2009). The communication of emotion via touch. *Emotion, 9*(4), 566–573.

Hertzog, C., Kramer, A. F., Wilson, R. S., & Lindenberger, U. (2009). Enrichment effects on adult cognitive development: Can the functional capacity of older adults be preserved and enhanced? *Psychological Science in the Public Interest, 9*, 1–65.

Hesse, E. (1999). The adult attachment interview: Historical and current perspectives. In J. Cassidy & P. Shaver (Eds.), *Handbook of attachment.* New York, NY: Guilford.

Hesse, E., & Main, M. (2000). Disorganized infant, child and adult attachment: Collapse in behavioral and attentional strategies. *Journal of the American Psychoanalytic Association, 48*(4), 1097–1127.

Hinz, L. (2009). *Expressive therapies continuum: A framework for using art in therapy.* New York, NY: Routledge, Chapman, and Hall.

Hoebel, B. G., Avena, N. M., & Rada, P. (2007). Accumbens dopamine–acetylcholine balance in approach and avoidance. *Current Opinion in Pharmacology, 7*, 617–627.

Hofmann, S. G., Sawyer, A. T., Witt, A. A., & Oh, D. (2010). The effect of mindfulness-based therapy on anxiety and depression: A meta-analytic review. *Journal of Counseling and Clinical Psychology, 78*(2), 169–183.

Hollins, S., Horrocks, C., & Sinason, V. (1998). *I can get through it.* London, U.K.: Gaskell/ St. George Hospital Medical School.

Hölzel, B. K., Carmody, J., Evans, K. C., Hoge, E. A., Dusek, J. A., Morgan, L., et al. (2010). Stress reduction correlates with structural changes in the amygdala. *Social Cognitive and Affective Neuroscience, 5*(1), 11–17.

Hölzel, B. K., Carmody, J., Vangel, M., Congleton, C., Yerramsetti, S. M., Gard, T., & Lazar, S. W. (2011). Mindfulness practice leads to increases in regional brain gray matter density. *Psychiatry Research: Neuroimaging, 191*(1), 36–43.

Hölzel, B. K., Ott, U., Hempel, H., Hackl, A., Wolf, K., & Stark, R. (2007). Differential engagement of anterior cingulate and adjacent medial frontal cortex in adept meditators and non-meditators. *Neuroscience Letters, 421*(1), 16–21.

Horner, P. J., & Gage, F. H. (2002). Regeneration in the adult and aging brain. *Archives of Neurology, 59*, 1717–1720.

Hosea, H. (2006). The brush's footmarks: Parents and infants paint together in a small community art therapy group. *International Journal of Art Therapy: Inscape, 11*(2), 69–78.

Hoshi, E., Tremblay, L., Feger, J., Carras, P. L., & Strick, P. L. (2005). The cerebellum communicates with the basal ganglia. *Nature Neuroscience, 8*(11), 1491–1493.

Howie, P., Burch, B., Conrad, S., & Shambaugh, S. (2002). Releasing trapped images: Children grapple with the reality of the September 11 attacks. *Art Therapy: Journal of the American Art Therapy Association, 19*(3), 100–105.

Hugdahl, K., & Davidson, R. J. (2002). Cerebral asymmetry, emotion, and affective style. In R. J. Davidson & K. Hugdahl (Eds.), *Brain asymmetry.* Cambridge, MA: MIT Press.

Hughes, A. E., Crowell, S. E., Uyeji, L., & Coan, J. A. (2012). An emotion dysregulation and social baseline theory. *Journal of Abnormal Child Psychology, 40*(1), 21–33.

Hughes, C., & Leekam, S. (2004). What are the links between theory of mind and social relations? Review, reflections and new directions for studies of typical and atypical development. *Social Development, 13*(4), 590–617.

Hughes, D. (2004). An attachment-based treatment of maltreated children and young people. *Attachment and Human Development, 6*(3), 263–278.

Husserl, E. (1970). *Logical investigations* (vols. 1–2, trans. J. N. Findlay). Atlantic Highlands, NJ: Humanities Press.

Husserl, E. (1989). *Ideas pertaining to a pure phenomenology and to a phenomenological philoso-*

phy. Second book: Studies in the phenomenology of constitution (trans. R. Rojcewicz & A. Schuwer). Dordrecht, Netherlands: Kluwer.

Hutcherson, C. A., Seppala, E. M., & Gross, J. J. (2008). Loving-kindness meditation increases social connectedness. *Emotion, 8*(5), 720–724.

Huttenlocher, P. R. (2002). *Neural plasticity: The effects of the environment on the development of the cerebral cortex.* Cambridge, MA: Harvard University Press.

Iacoboni, M., & Dapretto, M. (2006). The mirror neuron system and the consequences of its dysfunction. *Nature Reviews Neuroscience, 7*(12), 942–951.

Insel, T. R. (2003). Is social attachment an addictive disorder? *Physiology and Behavior, 79*(3), 351–357.

Ishizaki, J., Meguro, K., Ohe, K., Kimura, E., Tsuchiya, E., Ishii, H., Yasuyoshi, S., & Yamadori, A. (2002). Therapeutic psychosocial intervention for elderly subjects with very mild Alzheimer disease in a community: The Tajiri project. *Alzheimer Disease and Associated Disorders, 16*(4), 261–269.

Isserow, J. (2008). Looking together: Joint attention in art therapy. *International Journal of Art Therapy: Inscape, 13*(1), 34–42.

Ivanovski, B., & Malhi, G. S. (2007). The psychological and neurophysiological concomitants of mindfulness forms of meditation. *Acta Neuropsychiatrica, 19*(2), 76–91.

Ives-Deliperi, V. L., Solms, M., & Meintjes, E. M. (2011). The neural substrates of mindfulness: An fMRI investigation. *Social Neuroscience, 6*(3), 231–242.

Ivey, A., & Ivey, M. B. (2007). *Intentional interviewing and counseling* (6th ed.). Belmont, CA: Thomson-Brooks/Cole.

Jackson, P. L., Meltzoff, A. N., & Decety, J. (2005). How do we perceive the pain of others? A window into the neural processes involved in empathy. *Neuroimage, 24*(3), 771–779.

Jackson, P. L., Meltzoff, A. N., & Decety, J. (2006). Neural circuits involved in imitation and perspective-taking. *Neuroimage, 31*(1), 429–439.

Jameison, K., & Dinan, T. G. (2001). Glucocorticoids and cognitive function: From physiology to pathophysiology. *Human Psychopharmacology Clinical and Experimental, 16*, 293–302.

James, W. (1890). *The principles of psychology.* London, U.K.: Dover.

Janklowicz-Mann, D., & Mann, A. (Directors). (2002). *Shanghai ghetto* [DVD]. United States: Rebel Child Productions.

Jankowski, K. F., & Takahashi, H. (2014). Cognitive neuroscience of social emotions and implications for psychopathology: Examining embarrassment, guilt, envy, and schadenfreude. *Psychiatry Clinical Neuroscience, 68*(5), 319–336.

Jansari, A., & Parkin, A. J. (1996). Things that go bump in your life: Explaining the reminiscence bump in autobiographical memory. *Psychology and Aging, 1*, 85–91.

Jensen, E. (2001). *Arts with the brain in mind.* Alexandria, VA: Association for Supervision and Curriculum Development.

Jernberg, A., & Booth, P. (1999). *Theraplay: Helping parents and children build better relationships through attachment-based play.* New York, NY: Wiley.

Jessberger, S., & Gage, F. H. (2008). Stem-cell-associated structural and functional plasticity in the aging hippocampus. *Psychology and Aging, 23*(4), 684–691.

Jones, L. (2012). *Drawing Surrealism.* With contributions from Isabelle Dervaux and Susan Laxton. New York, NY: Prestel Publications.

Jones, R., & Bhattacharyaa, J. (2013). A role for the precuneus in thought–action fusion: Evidence from participants with significant obsessive–compulsive symptoms. *Neuroimage Clinical, 4*, 112–121.

Jones, S. E. (1994). *The right to touch: Understanding and using the language of physical contact.* Cresskill, NJ: Hampton.

Jørgensen, C. R., Berntsen, D., Bech, M., Kjølbye, M., Bennedsen, B. E., & Ramsgaard, S. B. (2012). Identity-related autobiographical memories and cultural life scripts in patients with borderline personality disorder. *Consciousness and Cognition, 21*, 788–798.

Josephson, B. R. (1996). Mood regulation and memory: Repairing sad moods with happy memories. *Cognition and Emotion, 10*(4), 437–444.

Jung, C. G. (1963). *Memories, dreams, reflections.* New York, NY: Crown/Random House.

Jung, R. E., Mead, B. S., Carrasco, J., & Flores, R. A. (2013). The structure of creative cognition in the human brain. *Frontiers in Human Neuroscience, 8*(7), 330.

Kaas, J. H. (2005). The evolution of visual cortex in primates. In J. Kremers (Ed.), *The primate visual system: A comparative approach* (pp. 267–283). Somerset, NJ: Wiley.

Kabat-Zinn, J. (1994). *Wherever you go there you are.* New York, NY: Hyperion.

Kabat-Zinn, J. (2005). *Full catastrophe living: Using the wisdom of your body and mind to face stress, pain, and illness* (15th anniversary ed.). New York, NY: Bantam Dell.

Kagan J. (2003). *Surprise, uncertainty and mental structures.* Cambridge, MA: Harvard University Press.

Kagan, J. (2007). *What is emotion? History, measures, and meaning.* New Haven, CT: Yale University Press.

Kaiser, D. H. (1996). Indications of attachment theory in a drawing task. *Arts in Psychotherapy, 23*(4), 333–340.

Kaiser, D. H., & Deaver, S. (2009). Assessing attachment with the bird's nest drawing: A review of the research. *Art Therapy: Journal of the American Art Therapy Association, 26*(1), 26–33.

Kalat, J. W. (2012). *Biological psychology* (11th ed.). Belmont, CA: Thomson/Wadsworth.

Kalmanowitz, D., & Lloyd, B. (1999). Fragments of art at work: Art therapy in the former Yugoslavia. *Arts in Psychotherapy, 25*(1), 15–25.

Kampe, K. K. W., Frith, C. D., & Frith, U. (2003). "Hey John": Signals conveying communicative intention toward the self activate brain regions associated with "mentalizing," regardless of modality. *Journal of Neuroscience, 23*(12), 5258–5263.

Kandel, E. R., Schwartz, J. H., & Jessell, T. M. (2001). *Principles of neural science* (4th ed.). New York, NY: McGraw-Hill.

Kang, C., & Whittingham, K. (2010). Mindfulness: A dialogue between Buddhism and clinical psychology. *Mindfulness, 1*(3), 161–173.

Kanwisher, N. (2000). Domain specificity in face perception. *Nature Neuroscience, 3*(8), 759–763.

Kanwisher, N., McDermott, J., & Chun, M. M. (1997). The fusiform face area: A module in human extrastriate cortex specialized for face perception. *Journal of Neuroscience, 17*(11), 4302–4311.

Kapitan, L. (2010). The empathic imagination of art therapy: Good for the brain? *Art Therapy, 27*(4), 158–159.

Kaplan, F. (2000). *Art, science, and art therapy: Repainting the picture.* Philadelphia, PA: Jessica Kingsley.

Kaufman, J., Plotsky, P. M., Nemeroff, C. B., & Charney, D. S. (2000). Effects of early adverse experiences on brain structure and function: Clinical implications. *Biological Psychiatry, 48*(8), 778–790.

Kawabata, H., & Zeki, S. J. (2004). Neural correlates of beauty. *Neurophysiology, 4*, 1699–1705.

Kays, J. L., Hurley, R. A., & Taber, K. H. (2012). The dynamic brain: Neuroplasticity and mental health. *Journal of Neuropsychiatry and Clinical Neurosciences, 24*(2), 118–124.

Kellogg, J. (1992). Color theory from the perspective of the great round of mandala. *Journal of Religion and Psychical Research, 15*(3), 138–146.

Kellogg, J. (2002). *Mandala: Path of beauty* (3rd ed.). Belleair, FL: ATMA.

Kempermann, G., Kuhn, H. G., & Gage, F. H. (1997). More hippocampal neurons in adult mice living in an enriched environment. *Nature, 3*(386), 493–495.

Kempermann, G., Kuhn, H. G., & Gage, F. H. (1998). Experience-induced neurogenesis in the senescent dentate gyrus. *Journal of Neuroscience, 18*(9), 3206–3212.

Kenny, M., & Williams, J. (2007). Treatment-resistant depressed patients show a good response to mindfulness-based cognitive therapy. *Behavior Research and Therapy, 45*, 617–625.

Kerr, C. E., Sacchet, M. D., Lazar, S. W., Moore, C. I., & Jones, S. R. (2013). Mindfulness starts with the body: Somatosensory attention and top-down modulation of cortical alpha rhythms in mindfulness meditation. *Frontiers in Human Neuroscience, 7*(12), 1–15.

Kersten, A., & van der Vennet, R. (2010). The impact of anxious and calm emotional states on color usage in pre-drawn mandalas. *Art Therapy, 27*(4), 184–189.

Keyes, C. L. M., & Ryff, C. D. (2000). Subjective change and mental health: A self-concept theory. *Social Psychology Quarterly, 63*, 264–279.

Keysers, C., & Gazzola, V. (2010). Social neuroscience: Mirror neurons recorded in humans. *Current Biology, 20*(8), R353–R354.

Ki, P. (2011). Exploring the experiences of participants in short-term art-based support groups for adults living with eating disorders. *Canadian Art Therapy Association Journal, 24*(2), 1–13.

Kilpatrick, L. A., Suyenobu, B. Y., Smith, S. R., Bueller, J. A., Goodman, T., Creswell, J. D., et al. (2011). Impact of mindfulness-based stress reduction training on intrinsic brain connectivity. *Neuroimage, 56*(1), 290–298.

Kim, K. J., Conger, R. D., Lorenz, F. O., & Elder Jr., G. H., (2001). Parent-adolescent reciprocity in negative affect and its relation to early adult social development. *Developmental Psychology, 37*(6), 775–790.

Kim, S., & Kochanska, G. (2012). Child temperament moderates effects of parent-child mutuality on self-regulation: A relationship-based path for emotionally negative infants. *Child Development, 83*(4), 1275–1289.

Kimonis, E. R., Cross, B., Howard, A., & Donoghue, K. (2012). Maternal care, maltreatment and callous-unemotional traits among urban male juvenile offenders. *Journal of Youth and Adolescence, 42*(2), 165–177.

Kindt, M., Soeter, M., & Vervliet, B. (2009). Beyond extinction: Erasing human fear responses and preventing the return of fear. *Nature Neuroscience, 12*(3), 256–258.

King, J. (Ed.). (2015). *Art therapy, trauma and neuroscience: Theoretical and practical perspectives.* New York, NY: Routledge.

Kingston, T., Dooley, B., Bates, A., Lawlor, E., & Malone, K. (2007). Mindfulness-based cognitive therapy for residual depressive symptoms. *Psychology and Psychotherapy: Theory, Research and Practice, 80*, 193–203.

King-West, E., & Hass-Cohen, N. (2008). Art therapy, neuroscience and complex PTSD. In N. Hass-Cohen & R. Carr (Eds.), *Art therapy and clinical neuroscience* (pp. 227–231). London, U.K.: Jessica Kingsley.

Kisilevsky, B. S., Hains, S. M., Brown, C. A., Lee, C. T., Cowperthwaite, B., Stutzman, S. S., Swansburg, M. L., Lee, K., Xie, X., Huang, H., Ye, H. H., Zhang, K., & Wang, Z. (2009). Fetal sensitivity to properties of maternal speech and language. *Infant Behavior and Development, 32*(1), 59–71.

Kitayama, N., Quinn, S., & Bremner, J. D. (2006). Smaller volume of anterior cingulate cortex in abuse-related posttraumatic stress disorder. *Journal of Affective Disorders, 90*, 171–174.

Klein, S. B., & Thorne, B. M. (2006). *Biological psychology*. New York, NY: Worth.

Klimecki, O. M., Leiberg, S., Lamm, C., & Singer, T. (2013). Functional neural plasticity and associated changes in positive affect after compassion training. *Cerebral Cortex, 23*(7), 1552–1561.

Klorer, P. G. (2005). Expressive therapy with severely maltreated children: Neuroscience contributions. *Art Therapy: Journal of the American Art Therapy Association, 22*(4), 213–220.

Knecht, S., Dräger, B., Deppe, M., Bobe, L., Lohmann, H., Flöel, A., Ringelstein, E. B., & Henningsen, H. (2000). Handedness and hemispheric language dominance in healthy humans. *Brain, 123*(12), 2512–2518.

Knez, I. (2014). Place and the self: An autobiographical memory synthesis. *Philosophical Psychology, 27*(2), 164–192.

Knight, D. C., Nguyen, H. T., & Bandettini, P. A. (2005). The role of the human amygdala in the production of conditioned fear responses. *Neuroimage, 26*(4), 1193–1200.

Kochanska, G., Philibert, R. A., & Barry, R. A. (2010). Interplay of genes and early mother–child relationship in the development of self-regulation from toddler to preschool age. *Journal of Child Psychology and Psychiatry, 50*(11), 1331–1338.

Koelsch, S., Skouras, S., Fritz, T., Herrera, P., Bonhage, C., Küssner, M. B., & Jacobs, A. M. (2013). Neural correlates of music-evoked fear and joy: The roles of auditory cortex and superficial amygdala. *NeuroImage, 1*(81), 49–60.

Koenigs, M., Huey, E. D., Raymont, V., Cheon, B., Solomon, J., Wassermann, E. M., & Grafman, J. (2008). Focal brain damage protects against post-traumatic stress disorder in combat veterans. *Nature Neuroscience, 11*(2), 232–237.

Kok, B. E., Coffey, K. A., Cohn, M. A., Catalino, L. I., Vacharkulksemsuk, T., Algoe, S. B., Brantley, M., & Fredrickson, B. L. (2013). How positive emotions build physical health: Perceived positive social connections account for the upward spiral between positive emotions and vagal tone. *Psychological Science, 24*, 1123–1132.

Kolb, A. Y., & Kolb, D. A. (2005). Learning styles and learning spaces: Enhancing experiential learning in higher education. *Academy of Management Learning and Education, 4*(2), 193–212.

Kolb, D. A. (1984). *Experiential learning: Experience as a source of learning and development*. Upper Saddle River, NJ: Prentice Hall.

Konarski, J. Z., McIntyre, R. S., Grupp, L. A., & Kennedy, S. H. (2005). Is the cerebellum relevant in the circuitry of neuropsychiatric disorders? *Review of Psychiatric Neuroscience, 30*(3), 178–186.

Konijn, E. A., & Van Vugt, H. C. (2008). Emotions in mediated interpersonal communication: Toward modeling emotion in virtual agents. In E. A. Konijn, S. Utz, M. Tanis, & S. B. Barnes (Eds.), *Mediated interpersonal communication* (p. 100). New York, NY: Taylor and Francis.

Kosfeld, M., Heinrichs, M., Zak, P. J., Fischbacher, U., & Fehr, E. (2005). Oxytocin increases trust in humans. *Nature, 435*(2), 673–676.

Kourtzi, Z., & Kanwisher, N. (2000). Activation in human MT/MST by static images with implied motion. *Journal of Cognitive Neuroscience, 12*(1), 48–55.

Kramer, A. F., & Erickson, K. I. (2007). Capitalizing on cortical plasticity: Influence of physical activity on cognition and brain function. *Trends in Cognitive Science, 11*(8), 342–348. doi:10.1016/j.tics.2007.06.009

Kramer, E. (1971). *Art as therapy with children*. New York, NY: Schocken.

Kramer, E. (1986). The art therapist's third hand: Reflections on art, art therapy, and society at large. *Art Therapy: Journal of the American Art Therapy Association, 24,* 71–86.

Kramer, E. (2000). *Art as therapy: Collected papers.* London, U.K.: Jessica Kingsley.

Kravits, K. (2008a). The neurobiology of relatedness: Attachment. In N. Hass-Cohen & R. Carr (Eds.), *Art therapy and clinical neuroscience* (pp. 137–140). London, U.K.: Jessica Kingsley.

Kravits, K. (2008b). The stress response and adaptation theory. In N. Hass-Cohen & R. Carr (Eds.), *Art therapy and clinical neuroscience* (pp. 116–120). London, U.K.: Jessica Kingsley.

Kringelbach, M. L., & Rolls, E. T. (2004). The functional neuroanatomy of the human orbitofrontal cortex: Evidence from neuroimaging and neuropsychology. *Progress in Neurobiology, 72*(5), 341–372.

Kruk, K. A. (2004). *Neural correlates of art therapy as indicated through electroencephalography* (Thesis, Eastern Virginia Medical School, Norfolk).

Kwiatkowska, H. (1978). *Family therapy and evaluation through art.* Springfield, IL: Charles C. Thomas.

Lahad, M. (1993). Tracing coping resources through a story in six parts—The "BASIC PH" model. In S. Levinson (Ed.), *Psychology at school and the community during peaceful and emergency times* (pp. 55–70). Tel-Aviv, Israel: Levinson-Hadar (in Hebrew).

Lahad, M. (2000). *Creative supervision.* London, U.K.: Jessica Kingsley Publishers.

Lambert, M. J. (1986). Implications of psychotherapy outcome research for eclectic psychotherapy. In J. C. Norcross (Ed.), *Handbook of eclectic psychotherapy* (pp. 436–462). New York, NY: Brunner/Mazel.

Lambert, M. J., Shapiro, D. A., & Bergin, A. E. (1986). The effectiveness of psychotherapy. In S. L. Garfield & A. E. Bergin (Eds.), *Handbook of psychotherapy and behavior change* (pp. 157–212). New York, NY: Wiley.

Lamm, C., Meltzoff, A. N., & Decety, J. (2010). How do we empathize with someone who is not like us? A functional magnetic resonance imaging study. *Journal of Cognitive Neuroscience, 22*(2), 362–376.

Lane, R. D., & Garfield, D. S. (2005). Becoming aware of feelings: Integration of cognitive-developmental, neuroscientific, and psychoanalytic perspectives. *Journal of Neuro-Psychoanalysis, 7*(1), 5–30.

Lane, R. D., Reiman, E. M., Axelrod, B., Yun, L. S., Holmes, A., & Schwartz, G. E. (1998). Neural correlates of levels of emotional awareness: Evidence of an interaction between emotion and attention in the anterior cingulate cortex. *Journal of Cognitive Neuroscience, 10*(4), 525–535.

Lane, R. D., Ryan, L., Nadel, L., & Greenberg, L. (2014). Memory reconsolidation, emotional arousal and the process of change in psychotherapy: New insights from brain science. *Behavioral and Brain Sciences,* 1–80.

Langer, L. L. (1993). *Holocaust testimonies: The ruins of memory.* New Haven, CT: Yale University Press.

Lanius, R. A., Bluhm, R. L., Coupland, N. J., Hegadoren, K. M., Rowe, B., Théberge, J., Neufeld, R. W., Williamson, P. C., & Brimson, M. (2010). Default mode network connectivity as a predictor of post-traumatic stress disorder symptom severity in acutely traumatized subjects. *Acta Psychiatrica Scandinavica, 121*(1), 33–40.

Lanius, R. A., Bluhm, R. L., & Frewen, P. A. (2011). How understanding the neurobiology of complex post-traumatic stress disorder can inform clinical practice: A social cognitive and affective neuroscience approach. *Acta Psychiatrica Scandinavica, 124,* 331–348.

Lanius, R. A., Frewen, P. A., Vermetten, E., & Yehuda, R. (2010). Fear conditioning and early life vulnerabilities: Two distinct pathways of emotional dysregulation and brain dysfunction in PTSD. *European Journal of Psychotraumatology, 1.*

Lanius, R. A., Hopper, J. W., & Menon, R. S. (2003). Individual differences in a husband and wife who developed PTSD after a motor vehicle accident: A functional MRI case study. *American Journal of Psychiatry, 160*(4), 667–669.

Lanius, R., Lanius, U., Fisher, J., & Ogden, P. (2006). Psychological trauma and the brain: Toward a neurobiological treatment model. In P. Ogden, K. Minton, & C. Pain (Eds.), *Trauma and the body.* New York, NY: Norton.

Lanius, R. A., Williamson, P. C., Bluhm, R. L., Densmore, M., Boksman, K., Neufeld, R. W. J., Gati, S. J., & Ravi, S. M. (2005). Functional connectivity of dissociative responses in post-traumatic stress disorder: A functional magnetic resonance imaging investigation. *Biological Psychiatry, 57*(8), 873–884.

Lanius, R. A., Williamson, P. C., Boksman, K., Densmore, M., Gupta, M., Neufeld, R. W., et al. (2002). Brain activation during script-driven imagery induced dissociative responses in PTSD: A functional magnetic resonance imaging investigation. *Biological Psychiatry, 52,* 305–311.

Lanius, R. A., Williamson, P. C., Densmore, M., Boksman, K., Neufeld, R. W., Gati, J. S., & Menon, R. S. (2004). The nature of traumatic memories: A 4.0 Tesla fMRI functional connectivity analysis. *American Journal of Psychiatry, 161*(1), 36–44.

Lau, G., Moulds, M. L., & Richardson, R. (2009). Ostracism: How much it hurts depends on how you remember it. *Emotion, 9*(3), 430.

Lazar, S. W., Kerr, C. E., Wasserman, R. H., Gray, J. R., Greve, D. N., Treadway, M. T., McGarvey, M., Quinn, B. T., Dusek, J. A., Benson, H., Rauch, S. L., Moore, C. I., & Fischl, B. (2005). Meditation experience is associated with increased cortical thickness. *Neuroreport, 16*(17), 1893–1897.

Lazarus, R. S. (1966). *Psychological stress and the coping process.* New York, NY: McGraw-Hill.

LeDoux, J. E. (1996). *The emotional brain.* New York, NY: Simon and Schuster.

LeDoux, J. E. (2000). Emotion circuits in the brain. *Annual Review of Neuroscience, 23,* 155–184.

LeDoux, J. E. (2003a). The emotional brain, fear, and the amygdala. *Cellular and Molecular Neurobiology, 23*(4–5), 727–738.

LeDoux, J. E. (2003b). *The synaptic self: How our brains become who we are.* New York, NY: Penguin.

LeDoux, J. E. (2007). The amygdala. *Current Biology, 17*(20), R868–R874.

LeDoux, J. E., & Muller, J. (1997). Emotional memory and psychopathology. *Philosophical Transactions of the Royal Society of London, 352,* 1719–1726.

Leserman, J., Petitto, J. M., Gu, H., Gaynes, B. N., Barroso, J., Golden, R. N., Perkins, D. O., Folds, J. D., & Evans, D. L. (2002). Progression to AIDS, a clinical AIDS condition, and mortality: Psychosocial and physiological predictors. *Psychological Medicine, 32,* 1059–1073.

Levine, P. (1997). *Waking the tiger: Healing trauma: The innate capacity to transform overwhelming experiences away from stress.* Berkeley, CA: North Atlantic.

Levine-Madori, L., & Alders, A. (2010).The effect of art therapy on cognitive performance of Hispanic/Latino adults. *Art Therapy: Journal of the American Art Therapy Association, 27*(3), 127–153.

Lev-Wiesel, R., & Al-Krenawi, A. (2000). Perception of family among Bedouin-Arab children of polygamous families as reflected in their family drawings *Art Therapy: Journal of the American Art Therapy Association, 38*(4), 98–106.

Libby, L. K., Eibach, R. P., & Gilovich, T. (2005). Here's looking at me: The effect of memory perspective on assessments of personal change. *Journal of Personality and Social Psychology, 88*(1), 50.

Lieberman, M. (2007). Social cognitive neuroscience: A review of core processes. *Annual Reviews of Psychology, 58*, 259–289.

Linden, D. J. (2008). *The accidental mind: How brain evolution has given us love, memory dreams and God.* Cambridge, MA: Belknap.

Linehan, M. M. (1993a). *Cognitive behavioral treatment of borderline personality disorder.* New York, NY: Guilford.

Linehan, M. M. (1993b). *Skills training manual for treating borderline personality disorder.* New York, NY: Guilford.

Longe, O., Senior, C., & Rippon, G. (2009). The lateral and ventromedial prefrontal cortex work as a dynamic integrated system: Evidence from FMRI connectivity analysis. *Journal of Cognitive Neuroscience, 21*(1), 141–154.

Lovden, M., Bacman, L., Lindenberger, U., Schaefer, S., & Schmiedek, F. (2010). A theoretical framework for the study of adult cognitive plasticity. *Psychological Bulletin, 136*(4), 659–676.

Lowenfeld, V. (1987). Therapeutic aspects of art education. *Art Therapy: Journal of the American Art Therapy Association, 25,* 111–146.

Lunkenheimer, E. (2007). Parent-child co-regulation of affect in early childhood pathways to children's externalizing behavior problems. *Dissertation Abstracts International, 67*(10-B).

Lupien, S. J., McEwen, B. S., Gunnar, M. R., & Heim, C. (2009). Effects of stress throughout the lifespan on the brain, behavior and cognition. *Nature Reviews, 10*, 434–445.

Luscher, M. (1971). *The Luscher color test.* Hamburg, Germany: Rowohlt.

Lusebrink, V. B. (2004). Art therapy and the brain: An attempt to understand the underlying processes of art expression in therapy. *Art Therapy: Journal of the American Art Therapy Association, 21*(3), 125–135.

Lusebrink, V. B. (2014). Neural basis of imagery. *Art Therapy: Journal of the American Art Therapy Association, 31*(2), 87–90.

Lutz, A., Brefczynski-Lewis, J., Johnstone, T., & Davidson, R. J. (2008). Regulation of the neural circuitry of emotion by compassion meditation: Effects of meditative expertise. *PLoS ONE, 26*(3), e1897.

MacDonald, A. W., Cohen, J. D., Stenger, V. A., & Carter, C. S. (2000). Dissociating the role of the dorsolateral prefrontal cortex and anterior cingulate cortex in cognitive control. *Science, 288*, 1835–1838.

Machin, A. J., & Dunbar, R. I. M. (2011). The brain opioid theory of social attachment: A review of the evidence. *Behavior, 148*, 9–10.

MacLean, P. D. (1990). *The triune brain in evolution: Role in paleocerebral functions.* New York, NY: Plenum.

MacNeilage, P. F., Rogers, L. J., & Vallortigara, G. (2009). Origins of the left and right brain. *Scientific American, 301*(1), 60–67.

Maguire, E. A., Gadian, D. G., Johnsrude, I. S., Good, C. D., Ashburner, J., Frackowiak, R. S., & Frith, C. D. (2000). Navigation-related structural change in the hippocampi of taxi drivers. *Proceedings of the National Academy of Sciences of the United States of America, 97*(8), 4398–4403.

Main, M. (2000). The organized categories of infant, child, and adult attachment: Flexible vs. inflexible attention under attachment-related stress. *Journal of the American Psychoanalytic Association, 48*(4), 1055–1096.

Main, M., & Goldwyn, R. (1998). *Adult attachment scoring and classification system* (version 6.3). Unpublished scoring manual, University of California at Berkeley, CA.

Main, M., & Solomon, J. (1990). Procedures for identifying infants as disorganized/disoriented during the Ainsworth Strange Situation. In M. T. Greenberg, D. Cicchetti, & E. M. Cummings (Eds.), *Attachment in the preschool years: Theory, research, and intervention* (pp. 121–160). Chicago, IL: University of Chicago Press.

Malchiodi, C. A. (1998a). *The art therapy sourcebook*. Los Angeles, CA: Lowell House.

Malchiodi, C. A. (1998b). *Understanding children's drawings*. New York, NY: Guilford.

Malchiodi, C. A. (Ed.). (2011). *Handbook of art therapy*. New York, NY: Guilford.

Malchiodi, C. A. (Ed.). (2013). *Expressive therapies*. New York, NY: Guilford.

Malchiodi, C. A., & Crenshaw, D. A. (Eds.). (2013). *Creative arts and play therapy for attachment problems*. New York, NY: Guilford.

Manders, E., & Chilton, G. (2013). Translating the essence of dance: Rendering meaning in artistic inquiry of the creative arts therapies. *International Journal of Education and the Arts, 14*(16), 1–17.

Mar, R. A. (2011). The neural bases of social cognition and story comprehension. *Annual Review of Psychology, 62*, 103–134.

Mars, R. B., Neubert, F., Noonan, M. P., Sallet, J., Toni, I., & Rushworth, M. F. S. (2012). On the relationship between the "default mode network" and the "social brain." *Frontiers in Human Neuroscience, 6*, 189.

May, A., & Gaser, C. (2006). Magnetic resonance-based morphometry: A window into structural plasticity of the brain. *Current Opinion in Neurology, 19*(4), 407–411.

McAdams, D. P., Diamond, A., de St. Aubin, E., & Mansfield, E. (1997). Stories of commitment: The psychosocial construction of generative lives. *Journal of Personality and Social Psychology, 72*(3), 678.

McAdams, D. P., Reynolds, J., Lewis, M., Patten, A. H., & Bowman, P. J. (2001). When bad things turn good and good things turn bad: Sequences of redemption and contamination in life narrative and their relation to psychosocial adaptation in midlife adults and in students. *Personality and Social Psychology Bulletin, 27*(4), 474–485.

McEwen, B. S. (2013). The brain on stress: Toward an integrative approach to brain, body, and behavior. *Perspectives on Psychological Science, 8*(6), 673–675.

McGoldrick, M., Gerson, R., & Petry, S. (2008). *Genograms: Assessment and intervention* (3rd ed.). New York, NY: Norton Professional Books.

McGoldrick, M., Giordano, J., & Garcia-Preto, N. (2005). *Ethnicity and family therapy* (3rd ed.). New York, NY: Guilford.

McIsaac, H. K., & Eich, E. (2004). Vantage point in traumatic memory. *Psychological Science, 15*(4), 248–253.

McLean, K. C., & Pratt, M. W. (2006). Life's little (and big) lessons: Identity statuses and meaning-making in the turning point narratives of emerging adults. *Developmental Psychology, 42*(4), 714.

McNamee, C. M. (2003). Bilateral art: Facilitating systemic integration and balance. *Arts in Psychotherapy, 30*, 283–292.

McNaughton, N., & Gray, J. A. (2000). Anxiolytic action on the behavioral inhibition system implies multiple types of arousal contribute to anxiety. *Journal of Affective Disorders, 61*, 161–176.

McNiff, S. (1986). *Educating the creative art therapist: A profile of the profession*. Springfield, IL: Charles C. Thomas.

McNiff, S. (1992). *Art as medicine: Creating a therapy of imagination*. Boston, MA: Shambhala.

Meaney, M. J. (2001). Maternal care, gene expression, and the transmission of individual differences in stress reactivity across generations. *Annual Reviews of Neuroscience, 24,* 1161–1192.

Mechelli, A., Crinion, J. T., Noppeney, U., O'Doherty, J., Ashburner, J., Frackowiak, R. S., & Price, C. J. (2004). Structural plasticity in the bilingual brain: Proficiency in a second language and age at acquisition affect grey-matter density. *Nature, 431,* 757.

Meekums, B. (1999). A creative model for recovery from child sexual abuse trauma. *Arts in Psychotherapy, 26*(4), 247–259.

Meltzoff, A. N., & Moore, M. K. (1983). Newborn infants imitate adult facial gestures. *Child Development, 54*(3), 702–709.

Menon, V., & Uddin, L. Q. (2010). Saliency, switching, attention and control: A network model of insula function. *Brain Structure and Function, 214*(5–6), 655–667.

Michael, G. A., & Buron, V. (2005). The human pulvinar and stimulus-driven attentional control. *Behavioral Neuroscience, 119*(5), 1353–1367.

Mikulincer, M., Gillath, O., Halevy, V., Avihou, N., Avidan, S., & Eshkoli, N. (2001). Attachment theory and reactions to others' needs: Evidence that activation of the sense of attachment security promotes empathic responses. *Journal of Personality and Social Psychology, 81*(6), 1205–1224.

Mikulincer, M., Gillath, O., & Shaver, P. R. (2002). Activation of the attachment system in adulthood: Threat-related primes increase the accessibility of mental representations of attachment figures. *Journal of Personality and Social Psychology, 83*(4), 881–895.

Mikulincer, M., & Shaver, P. R. (2001). Attachment theory and intergroup bias: Evidence that priming the secure base schema attenuates negative reactions to out-groups. *Journal of Personality and Social Psychology, 81,* 97–115.

Mikulincer, M., & Shaver, P. R. (2010). *Attachment in adulthood: Structure, dynamics, and change.* New York, NY: Guilford Press

Mikulincer, M., & Shaver, P. (2012). An attachment perspective on psychopathology. *World Psychiatry: Official Journal of the World Psychiatric Association (WPA), 11*(1), 11–15.

Mikulincer, M., Shaver, P. R., Gillath, O., & Nitzberg, R. A. (2005). Attachment, caregiving, and altruism: Boosting attachment security increases compassion and helping. *Journal of Personality Social Psychology, 89*(5), 817–839.

Miller, S., Duncan, B., Brown, J., Sparks, J., & Claud, D. (2003). The Outcome Rating Scale: A preliminary study of reliability, validity, and feasibility of a brief visual analogue measure. *Journal of Brief Therapy, 2,* 91–100.

Miller, W. R., & Rollnick, S. (2002). *Motivational interviewing: Preparing people for change.* New York, NY: Guilford.

Ming, G. L., & Song, H. (2011). Adult neurogenesis in the mammalian brain: Significant answers and significant questions. *Neuron, 70*(4), 687–702.

Mitrushina, M., Boone, K. B., Razani, J., & D'Elia, L. F. (2005). *Handbook of normative data for neuropsychological assessment* (2nd ed.). New York, NY: Oxford University Press.

Modinos, G., Ormel, J., & Aleman, A. (2009). Activation of anterior insula during self-reflection. *PLoS ONE, 4*(2), e4618.

Moffitt, P. (2012). *Emotional chaos to clarity: How to live more skillfully, make better decisions, and find purpose in life.* New York, NY: Hudson Street.

Monti, D. A., Peterson, C., Kunkel, E., Hauck, W. W., Pequignot, E., Rhodes, L., & Brainard, G. C. (2006). A randomized, controlled trial of mindfulness-based art therapy (MBAT) for women with cancer. *Psycho-Oncology, 15*(5), 363–373.

Moon, B. L. (2008). *Introduction to art therapy: Faith in the product* (2nd ed.). Springfield, IL: Charles C. Thomas.

Moon, B. L. (2009). *Existential art therapy: The canvas mirror* (3rd ed.). Springfield, IL: Charles C. Thomas.

Moon, C. H. (2001). *Studio art therapy: Cultivating the artist identity in the art therapist.* London, U.K.: Jessica Kingsley.

Moretti, M., Holland, R., Moore, K., & McKay, S. (2004). An attachment-based parenting program for caregivers of severely conduct disordered adolescents: Preliminary findings. *Journal of Child and Youth Care Work, 19,* 170–178.

Mortimer, J. A., Ding, D., Borenstein, A. R., DeCarli, C., Guo, Q., Wu, Y., Zhao, Q., & Chu, S. (2012). Changes in brain volume and cognition in a randomized trial of exercise and social interaction in a community-based sample of non-demented Chinese elders. *Journal of Alzheimer's Disease, 30*(4), 757–766.

Mukamel, R., Ekstrom, A. D., Kaplan, J., Iacoboni, M., & Fried, I. (2010). Single-neuron responses in humans during execution and observation of actions. *Current Biology, 20,* 750–756.

Murray, M. M., & Wallace, M. T. (Eds.). (2011). *The neural bases of multisensory processes.* Boca Raton, FL: CRC Press.

Nader, K., Schafe, G. E., & LeDoux, J. E. (2000). The labile nature of consolidation theory. *Biological Psychiatry, 76*(4), 274–280. doi: 10.1016/j.biopsych.2014.03.008.

Naito, E., & Ehrsson, H. H. (2006). Somatic sensation of hand-object interactive movement is associated with activity in the left inferior parietal cortex. *The Journal of Neuroscience, 26*(14), 3783–3790.

Naparstek, B. (1994). *Staying well with guided imagery: How to harness the power of your imagination for health and healing.* Lebanon, IN: Warner.

Naumburg, M. (1973). *An introduction to art therapy.* New York, NY: Teachers College Press.

Neff, K. D. (2003). Self-compassion: An alternative conceptualization of a healthy attitude toward oneself. *Self and Identity, 2,* 85–102.

Neff, K. D. (2009). Self-compassion. In M. R. Leary & R. H. Hoyle (Eds.), *Handbook of individual differences in social behavior* (pp. 561–573). New York, NY: Guilford.

Neff, K. D. (2011). *Self-compassion.* New York, NY: William Morrow.

Neff, K. D., & Germer, C. K. (2013). A pilot study and randomized controlled trial of the mindful self-compassion program. *Journal of Clinical Psychology, 69*(1), 28–44.

Nelson, K. (1993). The psychological and social origins of autobiographical memory. *Psychological Science, 1,* 7–14.

Neshat-Doost, H. T., Dalgleish, T., Yule, W., Kalantari, M., Ahmadi, S. J., Dyregrov, A., & Jobson, L. (2013). Enhancing autobiographical memory specificity through cognitive training: An intervention for depression translated from basic science. *Clinical Psychological Science, 1*(84), 84–92.

Newport, D. J., Heim, C., Bonsall, R., Miller, A. H., & Nemeroff, C. B. (2004). Pituitary-adrenal responses to standard and low-dose dexamethasone suppression tests in adult survivors of child abuse. *Biological Psychiatry, 55*(1), 10–20.

Niedenthal, P. M., Mermillod, M., Maringer, M., & Hess, U. (2010). The simulation of smiles (SIMS) model: A window to general principles in processing facial expression. *Brain and Behavioural Sciences, 33,* 417–480.

Nolte, T., Guiney, J., Fonagy, P., Mayes, L. C., & Luyten, P. (2011). Interpersonal stress regulation and the development of anxiety disorders: An attachment-based developmental framework. *Frontiers in Behavioral Neuroscience, 21*(5), 55.

Norcross, J., Beutler, L., & Levant, R. (2005). *Evidence-based practices in mental health: Debate and dialogue on the fundamental questions.* Oxford, U.K.: Oxford University Press.

Norris, C. J., Gollan, J., Berntson, G. G., & Cacioppo, J. T. (2010). The current status of research on the structure of evaluative space. *Biological Psychology, 84,* 422–436.

Nudo, R. J. (2011). Neural bases of recovery after brain injury. *Journal of Communication Disorders, 44*(5), 515–520.

Nunn, K., Frampton, I., Gordon, I., & Lask, B. (2008). The fault is not in her parents but in her insula—a neurobiological hypothesis of anorexia nervosa. *European Eating Disorders Review, 16,* 355–360.

Nuriddin, T. A. (2008). Weathering the storm: Self-efficacy, social support processes, and health-related coping strategies among the Detroit-area widowed. *Dissertation Abstracts International Section A: Humanities and Social Sciences, 68*(10-A), 4495.

Ochsner, K. N., & Gross, J. J. (2007). The neural architecture of emotion regulation. In J. J. Gross (Ed.), *Handbook of emotion regulation* (pp. 87–109). New York, NY: Guilford.

Ogden, P., Minton, K., & Pain, C. (2006). *Trauma and the body: A sensorimotor approach to psychotherapy.* New York, NY: Norton.

Onrust, S. A., & Cuijpers, P. P. (2006). Mood and anxiety disorders in widowhood: A systematic review. *Aging and Mental Health, 10*(4), 327–334.

O'Reilly, R. A. (2010). The what and how of prefrontal cortical organization. *Trends in Neuroscience, 33*(8), 355–361. doi:10.1016/j.tins.2010.05.002

Oster, G. D., & Crone, P. G. (2004). *Using drawings in assessment and therapy: A guide for mental health professionals* (2nd ed.). Oxford, U.K.: Routledge.

Oya, H., Kawasaki, H., Howard III, M. A., & Adolphs, R. (2002). Electrophysiological responses in the human amygdala discriminate emotion categories of complex visual stimuli. *Journal of Neuroscience 22*(21), 9502–9512.

Pace, T. W., Negi, L. T., Adame, D. D., Cole, S. P., Sivilli, T. I., Brown, T. D., et al. (2009). Effect of compassion meditation on neuroendocrine, innate immune and behavioral responses to psychosocial stress. *Psychoneuroendocrinology, 34*(1), 87–98.

Panksepp, J. (1998). *Affective neuroscience: The foundations of human and animal emotions.* New York, NY: Oxford University Press.

Panksepp, J. (2010). Emotions as natural kinds within the mammalian brain. In M. Lewis, J. M. Haviland-Jones, & L. F. Barrett (Eds.), *Handbook of emotions* (3rd ed., pp. 137–156). New York, NY: Guilford.

Panksepp, J., & Biven, L. (2012). *The archaeology of mind: Neuroevolutionary origins of human emotions.* New York, NY: Norton.

Panksepp, J., & Burgdorf, J. (2006). The neurobiology of positive emotions. *Neuroscience and Biobehavioral Reviews, 30*(2), 173–187.

Panzer, A., Viljoen, M., & Roos, J. L. (2007). The neurobiological basis of fear: A concise review. *South African Psychiatry Review, 10*(2), 71–75.

Park, C. L. (2010). Making sense of the meaning literature: An integrative review of meaning making and its effects on adjustment to stressful life events. *Psychological Bulletin, 136*(2), 257.

Parkin, A. J. (1996). *Explorations in cognitive neuropsychology.* Malden, MA: Blackwell.

Pascual-Leone, A., Amedi, A., Fregni, F., & Merabet, L. B. (2005). The plastic human brain cortex. *Annual Reviews of Neuroscience, 28,* 377–401.

Pascual-Leone, A., & Hamilton, R. (2001). The metamodal organization of the brain. *Progress in Brain Research, 134,* 427–445.

Pascual-Leone, A., Nguyet, D., Cohen, L. G., Brasil-Neto, J. P., Cammarota, A., & Hallett, M. (1995). Modulation of muscle responses evoked by transcranial magnetic stimulation during the acquisition of new fine motor skills. *Journal of Neurophysiology, 74*(3), 1037–1045.

Pasupathi, M., Mansour, E., & Brubaker, J. R. (2007). Developing a life story: Constructing relations between self and experience in autobiographical narratives. *Human Development, 50*(2–3), 85–110.

Pergola, G., & Suchan, B. (2013). Associative learning beyond the medial temporal lobe: Many actors on the memory stage. *Frontiers in Behavioral Science, 7*, 1–24.

Perrett, D. I., Smith, P. A., Potter, D. D., Mistlin, A. J., Head, A. S., Milner, A. D., & Jeeves, M. A. (1984). Neurones responsive to faces in the temporal cortex: Studies of functional organization, sensitivity to identity and relation to perception. *Human Neurobiology, 3*(4), 197–208.

Perry, B. D. (1997). Incubated in terror: Neurodevelopmental factors in the "cycle of violence." In J. Osofsky (Ed.), *Children, youth and violence: The search for solutions* (pp. 124–148). New York, NY: Guilford.

Perry, B. D. (2001). The neurodevelopmental impact of violence in childhood. In D. Schetky & E. Benedek (Eds.), *Textbook of child and adolescent forensic psychiatry* (pp. 221–238). Washington, DC: American Psychiatric Press.

Perry, B. D. (2002a). Childhood experience and the expression of genetic potential: What childhood neglect tells us about nature and nurture. *Brain and Mind, 3*(1), 79–100.

Perry, B. D. (2002b). Neurodevelopmental impact of violence in childhood. In D. H. Schetky & E. P. Benedek (Eds.), *Principles and practice of child and adolescent forensic psychiatry* (pp. 124–149). Washington, DC: American Psychiatric Publishing.

Perry, B. D. (2006). The neurosequential model of therapeutics. In N. B. Webb (Ed.), *Working with traumatized youth in child welfare* (pp. 27–52). New York, NY: The Guilford Press.

Perry, B. D., & Hambrick, E. (2006). The Neurosequential Model of Therapeutics (NMT). *Reclaiming Children and Youth, 17*(3), 38–43.

Perry, B. D., Pollard, R. A., Blakley, T. L., Baker, W. L., & Vigilante, D. (1995). Childhood trauma, the neurobiology of adaptation, and "use-dependent" development of the brain: How "states" become "traits." *Infant Mental Health Journal, 16*(4), 271–291.

Peterson, C. (2014). Mindfulness based art therapy: Applications for healing with cancer. In L. Rappaport (Ed.), *Mindfulness and the arts therapies* (pp. 64–80). Philadelphia, PA: Jessica Kingsley.

Peterson, C., Maier, S. F., & Seligman, M. E. P. (1993). *Learned helplessness.* Oxford, U.K.: Oxford University Press.

Petitto, L. A. (2008). Arts education, the brain, and language. In C. A. Asbury & B. Rich (Eds.), *Learning, arts, and the brain: The Dana Consortium report on arts and cognition* (pp. 93–104). New York, NY: Dana Press.

Phelps, E. A., Delgado, M. R., Nearing, K. I., & LeDoux, J. E. (2004). Extinction learning in humans: Role of the amygdala and vmPFC. *Neuron, 43*, 897–905. doi:10.1016/j.neuron.2004.08.042

Phelps, E. A., & LeDoux, J. E. (2005). Contributions of the amygdala to emotion processing: From animal models to human behavior. *Neuron, 48*(2), 175–187.

Philippe, F. L., Koestner, R., Beaulieu-Pelletier, G., & Lecours, S. (2011). The role of need satisfaction as a distinct and basic psychological component of autobiographical memories: A look at well-being. *Journal of Personality, 79*(5), 905–938.

Philippe, F. L., Koestner, R., Beaulieu-Pelletier, G., Lecours, S., & Lekes, N. (2012). The role of episodic memories in current and future well-being. *Personality and Social Psychology Bulletin, 38*(4), 505–519.

Phillips, M. L., Ladouceur, C. D., & Drevets, W. C. (2008). A neural model of voluntary and automatic emotion regulation: Implications for understanding the pathophysiology and neurodevelopment of bipolar disorder. *Molecular Psychiatry, 13*(9), 829–857.

Piaget, J., & Inhelder, B. (1973). *Memory and intelligence*. London, U.K.: Routledge and Kegan Paul.

Piefke, M., Weiss, P. H., Zilles, K., Markowitsch, H. J., & Fink, G. R. (2003). Differential remoteness and emotional tone modulate the neural correlates of autobiographical memory. *Brain, 126*(3), 650–668.

Pifalo, T. (2002). Pulling out the thorns: Art therapy with sexually abused children and adolescents. *Art Therapy: Journal of the American Art Therapy Association, 19*(1), 12–22.

Pillemer, D. (2001). Momentous events and the life story. *Review of General Psychology, 5*(2), 123–134.

Pillemer, D. (2003). Directive functions of autobiographical memory: The guiding power of the specific episode. *Memory, 11*(2), 193–202.

Pineda, J. A. (Ed.). (2009). *Mirror neuron systems: The role of mirroring processes in social cognition*. New York, NY: Hanumana Press.

Pizarro, J. (2004). The efficacy of art and writing therapy: Increasing positive mental health outcomes and participant retention after exposure to traumatic experience. *Art Therapy: Journal of the American Art Therapy Association, 21*(1), 5–12.

Pliszka, S. R. (2003). *Neuroscience for the mental health clinician*. New York, NY: Guilford.

Popoli, M., Yan, Z., McEwen, B. S., & Sanacora, G. (2011). The stressed synapse: The impact of stress and glucocorticoids on glutamate transmission. *Nature Reviews Neuroscience 13*(1), 22–37.

Porges, S. W. (1998). Love: An emergent property of the mammalian autonomic nervous system. *Psychoneuroimmunology, 23*(8), 837–861.

Porges, S. W. (2001). The polyvagal theory: Phylogenetic substrates of a social nervous system. *International Journal of Psychophysiology, 42*(2), 123–146.

Porges, S. W. (2011). *The polyvagal theory: Neurophysiological foundations of emotions, attachment, communication, and self-regulation*. New York, NY: Norton.

Posner, M., Rothbart, M. K., Sheese, B. E., & Kieras, J. (2008). How arts training influences cognition. In C. A. Asbury & B. Rich (Eds.), *Learning, arts, and the brain: The Dana Consortium report on arts and cognition* (pp. 1–10). New York, NY: Dana Press.

Praissman, S. (2008). Mindfulness-based stress reduction: A literature review and clinician's guide. *Journal of the American Academy of Nurse Practitioners, 20*, 212–216.

Premack, D., & Woodruff, G. (1978). Does the chimpanzee have a theory of mind? *Behavioral and Brain Sciences, 1*(4), 515–526.

Prochaska, J. O., Norcross, J. C., & DiClemente, C. C. (1994). *Changing for good: A revolutionary six-stage program for overcoming bad habits and moving your life positively forward*. New York, NY: Avon.

Proulx, L. (2002a). *Strengthening emotional ties through parent-child art therapy*. London, U.K.: Jessica Kingsley.

Proulx, L. (2002b). Strengthening ties, parent-child-dyad: Group art therapy with toddlers and their parents. *Art Therapy: Journal of the American Art Therapy Association, 40*(4), 238.

Proverbio, A. M., Riva, F., & Zani, A. (2009). Observation of static pictures of dynamic actions enhances the activity of movement-related brain areas. *PLoS ONE, 5*(4), e5389.

Qin, P., & Northoff, G. (2011). How is ourself related to midline regions and the default-mode network? *Neuroimage, 57*, 1221–1233.

Raes, F., Hermans, D., Williams, J. M. G., Beyers, W., Eelen, P., & Brunfaut, E. (2006). Reduced autobiographical memory specificity and rumination in predicting the course of depression. *Journal of Abnormal Psychology, 115*(4), 699.

Raes, F., Hermans, D., Williams, J. M. G., Demyttenaere, K., Sabbe, B., Pieters, G., & Eelen,

P. (2005). Reduced specificity of autobiographical memory: A mediator between rumination and ineffective social problem-solving in major depression? *Journal of Affective Disorders, 87*(2), 331–335.

Raichle, M. E., MacLeod, A. M., Snyder, A. Z., Powers, W. J., Gusnard, D. A., & Shulman, G. L. (2001). Inaugural article: A default mode of brain function. *Proceedings of the National Academy of Sciences, 98*(2), 676–682.

Raichle, M. E., & Snyder, A. Z. (2007). A default mode of brain function: A brief history of an evolving idea. *Neuroimage, 37*, 1083–1090.

Ramachandran, V. S., & Hirstein, W. (1999). The science of art: A neurological theory of aesthetic experience. *Journal of Consciousness Studies, 6*(6–7), 15–51.

Ramachandran, V. S., & Oberman, L. M. (2006). Broken mirrors: A theory of autism. *Scientific American, 295*(5), 62–69.

Ramachandran, V. S., & Rogers-Ramachandran, D. (2000). Phantom limbs and neural plasticity. *Archives of Neurology, 57*(3), 317–320.

Ranganath, C., & Ritchey, M. (2012). Two cortical systems for memory-guided behavior. *Nature Reviews Neuroscience, 13*, 713–726.

Rankin, A. B., & Taucher, L. C. (2003). A task-oriented approach to art therapy in trauma treatment. *Art Therapy: Journal of the American Art Therapy Association, 20*(3), 138–147.

Rappaport, L. (Ed.). (2014). *Mindfulness and the arts therapies.* London, U.K.: Jessica Kingsley.

Rasmussen, A. S., & Berntsen, D. (2009). Emotional valence and the functions of autobiographical memories: Positive and negative memories serve different functions. *Memory Cognition, 37*(4), 477–492.

Rasmussen, A. S., & Habermas, T. (2011). Factor structure of overall autobiographical memory usage: The directive, self and social functions revisited. *Memory, 19*(6), 597–605.

Ratey, J. J. (2008). *Spark: The revolutionary new science of exercise and the brain.* New York, NY: Little, Brown.

Ratey, J. J., & Hagerman, E. (2010). *Spark! How exercise will improve the performance of your brain.* London, U.K.: Quercus.

Ray, R., & Zald, D. H. (2012). Anatomical insights into the interaction of emotion and cognition in the prefrontal cortex. *Neuroscience and Biobehavioral Reviews, 36*(1), 479–501.

Regev, D. (2014). *Dyadic drawings.* Manuscript in preparation.

Riley, S. (1999). *Contemporary art therapy with adolescents.* London, U.K.: Jessica Kingsley.

Riley, S. (2001). *Group process made visible.* New York, NY: Routledge.

Rizzolatti, G., & Arbib, M. A. (1998). Language within our grasp. *Trends in Neuroscience, 21*, 188–194.

Rizzolatti, G., & Craighero, L. (2004). The mirror-neuron system. *Annual Review of Neuroscience, 27*(1), 169–C-4.

Rizzolatti, G., Fadiga, L., Gallese, V., & Fogassi, L. (1996). Premotor cortex and the recognition of motor actions. *Cognitive Brain Research 3*, 131–141.

Rizzolatti, G., Fogassi, L., & Gallese, V. (2001). Neurophysiological mechanisms underlying the understanding and imitation of actions. *Nature Reviews Neuroscience, 2*, 661–670.

Robinson, J. A., & Swanson, K. L. (1990). Autobiographical memory: The next phase. *Applied Cognitive Psychology, 4*(4), 321–335.

Rodrigues, S. M., Schafe, G. E., & LeDoux, J. E. (2004). Molecular mechanisms underlying emotional learning and memory in the lateral amygdala. *Neuron, 44*(1), 75–91.

Roisman, G. I., Padrón, E., Sroufe, L. A., & Egeland, B. (2002). Earned-secure attachment status in retrospect and prospect. *Child Development, 73*(4), 1204–1219.

Rorschach, H. (1951). *Psychodiagnostics* (5th ed.). Bern, Switzerland: Hans Huber.

Rosnick, C. B., Small, B. J., & Burton, A. M. (2010). The effect of spousal bereavement on cognitive functioning in a sample of older adults. *Aging, Neuropsychology and Cognition, 17*(3), 257–269.

Rothschild, B. (2000). *The body remembers.* New York, NY: Norton.

Rubin, D. C., & Berntsen, D. (2003). Life scripts help to maintain autobiographical memories of highly positive, but not highly negative, events. *Memory and Cognition, 31*(1), 1–14.

Rubin, J. A. (2012). *The art of art therapy: What every art therapist needs to know.* New York, NY: Routledge.

Russell, J. A. (2003). Core affect and the psychological construction of emotion. *Psychological Review, 110,* 145–172.

Salimi, I., Friel, K. M., & Martin, J. H. (2008). Pyramidal tract stimulation restores normal corticospinal tract connections and visuomotor skill after early postnatal motor cortex activity blockade. *Journal of Neuroscience, 28*(29), 7426–7434.

Salzman, S., & Fusi, S. (2010). Emotion, cognition, and mental state representation in amygdala and prefrontal cortex. *Annual Review of Neuroscience, 33,* 173–202. doi:10.1146/annurev.neuro.051508.135256

Sapolsky, R. M. (1992). *Stress, the aging brain, and the mechanisms of neuron death.* Cambridge, MA: MIT Press.

Sapolsky, R. M. (2004). *Why zebras don't get ulcers: An updated guide to stress, stress-related diseases, and coping* (3rd ed.). New York, NY: W. H. Freeman.

Sapolsky, R. M. (2005). The influence of social hierarchy on primate health. *Science, 308,* 648–652.

Sarid, O., & Huss, E. (2010). Trauma and acute stress disorder: A comparison between cognitive behavioral intervention and art therapy. *Arts in Psychotherapy, 37*(1), 8–12. doi:10.1016/j.aip.2009.11.004

Sarid, O., & Huss, E. (2011). Image formation and image transformation. *The Arts in Psychotherapy, 38,* 252–255.

Satir, V. (1988). *The new peoplemaking.* Palo Alto, CA: Science and Behavior.

Satz, P. (1993). Brain reserve capacity on symptom onset after brain injury: A formulation and review of evidence for threshold theory. *Neuropsychology, 7,* 273–295.

Saxe, R. (2006). Uniquely human social cognition. *Current Opinion in Neurobiology, 16,* 235–239. doi:10.1016/j.conb.2006.03.001

Saxe, R., & Kanwisher, N. (2003). People thinking about thinking people: The role of the temporo-parietal junction in "theory of mind." *NeuroImage, 19*(4), 1835–1842.

Sbarra, D. A., & Hazan, C. (2008). Coregulation, dysregulation, self-regulation: An integrative analysis and empirical agenda for understanding adult attachment, separation, loss, and recovery. *Personality and Social Psychology Review, 12,* 141.

Scaer, R. (2001). *The body bears the burden: Trauma, dissociation and disease.* Binghamton, NY: Haworth.

Schachter, D. L., Addis, D. R., Hassabis, D., Martin, V. C., Spreng, R. N., & Szpunar, K. K. (2012). The future of memory: Remembering, imagining, and the brain. *Neuron, 76,* 677–694.

Scheiby, B. B. (2005). An intersubjective approach to music therapy: Identification and processing of musical countertransference in a music psychotherapeutic context. *Music Therapy Perspectives, 23,* 8–17.

Schelling, G., Roozendaal, B., Krauseneck, T., Schmoelz, M. D. E., Quervain, D., & Briegel,

J. (2006). Efficacy of hydrocortisone in preventing posttraumatic stress disorder following critical illness and major surgery. *Annals of the New York Academy of Sciences, 1071,* 46–53.

Schilbach, L., Timmermans, B., Reddy, V., Costall, A., Bente, G., Schlicht, T., & Vogeley, K. (2013). Toward a second-person neuroscience. *Behavioral and Brain Sciences, 36*(4), 393–414.

Schmahmann, J. D., Weilburg, J. B., & Sherman, J. C. (2007). The neuropsychiatry of the cerebellum: Insights from the clinic. *Cerebellum, 6,* 254–267.

Schoenfeld, T. J., & Gould, E. (2012). Stress, stress hormones, and adult neurogenesis. *Experimental Neurology, 233*(1), 12–21.

Schore, A. N. (1994). *Affect regulation and the origin of the self: The neurobiology of emotional development.* Hillsdale, NJ: Lawrence Erlbaum.

Schore, A. N. (2000). Attachment and the regulation of the right brain. *Attachment and Human Development, 2*(1), 23–47.

Schore, A. N. (2001a). Effects of a secure attachment relationship on right brain development, affect regulation, and infant mental health. *Infant Mental Health Journal, 22*(1–2), 7–66.

Schore, A. N. (2001b). The effects of early relational trauma on right brain development, affect regulation, and infant mental health. *Infant Mental Health Journal, 22*(1–2), 201–269.

Schore, A. N. (2003). *Affect dysregulation and disorders of the self* (vol. 2). New York, NY: Norton.

Schore, A. N. (2008). Paradigm shift: The right brain and the relational unconscious. Invited plenary address to the American Psychological Association 2009 Convention, Toronto, Canada.

Schore, A. N. (2009). Right brain affect regulation: An essential mechanism of development, trauma, dissociation, and psychotherapy. In D. Fosha, D. Siegel, & M. Solomon (Eds.), *The healing power of emotion: Affective neuroscience, development, and clinical practice* (pp. 112–144). New York, NY: Norton.

Schupp, H. T., Stockburger, J., Bublatzky, F., Junghöfer, M., Weike, A. I., & Hamm, A. O. (2007). Explicit attention interferes with selective emotion processing in human extrastriate cortex. *BMC Neuroscience, 8,* 16–28.

Schwabe, L., Nader, K., & Pruessner, J. C. (2014). Reconsolidation of human memory: Brain mechanisms and clinical relevance. *Biological Psychiatry, 76*(4), 274–280.

Segal, Z. V., Williams, J. M. G., & Teasdale, J. D. (2012). *Mindfulness-based cognitive therapy for depression.* New York, NY: Guilford.

Selman, R. L. (1980). *The growth of interpersonal understanding.* New York, NY: Academic Press.

Sestieri, C., Corbetta, M., Romani, G., & Shulman, G. L. (2011). Episodic memory retrieval, parietal cortex, and the default mode network: Functional and topographic analyses. *Journal of Neuroscience, 31*(12), 4407–4420.

Shah, G. S., Klumpp, H., Angstadt, M., Nathan, P. J., & Phan, K. L. (2009). Amygdala and insula response to emotional images in patients with generalized social anxiety disorder. *Journal of Psychiatry Neuroscience, 34*(4), 296–302.

Shaw, P., Bramham, J., Lawrence, E. J., Morris, R., Baron-Cohen, S., & David, A. S. (2005). Differential effects of lesions of the amygdala and prefrontal cortex on recognizing facial expressions of complex emotions. *Journal of Cognitive Neuroscience, 17*(9), 1410–1419.

Shea, A., Walsh, C., MacMillan, H., & Steiner, M. (2005). Child maltreatment and HPA axis dysregulation: Relationship to major depressive disorder and post-traumatic stress disorder in females. *Psychoneuroendocrinology, 30*(2), 162–178.

Shearin, E. N., & Linehan, M. M. (1994). Dialectical behavior therapy for borderline personality disorder: Theoretical and empirical foundations. *Acta Psychiatra Scandinavica Supplementum, 379,* 61–68.

Shelley, B., & Trimble, M. (2004). The insular lobe of Reil: Its anatomico-functional, behavioral and neuropsychiatric attributes in humans—a review. *World Journal of Biological Psychiatry, 5,* 176–200.

Sherman, S. M. (2012). Thalamocortical interactions. *Current Opinion in Neurobiology, 22,* 575–579.

Sherman, S. M., & Guillery, R. W. (2011). Distinct functions for direct and transthalamic corticocortical connections. *Journal of Neurophysiology, 106,* 1068–1077.

Shin, L. M., & Liberzon, I. (2010). The neurocircuitry of fear, stress, and anxiety disorders. *Neuropsychopharmacology, 35*(1), 169–191.

Shin, L. M., Rauch, S. L., & Pitman, R. K. (2006). Amygdala, medial prefrontal cortex, and hippocampal function in PTSD. *Annals of the New York Academy of Sciences, 1071,* 67–79.

Sholt, M., & Gavron, T. (2006). Therapeutic qualities of clay-work in art therapy and psychotherapy: A review. *Art Therapy: Journal of the American Art Therapy Association, 23*(2), 66–72.

Siegel, D. J. (2001). Toward an interpersonal neurobiology of the developing mind: Attachment relationships, "mindsight," and neural integration. *Infant Mental Health Journal, 22*(1–2), 67–94.

Siegel, D. J. (2003). *Parenting from the inside out.* New York, NY: Penguin Putnam.

Siegel, D. J. (2006). An interpersonal neurobiology approach to psychotherapy: Awareness, mirror neurons, and neural plasticity in the development of well-being. *Psychiatric Annals, 36*(4), 248–256.

Siegel, D. J. (2007). *The mindful brain.* New York, NY: Norton.

Siegel, D. J. (2010). *The mindful therapist: A clinician's guide to mindsight and neural integration.* New York, NY: Norton.

Siegel, D. J. (2012). *The developing mind: How relationships and the brain interact to shape who we are* (2nd ed.). New York, NY: Guilford.

Siegel, D. J. (2013). *Brainstorm: The power and purpose of the teenage brain.* New York, NY: Penguin.

Siegel, D. J., & Hartzell, M. (2003). *Parenting from the inside out: How a deeper self understanding can help you raise children who thrive.* New York, NY: Tarcher/Penguin.

Siegel, D. J., & Payne Bryson, T. (2012). *The whole-brain child: 12 revolutionary strategies to nurture your child's developing mind.* New York, NY: Bantam.

Silananda, S. U. (2002). *The four foundations of mindfulness.* Boston, MA: Wisdom.

Singer, J. A. (2004). Narrative identity and meaning making across the adult lifespan: An introduction. *Journal of Personality, 72*(3), 437–460.

Singer, J. A., Blagov, P., Berry, M., & Oost, K. M. (2013). Self-defining memories, scripts, and the life story: Narrative identity in personality and psychotherapy. *Journal of Personality, 81*(6), 569–582.

Singer, T., Seymour, B., O'Doherty, J., Kaube, H., Dolan, R. J., & Frith, C. D. (2004). Empathy for pain involves the affective but not sensory components of pain, *Science, 303*(20), 1157–1161.

Singleton, O., Hölzel, B. K., Vangel, M., Brach, N., Carmody, J., & Lazar, S. W. (2014). Change in brainstem gray matter concentration following a mindfulness-based intervention is correlated with improvement in psychological well-being. *Frontiers in Human Neuroscience, 18*(8), 33.

Small, B. J., Herlitz, A., & Backman, L. (2004). Neurobiological changes in Alzheimer's disease: Structural, genetic and functional correlates of cognitive dysfunction. In R. Morris & J. Becker (Eds.), *Cognitive neuropsychology of Alzheimer's disease* (pp. 63–80). New York, NY: Oxford University Press.

Smith, D., Crocker, L., Staton, C., Gillaspy, A., & Charlton, S. (2010). *Psychometric properties of the Outcome Rating Scale in a non-clinical sample.* Poster presentation at the Heart and Soul of Change Conference, New Orleans, LA.

Snir, S., & Hazut, T. (2012). Observing the relationship: Couple patterns reflected in joint paintings. *Arts in Psychotherapy, 39*(1), 11–18.

Snir, S., & Regev, D. (2013a). A dialogue with five art materials: Creators share their art making experiences. *Arts in Psychotherapy, 40*(1), 94–100.

Snir, S., & Regev, D. (2013b). ABI–Art-Based Intervention Questionnaire. *Arts in Psychotherapy, 40*(3), 338–346.

Sohn, M. H., Albert, M. V., Jung, K., Carter, C. S., & Anderson, J. R. (2007). Anticipation of conflict monitoring in the anterior cingulate cortex and the prefrontal cortex. *Proceedings of the National Academy of Sciences, 104*(25), 10330–10334.

Spangler, G., Johann, M., Ronai, Z., & Zimmermann, P. (2009). Genetic and environmental influence on attachment disorganization. *Journal of Child Psychology and Psychiatry, 50*(8), 952–961.

Spreng, R., & Grady, C. L. (2010). Patterns of brain activity supporting autobiographical memory, prospection, and theory of mind, and their relationship to the default mode network. *Journal of Cognitive Neuroscience, 22*(6), 1112–1123.

Spreng, R. N., & Levine, B. (2012). Doing what we imagine: Completion rates and frequency attributes of imagined future events one year after prospection. *Memory, 21*(4), 458–466.

Spreng, R. N., Mar, R. A., & Kim, A. S. (2009). The common neural basis of autobiographical memory, prospection, navigation, theory of mind, and the default mode: A quantitative meta-analysis. *Journal of Cognitive Neuroscience, 21*(3), 489–510.

Sripada, R. K., King, A. P., Welsh, R. C., Garfinkel, S. N., Wang, X., Sripada, C. S., & Liberzon, I. (2012). Neural dysregulation in posttraumatic stress disorder: Evidence for disrupted equilibrium between salience and default mode brain networks. *Psychosomatic Medicine, 74*(9), 904–911.

Sroufe, L. A. (2000). Early relationships and the development of children. *Infant Mental Health Journal, 21*(1–2), 67–74.

Staff, R. T., Murray, A. D., Deary, I. J., & Whalley, L. J. (2004). What provides cerebral reserve? *Brain, 127,* 1191–1199.

Stanley, B., & Siever, L. J. (2010). The interpersonal dimension of borderline personality disorder: Toward a neuropeptide model. *American Journal of Psychiatry, 167,* 24–39. doi: 10.1176/appi.ajp.2009.09050744

Steckler, T., & Risbrough, V. (2012). Pharmacological treatment of PTSD: Established and new approaches. *Neuropharmacology, 62*(2), 617–627.

Steinhardt, L. (2006). The eight frame colored squiggle technique. *Art Therapy: Journal of the American Art Therapy Association, 23*(3), 112–118.

Stern, D. (2004). *The present moment in psychotherapy and everyday life.* New York, NY: W. W. Norton.

Stern, D. N. (1985). *The interpersonal world of the infant: A view from psychoanalysis and developmental psychology.* New York, NY: Basic Books.

Stern, E. (1955). Der Farbpyramidentest von Pfister-Heiss. In E. Stern (Ed.), *Die tests in der lininischen psychologie* (pp. 462–485). Zurich, Switzerland: Rascher Verlag.

Stevens, C., & Neville, H. (2009). Profiles of development and plasticity in human neurocognition. In M. Gazzaniga (Ed.), *The cognitive neurosciences* (4th ed., pp. 165–181). Cambridge, MA: MIT Press.

Stiles, J., Reilly, J., Paul, B., & Moses, P. (2005). Cognitive development following early brain injury: Evidence for neural adaptation. *Trends in Cognitive Sciences, 9*(3), 136–143.

St. Jacques, P. L. (2012). Functional neuroimaging of autobiographical memory. In D. Bernsten & D. C. Rubin (Eds.), *Understanding autobiographical memory: Theories and approaches* (pp. 114–138). Cambridge, MA: Cambridge University Press.

Stocco, A., Lebiere, C., & Anderson, J. R. (2010). Conditional routing of information to the cortex: A model of the basal ganglia's role in cognitive coordination. *Psychological Review, 117*(2), 541–574.

Strauch, B. (2003). *The primal teen.* New York, NY: Doubleday.

Strick, M., Dijksterhuis, A., Bos, M. W., Sjoerdsma, A., van Baaren, R. B., & Nordgren, L. F. (2011). A meta-analysis on unconscious thought effects. *Social Cognition, 29*(6), 738–762.

Strick, P. L. (2002). Stimulating research on motor cortex. *Nature Neuroscience, 5,* 714–715.

Strick, P. L., Dum, R. P., & Fiez, J. A. (2009). Cerebellum and nonmotor function. *Annual Review of Neuroscience, 32,* 413–434.

Stroebe, M., Schut, H., & Stroebe, W. (2007). Health outcomes of bereavement. *Lancet, 370*(9603), 1960–1973.

Ströhle, A., & Holsboer, F. (2003). Stress responsive neurohormones in depression and anxiety. *Pharmacopsychiatry, 36*(3), S207–S214.

Sullivan, E. V., Rosenbloom, M. J., Desmond, J. E., & Pfefferbaum, A. (2001). Sex differences in corpus callosum size: Relationship to age and intracranial size. *Neurobiology of Aging, 22*(4), 603–611.

Summerfield, J. J., Hassabis, D., & Maguire, E. A. (2009). Cortical midline involvement in autobiographical memory. *Neuroimage, 44*(3), 1188–1200.

Sutin, A. R., & Gillath, O. (2009). Autobiographical memory phenomenology and content mediate attachment style and psychological distress. *Journal of Counseling Psychology, 56*(3), 351.

Sutin, A. R., & Robins, R. W. (2008). Going forward by drawing from the past: Personal strivings, personally meaningful memories, and personality traits. *Journal of Personality, 76*(3), 631–664.

Sutin, A. R., & Robins, R. W. (2010). Correlates and phenomenology of first and third person memories. *Memory, 18*(6), 625–637.

Suzuki, S., Niki, K., Fujisaki, S., & Akiyama, E. (2011). Neural basis of conditional cooperation. *Social Cognitive and Affective Neuroscience, 6*(3), 338–347.

Takeuchi, H., Taki, Y., Sassa, Y., Hashizume, H., Sekiguchi, A., Fukushima, A., & Kawashima, R. (2010). White matter structures associated with creativity: Evidence from diffusion tensor imaging. *Neuroimage, 51,* 11–18. doi:10.1016/j.neuroimage.2010.02.035

Talwar, S. (2007). Accessing traumatic memory through art making: An art therapy trauma protocol (ATTP). *Arts in Psychotherapy, 34*(1), 22–35.

Tanaka, Y., Fukushima, H., Okanoya, K., & Myowa-Yamakoshi, M. (2014). Mothers' multimodal information processing is modulated by multimodal interactions with their infants. *Scientific Reports, 4,* 6623.

Tang, Y. Y., & Posner, M. I. (2012). Special issue on mindfulness neuroscience. *Social Cognitive and Affective Neuroscience*, nss104.

Taub, E., Uswatte, G., King, D. K., Morris, D., Crago, J. E., & Chatterjee, A. (2006). A placebo-controlled trial of constraint-induced movement therapy for upper extremity after stroke. *Stroke, 37*(4), 1045–1049.

Taubert, M., Draganski, B., Anwander, A., Müller, K., Horstmann, A., Villringer, A., & Ragert, P. (2010). Dynamic properties of human brain structure: Learning-related changes in cortical areas and associated fiber connections. *Journal of Neuroscience, 35,* 11670–11677.

Taylor, S. E., Klein, L. C., Lewis, B. P., Gruenewald, T. L., Gurung, R. A., & Updegraff, J. A. (2000). Biobehavioral responses to stress in females: Tend-and-befriend, not fight-or-flight. *Psychological Review, 107*(3), 411.

Teicher, M. H., Andersen, S. L., Polcari, A., Anderson, C. M., & Navalta, C. P. (2002). Developmental neurobiology of childhood stress and trauma. *Psychiatric Clinics of North America, 25*(2), 397–426.

Teicher, M. H., Tomoda, A., & Andersen, S. L. (2006). Neurobiological consequences of early stress and childhood maltreatment: Are results from human and animal studies comparable? *Annals of the New York Academy of Sciences, 1071,* 313–323.

Tessler, M., & Nelson, K. (1994). Making memories: The influence of joint encoding on later recall by young children. *Consciousness and Cognition, 3*(3), 307–326.

Tettamanti, M., Buccino, G., Saccuman, M. C., Gallese, V., Danna, M., Scifo, P., et al. (2005). Listening to action-related sentences activates fronto-parietal motor circuits. *Journal of Cognitive Neuroscience, 17*(2), 273–281.

Thaut, M. H. (2008). *Rhythm, music, and the brain: Scientific foundations and clinical applications.* New York, NY: Taylor and Francis.

Thompson, P. M., Giedd, J. N., Woods, R. P., MacDonald, D., Evans, A. C., & Toga, A. W. (2000). Growth patterns in the developing brain detected by using continuum mechanical tensor maps. *Nature, 404*(9), 190–193.

Timmann, D., & Daum, I. (2007). Cerebellar contributions to cognitive functions: A progress report after two decades of research. *Cerebellum, 6*(3), 159–162.

Toga, A. W., Thompson, P. M., & Sowell, E. R. (2006). Mapping brain maturation. *Trends in Neurosciences, 29*(3), 148–159.

Tomarken, A. J., Davidson, R. J., Wheeler, R. E., & Doss, R. C. (1992). Individual differences in anterior brain asymmetry and fundamental dimensions of emotion. *Journal of Personality and Social Psychology, 62,* 676–687.

Tong, F., Nakayama, K., Moscovitch, M., Weinrib, O., & Kanwisher, N. (2000). Response properties of the human fusiform face area. *Cognitive Neuropsychology, 17*(1/2/3), 257–280.

Touryan, S. R., Johnson, M. K., Mitchell, K. J., Farb, N., Cunningham, W. A., & Raye, C. L. (2007). The influence of self-regulatory focus on encoding of, and memory for, emotional words. *Society of Neuroscience, 2*(1), 14–27.

Treadway, M. T., & Lazar, S. W. (2009). The neurobiology of mindfulness. In F. Didonna (Ed.), *Clinical handbook of mindfulness* (pp. 45–58). New York, NY: Springer.

Trevarthen, C. (2006). The concept and foundations of infant intersubjectivity. In S. Braten (Ed.), *Intersubjective communication and emotion in early ontogeny* (pp. 15–46). Cambridge, MA: Cambridge University Press.

Tripp, T. (2007). A short-term therapy approach to processing trauma: Art therapy and bilateral stimulation. *Art Therapy: Journal of the American Art Therapy Association, 24*(4), 176–183.

Tronick, E. (1989). Emotions and emotional communication in infants. *Psychologist, 44,* 112–119.

Tronick, E. (2001). Emotional connections and dyadic consciousness in infant–mother and patient–therapist interactions. *Psychoanalytic Dialogues, 11*(2), 187–194.

Tronick, E. (2007). *The neurobehavioral and social-emotional development of infants and children.* New York, NY: W. W. Norton.

Tronick, E., & Beeghly, M. (2011). Infants' meaning-making and the development of mental health problems. *American Psychologist, 66*(2), 107–119.

Tronick, E., Bruschweiler-Stern, N., Harrison, M. A., Lyons-Ruth, K., Morgan, A. C., Nahum, J. P., Sander, L., & Stern, D. N. (1998). Dyadically expanded states of consciousness and the process of therapeutic change. *Infant Mental Health Journal, 19*(3), 290–299.

Turner, B. M., Paradiso, S., Marvel, C. L., Pierson, R., Boles Ponto, L. L., Hichwa, R. D., & Robinson, R. G. (2007). The cerebellum and emotional experience. *Neuropsychologia, 45*(6), 1331–1341.

Underwood, M. K., & Rosen, L. H. (2011). *Social development: Relationships in infancy, childhood and adolescence.* New York, NY: Guilford.

Urgesi, C., Moro, V., Candidi, M., & Aglioti, S. M. (2006). Mapping implied body actions in the human motor system. *Journal of Neuroscience, 26,* 7942–7949.

Vallar, G. (2007). Spatial neglect, Balint-Homes' and Gerstmann's syndrome, and other spatial disorders. *CNS Spectrums, 12*(7), 527–536.

Vance, R., & Wahlin, K. (2008). Memory and art. In N. Hass-Cohen & R. Carr (Eds.), *Art therapy and clinical neuroscience* (pp. 159–173). London, U.K.: Jessica Kingsley.

van der Kolk, B. A. (2001). The psychobiology and psychopharmacology of PTSD. *Human Psychopharmacology, 16*(1), 49–64.

van der Kolk, B. A. (2005). Developmental trauma disorder: Towards a rational diagnosis for children with complex trauma histories. *Psychiatric Annals, 33*(5), 401–408.

van der Kolk, B. A., & Fisler, R. (1995). Dissociation and the fragmentary nature of traumatic memories: Overview and exploratory study. *Journal of Traumatic Stress, 5,* 505–525.

van der Kolk, B. A., Roth, S., Pelcovitz, D., Sunday, S., & Spinazzola, J. (2005). Disorders of extreme stress: The empirical foundation of a complex adaptation to trauma. *Journal of Traumatic Stress, 18*(5), 389–399.

van IJzendoorn, M. (1995). Adult attachment representations, parental responsiveness, and infant attachment: A meta-analysis on the predictive validity of the Adult Attachment Interview. *Psychological Bulletin, 117,* 387–403.

Vanni-Mercier, G., Mauguiere, F., Isnard, J., & Dreher, J. (2009). The hippocampus codes the uncertainty of cue-outcome associations: An intracranial electrophysiological study in humans. *Journal of Neuroscience, 29*(16), 5287–5294.

van Praag, H., Schinder, A. F., Christie, B. R., Toni, N., Palmer, T. D., & Gage, F. H. (2002). Functional neurogenesis in the adult hippocampus. *Nature, 415*(6875), 1030.

Vartanian, O., & Goel, V. (2009). Neuroanatomical correlates of aesthetic preference for paintings. *Neuroreport, 15,* 893–897.

Vasterling, J. J., & Brewin, C. R. (Eds.). (2005). *Neuropsychology of PTSD: Biological, cognitive, and clinical perspectives.* New York, NY: Guilford.

Vermetten, E., & Bremner, J. D. (2002). Circuits and systems in stress: Preclinical studies. *Depression and Anxiety, 15,* 126–147.

Völlm, B. A., Taylor, A. N., Richardson, P., Corcoran, R., Stirling, J., McKie, S., Deakin, J. F., & Elliott, R. (2006). Neuronal correlates of theory of mind and empathy: A functional magnetic resonance imaging study in a nonverbal task. *Neuroimage, 29*(1), 90–98.

Vrticka, P., & Vuilleumier, P. (2012). Neuroscience of human social interactions and adult attachment style. *Human Neuroscience, 6,* 212.

Vuilleumier, P. (2005). How brains beware: Neural mechanisms of emotional attention. *Trends in Cognitive Sciences, 9*(12), 585–594.

Wager, T. D., Phan, K. L., Liberzon, I., & Taylor, S. F. (2003). Valence, gender, and lateralization of functional brain anatomy in emotion: A meta-analysis of findings from neuroimaging. *Neuroimage, 19*(3), 513–531.

Walrond-Skinner, S. (1986). *Dictionary of psychotherapy.* New York, NY: Routledge Publishers.

Waller, D. (2014). *Group interactive art therapy: Its use in training and treatment* (2nd ed.). New York, NY: Routledge.

Wallin, D. (2007). *Attachment in psychotherapy.* New York, NY: Guilford.

Ward, L., Mathias, J. L., & Hitchings, S. E. (2007). Relationships between bereavement and cognitive functioning in older adults. *Gerontology, 53*(6), 362–372.

Warren, Z., & Haslam, C. (2007). Overgeneral memory for public and autobiographical events in depression and schizophrenia. *Cognitive Neuropsychiatry, 12*(4), 301–321.

Waters, T. E. A. (2013). Relations between the functions of autobiographical memory and psychological wellbeing. *Memory, 22*(3), 265–275.

Watkins, K. E., Strafella, A. P., & Paus, T. T. (2003). Seeing and hearing speech excites the motor system involved in speech production. *Neuropsychologia, 41*(8), 989–994.

Watt, D. F. (2005). Social bonds and the nature of empathy. *Journal of Consciousness Studies, 12*, 185–209.

Weaver, I. G. (2011). Toward an understanding of the dynamic interdependence of genes and environment in the regulation of phenotype. In A. Petronis & J. Mill (Eds.), *Brain, behavior and epigenetics* (pp. 209–243). New York, NY: Springer-Verlag.

Wells, A., Fisher, P., Myers, S., Wheatley, J., Patel, T., & Brewin, C. R. (2009). Metacognitive therapy in recurrent and persistent depression: A multiple-baseline study of a new treatment. *Cognitive Therapy and Research, 33*(3), 291–300.

Wessberg, J., Olausson, H., Fernström, K. W., & Vallbo, Å. B. (2013). Receptive field properties of unmyelinated tactile afferents in the human skin. *Journal of Neurophysiology, 89*(3), 1567–1575.

Wicker, B., Keysers, C., Plailly, J., Royet, J. P., Gallese, V., & Rizzolatti, G. (2003). Both of us disgusted in my insula: The common neural basis of seeing and feeling disgust. *Neuron, 40*, 655–664.

Williams, J. M. G., Barnhofer, T., Crane, C., Herman, D., Raes, F., Watkins, E., & Dalgleish, T. (2007). Autobiographical memory specificity and emotional disorder. *Psychological Bulletin, 133*(1), 122.

Williams, J. M. G., Teasdale, J. D., Segal, Z. V., & Soulsby, J. (2000). Mindfulness-based cognitive therapy reduces overgeneral autobiographical memory in formerly depressed patients. *Journal of Abnormal Psychology, 109*(1), 150–155.

Wilson, A., & Ross, M. (2003). The identity function of autobiographical memory: Time is on our side. *Memory, 11*(2), 137–149.

Wilson, K. G. (2003). *Acceptance and commitment therapy: An experiential approach to behavior change.* New York, NY: Guilford.

Wismer Fries, A. B., Ziegler, T. E., Kurian, J. R., Jacoris, S., & Pollak, S. D. (2005). Early experience in humans is associated with changes in neuropeptides critical for regulating social behavior. *Proceedings of the National Academy of Sciences, 102*(47), 17237–17240. doi:10.1073/pnas.0504767102

Withrow, R. L. (2004). The use of color in art therapy. *Journal of Humanistic Counseling, Education and Development, 43*(1), 33–40.

Wolpe, J., & Lazarus, A. A. (1966). *Behavior therapy techniques: A guide to the treatment of neuroses.* Oxford, U.K.: Pergamon.

Wood, J. N., & Grafman, J. (2003). Human prefrontal cortex: Processing and representational perspectives. *Nature Reviews Neuroscience, 4*(2), 139–147.

Woon, F. L., Sood, S., & Hedges, D. W. (2010). Hippocampal volume deficits associated with exposure to psychological trauma and posttraumatic stress disorder in adults: A meta-analysis. *Progress in Neuro-Psychopharmacology and Biological Psychiatry, 34*(7), 1181–1188.

Wu, F., Chang, E., & Chen, C. (2009). Depressive tendency of design major freshman students explored through the use of color in mosaic creations. *Arts in Psychotherapy, 36*(4), 185–190. doi:10.1016/j.aip.2009.01.002

Wupperman, P., Neumann, C. S., Whitman, J. B., & Axelrod, S. R. (2009). The role of mindfulness in borderline personality disorder features. *Journal of Nervous and Mental Disease, 197*(10), 766–771.

Wynne, A. (2007). *The origin of Buddhist meditation.* London, U.K.: Routledge.

Xavier, F. F., Ferraz, M. T., Trentini, C. M., Freitas, N. K., & Moriguchi, E. H. (2002). Bereavement-related cognitive impairment in an oldest-old community-dwelling Brazilian sample. *Journal of Clinical and Experimental Neuropsychology, 24*(3), 294.

Yalom, I., & Leszcz, M. (2005). *Theory and practice of group psychotherapy* (5th ed.). New York, NY: Basic Books.

Yaxley, R. H., Van Voorhees, E. E., Bergman, S., Hooper, S. R., Huettel, S. A., & De Bellis, M. D. (2011). Behavioral risk elicits selective activation of the executive system in adolescents: Clinical implications. *Frontiers in Psychiatry, 2*(68).

Yehuda, R., Halligan, S. L., & Grossman, R. (2001). Childhood trauma and risk for PTSD: Relationship to intergenerational effects of trauma, parental PTSD, and cortisol excretion. *Development and Psychopathology, 13,* 733–753.

Yu, J. (Producer, Director). (1999). *The living museum* [Motion picture]. New York, NY: Living Filmworks.

Yucel, M., Wood, S. J., Phillips, L. J., Stuart, G. W., Smith, D., Yung, A. R., Velakoulis, D., McGorry, P. D., & Pantelis, C. (2003). Morphological anomalies of the anterior cingulate cortex in young individuals at ultra high risk of developing a psychotic illness. *British Journal of Psychiatry, 182,* 518–524.

Zeki, S. (1999). *Inner vision: An exploration of art and the brain.* Oxford, U.K.: Oxford University Press.

Zeki, S., & Bartels, A. (1998). The autonomy of the visual systems and the modularity of conscious vision. *Philosophical Transactions of the Royal Society of London. Series B: Biological Sciences, 353*(1377), 1911–1914.

Zelazo, P. D., & Muller, U. (2002). Executive function in typical and atypical development. In U. Goswami (Ed.), *Blackwell handbook of child cognitive development* (pp. 445–469). Oxford, U.K.: Blackwell.

Zhang, S., & Li, C. S. (2013). Functional connectivity mapping of the human precuneus by resting state fMRI. *Neuroimage, 59*(4), 3548–3562.

Zieliński, K. (2006). Jerzy Konorski on brain associations. *Acta Neurobiologiae, Experimentalis, 66*(1), 75–84.

Zur, O., & Nordmarken, N. (2011). To touch or not to touch: Exploring the myth of prohibition on touch in psychotherapy and counseling. Retrieved from http://www.zurinstitute.com/touchintherapy.html

Zylowska, L., Ackerman, D. L., Yang, M. H., Futrell, J. L., Horton, N. L., Hale, T. S., & Smalley, S. L. (2008). Mindfulness meditation training in adults and adolescents with ADHD: A feasibility study. *Journal of Attention Disorders, 11*(6), 737–746.

Index